£2·00

Requisites in Gastroenterology
Anil K. Rustgi (ed.)

Books in the series:

Volume 1: Esophagus and Stomach, David A. Katzka, David C. Metz (eds)
Volume 2: Small and Large Intestine, Gary R. Lichtenstein, Gary D. Wu (eds)
Volume 3: Hepatobiliary Tract and Pancreas, K. Rajender Reddy, William B. Long
(eds)
Volume 4: Endoscopy and Gastrointestinal Radiology, Gregory G. Ginsberg,
Michael L. Kochman (eds)

Commissioning Editor: *Rolla Couchman*
Project Development Manager: *Joanne Scott*
Project Manager: *Alan Nicholson*
Illustration Manager: *Mick Ruddy*
Designer: *Andy Chapman*

The Requisites in
Gastroenterology

Anil K. Rustgi MD (ed.)
T. Grier Miller Professor of Medicine and Genetics
Chief, Division of Gastroenterology
University of Pennsylvania School of Medicine
Philadelphia, PA
USA

Volume 3: Hepatobiliary Tract and Pancreas

Edited by
K. Rajender Reddy, MD
Professor of Medicine and Surgery
Director of Hepatology
Medical Director, Transplantation Hepatology
University of Pennsylvania School of Medicine
Philadelphia, PA
USA

William B. Long, MD
Associate Professor of Medicine
Division of Gastroenterology
University of Pennsylvania School of Medicine
Philadelphia, PA
USA

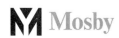 Mosby
An Affiliate of Elsevier Inc.
Edinburgh • London • New York • Oxford • Philadelphia • St Louis • Sydney • Toronto 2004

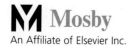

An Affiliate of Elsevier Inc.

First published 2004

ISBN 0-3230-1837-8

British Library Cataloguing in Publication Data
A catalogue record for this book is available from the British Library

Library of Congress Cataloging in Publication Data
A catalog record for this book is available from the Library of Congress

Note
Medical knowledge is constantly changing. As new information becomes available, changes in treatment, procedures, equipment and the use of drugs become necessary. The editors/contributors and the publishers have taken care to ensure that the information given in this text is accurate and up to date. However, readers are strongly advised to confirm that the information, especially with regard to drug usage, complies with the latest legislation and standards of practice.

Printed in the USA

The
publisher's
policy is to use
**paper manufactured
from sustainable forests**

Contents

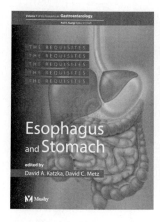
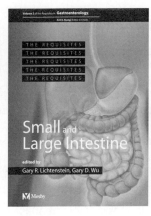
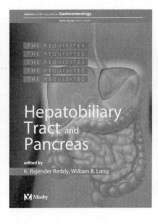
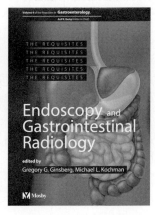
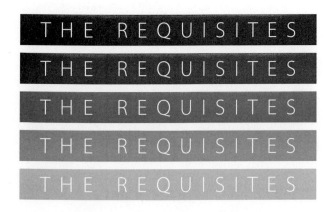

Series Foreword

This exciting and innovative *Requisites in Gastro-enterology* series takes a broad-based and fundamental approach to the pathophysiology, diagnosis and management of gastrointestinal, hepatic and pancreatic diseases and disorders. The series is divided into 4 interrelated volumes, each of which in turn is edited by nationally and internationally renowned editors who are supported by excellent contributors. The contributors represent a breadth of disciplines and expertise, and are drawn from a number of different institutions and academic medical centers. At the same time, the University of Pennsylvania provides a 'home' base for the series, and indeed, its gastroenterology, surgery, radiology and pathology departments have been a foundation for clinical care, teaching and investigation for several generations.

Volume 1 deals with diseases and disorders of the esophagus and stomach, edited by Drs David Katzka and David Metz. Volume 2 covers small and large intestinal diseases and disorders, edited by Drs Gary Lichtenstein and Gary Wu. Volume 3 delineates hepatobiliary and pancreatic diseases and disorders, edited by Drs Rajender Reddy and William Long. Finally, Volume 4, edited by Drs Gregory Ginsberg and Michael Kochman, brings together the important diagnostic and therapeutic modalities of endoscopy, interventional endoscopy and radiological imaging that are of direct relevance to topics covered in Volumes 1,2 and 3. While each volume is self-sufficient, all volumes provide the reader with a focused, cohesive and integrated view of the principles and practice of gastroenterology, hepatology and pancreatology. Each volume is well illustrated and contains tables and figures that highlight salient features of different topics. Of note, boxes are provided that encapsulate key information covered in each chapter. These collective features are meant to assist the reader. The references are pivotal ones from the literature, and are not meant to be exhaustive.

In the evolution of this series, our collective thinking was to target the audience of medical students, residents, gastrointestinal fellows, allied health professionals (nurses, nurse practitioners, physician assistants), and those physicians (gastroenterologists, hepatologists, oncologists, surgeons, pathologists, radiologists) who require overviews for certifying examinations. The series is unique in the library of books that span the discipline of gastroenterology. The reader will find the volumes 'user-friendly' and will be imparted with expert knowledge and insights, making this an engaging overview and refresher course. We hope and trust that we will succeed in this mission.

The volumes that form the kernel of this series were profoundly influenced on the one hand by students, residents and fellows, and on the other hand, by the pioneering advances of T. Grier Miller, Thomas Machella, Frank Brooks, Sidney Cohen, Richard McDermott, Peter Traber and Ed Raffensperger. It is to these past and future leaders to whom I wish to give my special gratitude.

Anil K. Rustgi, MD
Editor-in-Chief

Preface

This comprehensive volume is dedicated to the liver, biliary tree, gallbladder and pancreas. Given the importance of these organs and their central role in many aspects of clinical medicine, we have dedicated the first two-thirds of the volume to hepatobiliary diseases and disorders, and the remaining one-third to pancreatic diseases and disorders. We start off with evaluation of the liver and then review histopathology. Thereafter, there are three consecutive chapters covering viral hepatitis, alcoholic and nonalcoholic liver disease, and metabolic liver diseases (e.g. hemachromatosis, Wilson's disease, and alpha–1 antitrypsin deficiency). These chapters provide a platform for the chapters on autoimmune diseases, vascular disorders, and liver failure. Given the importance and emergence of liver tumors, both benign and malignant, we delve into these malignancies thoroughly. We then conclude the hepatobiliary section with chapters on non-viral liver infections and liver transplantation.

The chapters on pancreatic diseases deal with etiology, pathophysiology, diagnosis, and management of both acute and chronic pancreatitis. We conclude with pancreatic neoplasms and surgical approaches to pancreatic diseases.

We believe the reader will find this volume to be balanced between reviewing essential features and giving up-to-the-minute information on current developments. This will permit the reader to integrate knowledge gained from this volume to the principles and practice of hepatology and pancreatology. Recognizing the complexities of this undertaking, we are most appreciative to our contributing authors, all of whom represent experts in their respective fields.

K. Rajender Reddy, MD
William B. Long, MD

Contributors

Peter L. Abt, MD
Fellow in Transplantation
Division of transplantation
Department of Surgery
University of Pennsylvania
Philadelphia, PA
USA

Nuzhat A. Ahmad MD
Assistant Professor of Medicine
Director, Gastroenterology Section, PVAMC
Division of Gastroenterology
University of Pennsylvania School of Medicine
Philadelphia, PA
USA

Alphonso Brown MD
Clinical Assistant Professor of Medicine
School of Medicine
University of North Carolina at Chapel Hill
Division of Digestive Diseases
Chapel Hill, North CA
USA

Anne Burke MD
Assistant Professor of Medicine
Division of Gastroenterology
University of Pennsylvania School of Medicine
Philadelphia, PA
USA

Kyong-Mi Chang MD
Assistant Professor of Medicine
Director, Hepatitis Clinic
Division of Gastroenterology
Hospital of the University of Pennsylvania
Philadelphia, PA
USA

Stanley Martin Cohen MD
Assistant Professor of Medicine
Center for Liver Diseases
Section of Gastroenterology
Department of Medicine
The University of Chicago Hospitals and Clinics
Chicago, IL
USA

Thomas W. Faust MD
Assistant Professor of Medicine
Division of Gastroenterology
University of Pennsylvania School of Medicine
Philadelphia, PA
USA

Lisa M. Forman MD, MSCE
Assistant Professor of Medicine
Section of Hepatology
University of Colorado Health Sciences Center
Denver, CO
USA

Emma E. Furth MD
Professor
Department of Pathology and Laboratory Medicine
University of Pennsylvania School of Medicine
Philadelphia, PA
USA

Linda Greenbaum MD
Assistant Professor of Medicine
Division of Gastroenterology
University of Pennsylvania School of Medicine
Philadelphia, PA
USA

T. Sloane Guy MD
Fellow, Department of Surgery
University of Pennsylvania School of Medicine
Philadelphia, PA
USA

Umaprasanna S. Karnam MD
Consultant, Gastroenterology and Hepatology
Central Utah Medical Clinic American Fork,
Utah, UT
USA

William B. Long MD
Associate Professor of Medicine
Division of Gastroenterology
University of Pennsylvania School of Medicine
Philadelphia, PA
USA

Kim M. Olthoff MD
Associate Professor of Surgery
Division of Transplantation
Associate Director, Liver Transplant Program
University of Pennsylvania School of Medicine
Director, Liver Transplant Program
The Children's Hospital of Pennsylvania
Philadelphia, PA
USA

Barbara Piasecki MD
Instructor of Medicine
Division of Gatroenterology
Hospital of the University of Pennsylvania
Philadelphia, PA
USA

Steven B. Porter BA
Department of Medicine
University of Pennsylvania School of Medicine
Philadelphia, PA
USA

K. Rajender Reddy MD
Professor of Medicine and Surgery
Director of Hepatology
Medical Director, Transplantation Hepatology
University of Pennsylvania School of Medicine
Philadelphia, PA
USA

Arie Regev MD
Assistant Professor of Medicine
Division of Hepatology
Center for Liver Diseases
University of Miami School of Medicine
Miami, FL
USA

Ernest F. Rosato MD
Professor of Surgery
Department of Surgery
Chief, Division of Gastrointestinal Surgery
University of Pennsylvania School of Medicine
Philadelphia, PA
USA

Kia Saeian MD, MSC EPI
Assistant Professor of Medicine
Division of Gastroenterology and Hepatology
Medical College of Wisconsin
Milwaukee, WI
USA

Jeremy J. Schwartz MD
Fellow in Gastroenterology
Division of Gastroenterology
University of Pennsylvania School of Medicine
Philadelphia, PA
USA

Abraham Shaked MD, PhD
Professor of Surgery
Department of Surgery
Director, PENN Transplant Center
University of Pennsylvania School of Medicine
Philadelphia, PA
USA

Kirti Shetty MD
Assistant Professor of Medicine
Division of Gastroenterology
Ground Gates, Liver Transplantation
University of Pennsylvania School of Medicine
Philadelphia, PA
USA

Abhasnee Sobhonslidsuk MD
Assistant Professor
Department of Medicine
Ramathibodi Hospital
Mahidol University
Bangkok
Thailand

Dedication

To our respective families for their support.

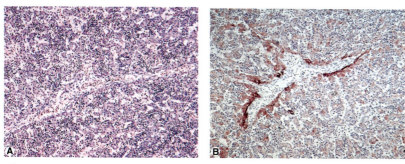

Figure 2.1   A. The beginning bile ducts B. These cells express high molecular weight cytokeratin

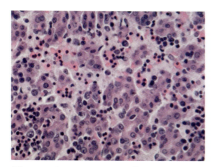

Figure 2.2   Extramedullary hematopoiesis.

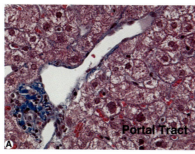

Figure 2.5   Trichrome staining of normal liver.

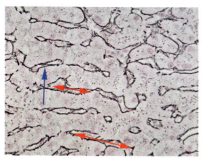

Figure 2.6   Reticulin stain of normal liver. Red arrows show sinusoidal spaces, which are bounded by the endothelial cells, and space of Disse (blue arrow).

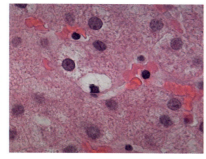

Figure 2.7   The hepatic stellate cells

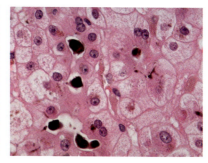

Figure 2.8   Cholestatic injury.

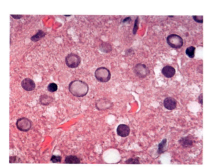

Figure 2.10   Glycogenated hepatocellular nuclei

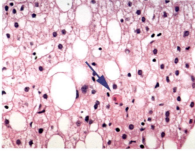

Figure 2.13   Apoptotic hepatocytes (arrow)

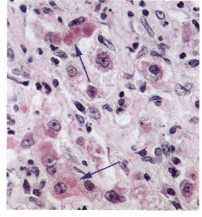

Figure 2.16   Mallory's hyaline in steatohepatitis

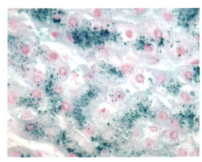

Figure 2.17 Prussian Blue iron stain showing intrahepatocellular hemosiderin

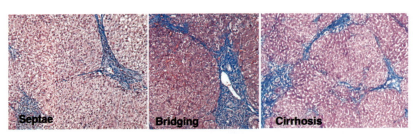

Figure 2.25 Trichrome staining of differing stages of fibrosis

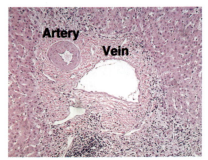

Figure 2.21 Ductopenia.

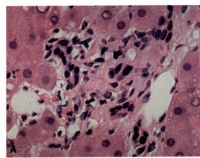

Figure 2.28 Portal tract venopathy

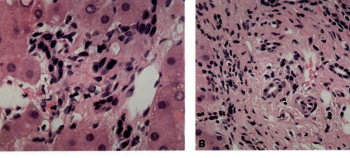

Figure 2.29 Trichrome stain of portal tracts in portal tract venopathy. A. Normal portal tract for comparison.

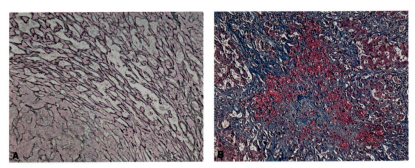

Figure 2.30 Vascular injury. A. Highlighted by a reticulin stain. B. Venous outflow obstruction will lead to perivenular fibrosis as shown by the trichrome stain.

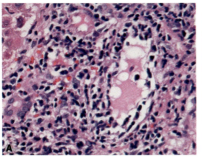 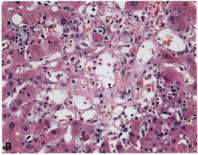

Figure 2.31   Acute cellular rejection. A. ductitis and endothelietitis in a portal tract. B. terminal venule involvement by cellular rejection ('central venulitis').

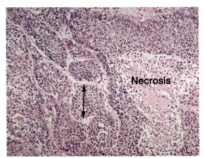

Figure 2.37   Cytology of hepatocellular carcinoma and normal hepatocytes.

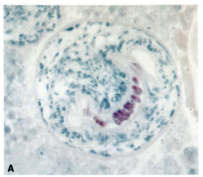 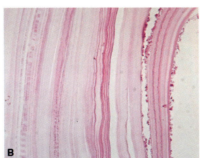

Figure 2.32   Echinococcal cyst. The hooklets stain red with acid-fast stain. A.The membrane of the cyst contains a layered, acellular material, which is pink with hemaotyxylin and eosin stain.

Figure 2.38   Poorly differentiated hepatocellular carcinoma.

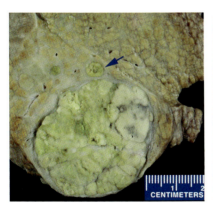 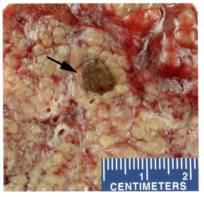

Figure 2.35   Hepatocellular carcinoma.

Figure 2.36   Macroregenerative nodule.

Figure 2.39   Macrotrabecular architecture of hepatocellular carcinoma.

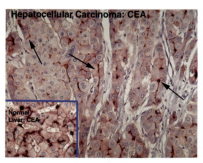

Figure 2.40 Immunohisto-chemistry using a polyclonal antibody to CEA.

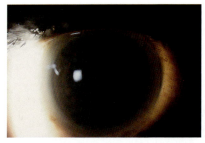

Figure 5.2 Kayser–Fleisher ring.

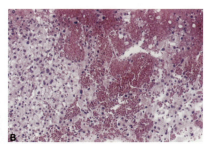

Figure 7.4B Budd–Chiari syndrome.

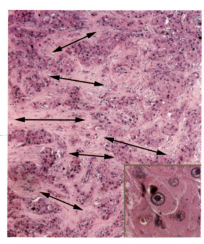

Figure 2.41 Fibrolamellar carcinoma.

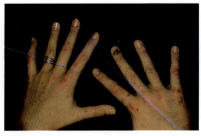

Figure 5.4 Porphyria cutanea tarda.

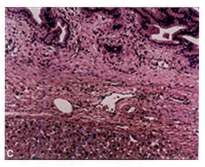

Figure 9.8C Hepatobiliary cystadenoma. (C) Histologic appearance.

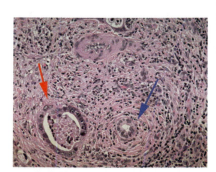

Figure 2.43 Cholangiocarcinoma. Cholangiocarcinomas form glands (red arrow) recapitulating the formation of the bile duct (blue arrow).

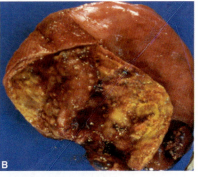

Figure 9.9 Cystadenocarcinoma. (B) Gross pathological examination. (D) Histologic examination.

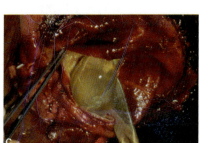

Figure 9.10 Echinococcal cyst. (C) Post-resection. (D) Histologic appearance.

Chapter 1

Evaluation of the Liver

Umaprasanna S. Karnam and K. Rajender Reddy

Introduction

The importance of the liver was recognized at the time of the Mesopotamians who considered the liver to be the seat of life as it appeared to be the collecting point of blood. The liver is the second largest organ in the body and is the "conductor of a complex symphony" which enables the human body to function well. It is a warehouse for several metabolic fuels and has numerous biochemical pathways for the modification of compounds that are absorbed from the small intestine.

Anatomy

Surface anatomy

The liver occupies the right upper quadrant, extending from the fifth intercostal space in the midclavicular line down to the right costal margin. It measures 12 to 15 cm in the coronal plane and 15 to 20 cm in the transverse plane, and its median weight is 1400 g in women and 1800 g in men. The adult liver weight is between 1.8% and 3.1% of body weight in 80% of individuals. The lower margin of the liver can usually be felt below the costal margin during inspiration.

The liver is wedge shaped, the superior, anterior, and lateral surfaces being smooth, and the posterior surface having indentations from the colon, kidney, stomach, and duodenum. The liver is covered by the fibrous capsule of Glisson or Walaeus. This capsule reflects onto the diaphragm and the posterior abdominal wall, leaving a "bare" area where the liver is in continuity with the retroperitoneum. The peritoneal reflections which form the coronary ligaments, right and left triangular ligaments, and the falciform ligament hold the liver in its place. The falciform ligament connects the liver to the diaphragm and anterior abdominal wall. The round ligament is the lower free edge of the falciform ligament and it contains the obliterated umbilical vein. The hepatoduodenal ligament (which is part of the lesser omentum) connects the liver to the superior part of the duodenum. The free margin of this ligament contains the hepatic artery, portal vein, bile duct, nerves, and lymphatic vessels. These structures connect with the liver in the transverse portal fissure. The quadrate lobe is anterior to the fissure, and the caudate lobe is posterior. The quadrate lobe is further demarcated by the gallbladder on the right and the umbilical fissure on the left.

Transcutaneous liver biopsies are obtained in the midaxillary line through the third interspace below the upper limit of liver dullness during full expiration. This is usually in the ninth intercostal space.

Several variations in the gross anatomy and topography of the liver are encountered.

- Riedel's lobe is a caudal prolongation of the right lobe, which gives a false impression of hepatomegaly.
- Extreme atrophy of the left lobe may be the result of vascular anomalies occurring early in life or extinction of parenchyma occurring after acquired vascular obstruction.
- Accessory livers may be found in the ligaments or mesentery or on the surface of the spleen, adrenals, or gallbladder.
- Hepar lobatum results in coarse lobulations on the surface of the liver as a result of obliterative lesions in medium and/or large vessels.
- Falciform left lobe is an elongated lobe that extends laterally and posteriorly like a scythe.

Segmental anatomy

The classic division of the liver into the left and right lobes is based on the location of the falciform

ligament and umbilical fissure. However, this is of no surgical or functional relevance as it does not correspond to the branch points in the vascular supply. Hjortso and Couinaud's nomenclature is a functional system based on the distribution of vessels and ducts in the liver. The Cantlie's line, extending between the vena cava and the gallbladder, is a relatively bloodless plane which demarcates the right (50% to 70% of liver mass) and left hemi-livers, each with independent vascular and duct supplies. The liver can be further divided into eight segments, each containing a pedicle of portal vessels and ducts, and drained by hepatic veins situated in the scissura between the segments. The segments have no surface fissures to allow their accurate identification. The left hemi-liver is composed of the classic left lobe, plus the caudate and quadrate lobe with its superior extension. (Figure 1.1).

Microanatomy

Hepatocytes, which are polyhedral with a central spherical nucleus, comprise 65% of the cells in the liver and are arranged in plates that are one cell thick. Blood-filled sinusoids lie on each side of these plates. The sinusoidal surface is covered with a layer of endothelial cells to enclose the extravascular space of Disse. Stellate cells of Ito and liver-associated lymphocytes are found in the space of Disse. Kuppfer cells are hepatic macrophages located in sinusoids with pseudopodia attached to subendothelial structures.

The *acinus* and the *lobule* are the two conceptual models of the three-dimensional organization of the liver. The central vein occupies the center of the lobule, and the functional portal triad occupies the center of the acinus. The dividing line between the acini is the watershed of biliary drainage and each acinus empties its biliary secretion into the axial bile ductile.

The location of the hepatocyte within the acinus determines its predominant function. Zone 1 hepatocytes (periportal), which have large mitochondria and high oxidative activities, play a dominant role in gluconeogenesis, beta-oxidation of fatty acids, cholesterol synthesis and bile-acid secretion. Zone 3 hepatocytes (perivenular) are involved in glycolysis, lipogenesis, and detoxification/biotransformation of drugs. This metabolic zonation is lost in cirrhosis and in certain genetic disorders (Figure 1.2).

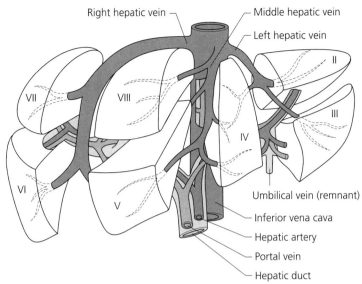

Figure 1.1 Diagram of the functional segments of the liver as per Couinaud's nomenclature (figure drawn by M.Thompson; reproduced with permission from Rappaport AM and Wanless IR. Physioanatomic considerations. In L Schiff and ER Schiff (eds), *Diseases of the Liver* 7th edn. Philadelphia PA, JB Lippincott, 1993).

Physiology

Hepatocytes are polarized epithelial cells which have three distinct membrane domains

- the sinusoidal or basolateral membrane
- the canalicular or apical membrane
- the lateral hepatic membrane between adjacent hepatocytes.

Complex arrays of transport proteins help in moving molecules into and out of the hepatocyte. The **A**denosine triphosphate **B**inding **C**assette (ABC) proteins represent a large family of transport proteins that share a common nucleotide-binding domain and are located on the canalicular membrane. These include MDR1, MDR2, MOAT, and other ABC proteins. The liver plays a central role in carbohydrate and fatty acid metabolism, lipid trans-

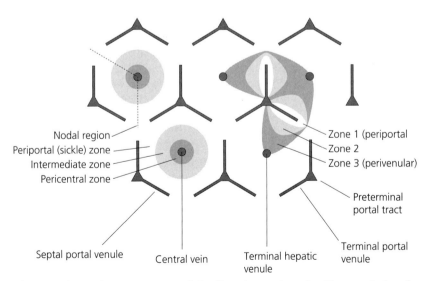

Figure 1.2 Acinar structure of the liver (reproduced with permission from Wanless IR. Anatomy and developmental anomalies of the liver. In M Feldman, BF Scharschmidt, Sleisenger MH (eds), *Sleisinger and Fordtran's Gastrointestinal and Liver Disease* 6th edn. Philadelphia PA: WB Saunders, 1997).

port, serum protein synthesis, and in the metabolism of fat-soluble vitamins.

Carbohydrate metabolism

The liver is the primary site for gluconeogenesis by which up to 240 mg of glucose a day can be produced. This is approximately twice the metabolic needs of the retina, red blood cells, and the brain. The liver can store a 2-day supply of glycogen. Glucose enters the liver via glucose transporter 2, the activity of which is independent of metabolic conditions or levels. This transporter has a Km of 60 mmol and is a low-affinity, but high-capacity transporter. Glucose is rapidly converted to glucose-6-phosphate which can then enter three independent metabolic pathways

1. glycogen synthesis
2. anaerobic glycolysis by means of the Embden–Meyerhof pathway
3. the pentose–phosphate shunt.

A detailed description of the various pathways and of disorders due to enzyme defects is beyond the scope of this chapter.

Fructose is the second most abundant carbohydrate in the western diet. It is absorbed by a sodium-independent carrier and is converted to fructose-1-phosphate by fructokinase using either adenosine triphosphate (ATP) or guanosine triphosphate (GTP) as cofactor. Fructose-1-phosphate is metabolized by an aldolase to form dihydroxyacetone phosphate and glyceraldehyde-3-phosphate. The former can enter the glycolytic pathway or provide the glycerol backbone for triacylglycerol and phospholipids. Glyceraldehyde-3-phosphate may be combined with dihydroxyacetone phosphate by aldolase B to ultimately form fructose-1,6-diphosphate which can partake in either glycolysis or gluconeogenesis.

Galactose is a component of lactose, which is present in high concentration in human milk (7%) and cow milk (5%). Galactose is converted to glucose-6-phosphate, which can be utilized for glycogen synthesis, or can be further oxidized to pyruvate or acetyl-CoA for additional energy generation or fatty acid synthesis.

Fatty acid synthesis and metabolism

Oxidation of fatty acids to carbon dioxide and water has the highest ATP production of any metabolic fuel and is the most efficient long-term storage form of energy. The liver is also involved in the beta-oxidation of fatty acids and the transport of fatty acids to other organs as lipoproteins.

Fatty acid synthesis occurs in the cytosol and is regulated by the availability of its precursors. Upon achieving the appropriate chain length, the fatty acid is esterified with glycerol to form triglycerides. Acetyl-CoA is synthesized predominantly in the mitochondrion, combines with oxaloacetate to form citrate, which is exported outside the mitochondrion. Cytosolic ATP citrate lyase (citrate cleavage enzyme) cleaves citrate to yield acetyl-CoA and oxaloacetate. Acetyl-CoA carboxylase converts acetyl-CoA to malonyl-CoA, which is the first step in fatty acid synthesis. Two nicotine adenine diphosphonucleotide, reduced (NADPH) molecules are required for each two-carbon unit that is added to the growing fatty acid chain. The complex fatty acid synthetic chain continues until a palmitate (carbon 16) or stearate (carbon 18) is formed.

Beta-oxidation of fatty acids provides a significant fuel source for multiple organs, including the liver. It can occur in both the mitochondria and peroxisomes. Acetyl-CoA is produced in large quantities during beta-oxidation. Beta-oxidation in the mitochondria starts with the translocation of fatty acids by first undergoing fatty acyl-CoA formation in the presence of fatty acyl-CoA synthetase in the cytosol. Carnitine palmitoyltransferase I located within the mitochondrial membrane helps in the formation of fatty acylcarnitine, which is then translocated into the mitochondrion by a fatty acyl carnitine, carnitine translocase, in exchange for free carnitine. The reverse reaction occurs in the mitochondrion through carnitine palmitoyltransferase II releasing fatty acyl-CoA. Fatty acyl-CoA is converted to trans-enol fatty acid by acyl-CoA dehydrogenase and in the process two electrons are transferred to the electron transport chain in the mitochondria.

A series of sequential reactions converts 3 keto fatty acyl-CoA to acetyl-CoA and fatty acyl-CoA, which then undergo another cycle of beta-oxidation. Acetyl-CoA can enter into the tricarboxylic acid cycle and generate 12 ATP, or it can enter the 3-hydroxyl-methyl-glutaryl-CoA cycle to form ketone bodies. Only hepatic mitochondria are capable of ketone-body formation. Unlike mitochondrial beta-oxidation, peroxisomes can only metabolize long-chain fatty acids with a minimum of 10-carbon chain length and up to 24-carbon chain length. In addition hydrogen peroxide is formed and overall fatty acid oxidation is less efficient. This provides a means of eliminating fatty acids with energy loss.

This lends to the therapeutic role of hypolipidemic drugs such as clofibrate.

Lipid transport

The liver plays a key role in lipid transport by receiving fatty acids and cholesterol from the diet and from peripheral tissues, the fatty acids and cholesteral are then packaged into lipoprotein complexes and released into the circulation. The liver synthesizes and extracts a large number of apolipoproteins (which in combination with lipids form lipoproteins). Fatty acids released from adipocytes by the action of intracellular hormone-sensitive lipase are bound to serum albumin and transported to other tissues, including the liver, where they are used for the synthesis of phospholipids and triglycerides. Lipids can be temporarily stored in the liver as fat droplets or cholesterol esters, directly excreted into bile, or metabolized into bile acids. Lipids are transported out of the liver by very low-density lipoprotein particles.

Serum protein synthesis

The liver is the major synthetic site for serum proteins involved in coagulation, iron-binding proteins, transport proteins, and protease inhibitors. In addition it is also the site of synthesis of acute-phase reactants such as fibrinogen. Alterations in serum levels may be caused by liver failure, or genetic mutations involving specific proteins.

The liver synthesizes factor II, VII, IX, X, and proteins C and S. All these proteins undergo a unique, vitamin K-dependent, post-translational modification involving gamma-carboxylation of specific glutamic-acid residues, which are essential for normal activity. These modified glutamic-acid residues bind to divalent cations, such as calcium, and subsequently to phospholipids or plasma membrane, which are required for their activity. These proteins are secreted into serum as proenzymes, which are activated to form serine proteases that function in the coagulation pathway.

The liver contains approximately 10% of total body iron stores, predominantly bound to ferritin in the hepatocyte. Each ferritin particle may contain up to 4000 molecules of iron. Release of iron from ferritin requires one electron reduction from the ferric to the ferrous state. Iron stored in the liver can exchange with iron bound to transferrin, which exchanges with iron in peripheral tissue, especially proliferating or malignant cells.

Serum albumin is the predominant serum-binding protein which is synthesized by the liver. It functions as a non-specific carrier protein that binds fatty acids, bile acids, and numerous exogenous compounds. It also provides serum oncotic pressure. Hepatic synthesis rates of albumin are regulated in part by the serum oncotic pressure.

Alpha-1-antitrypsin is a hepatic secretory protein whose major target is pulmonary elastin. Absence or reduced activity of this enzyme results in early onset emphysema. In addition, specific point mutations can alter the normal processing of the protein which accumulates in hepatocytes causing liver injury. An abnormality in another acute-phase reactant, ceruloplasmin, is associated with Wilson's disease.

Metabolism of fat-soluble vitamins

The liver plays a major role in the metabolism of fat-soluble vitamins A, D, E, and K. Vitamin A belongs to the retinoid family of chemicals that are members of natural and synthetic analogs of retinols and the provitamin A carotenoids. Approximately 80% of the vitamin A that is consumed is absorbed, and up to 50% of the absorbed vitamin A is excreted within 1 week as oxidized or biotransformed product. Retinoids are stored as retinyl esters in the non-parenchymal Ito cell or stellate cell. Vitamin D_2 (ergocalciferol) is a fat-soluble vitamin present in egg yolk, fish liver, and fish-liver oil. It plays a very important role in calcium homeostasis. In the liver vitamin D is hydroxylated to form 25-hydroxyl vitamin D by a microsomal P450 NADPH oxidase. Then 25-hydroxyl vitamin D undergoes hydroxylation at the first position to form the most potent metabolite in the kidney. Vitamin E is the term used to describe eight related compounds called tocopherols and tocotrienols. Vitamin E is a potent antioxidant and is contained in oil-containing grains. Most tocopherol is taken up by hepatocytes by way of the chylomicron remnant receptor. In the liver, selective retention of only the D-alpha-tocopherol isoform occurs, with gamma-tocopherol being either metabolized or excreted into bile. Retained D-alpha-tocopherol is packaged with very low-density lipoprotein and secreted into plasma. Vitamin K is a fat-soluble vitamin that requires adequate micelle formation for absorption. Coagulation proteins and osteocalcin (secreted by osteoblasts) are dependent on vitamin K for their synthesis.

Bilirubin metabolism

Bilirubin is the end product of the degradation of heme, the prosthetic group of hemoglobin, myoglobin, the cytochrome P450s, and various hemoproteins. The initial step in the conversion of heme to bilirubin is the opening of the heme molecule at its alpha-bridge carbon by the microsomal enzyme heme oxygenase, resulting in the formation of carbon monoxide and of the green tetrapyrrole biliverdin. Biliverdin is then reduced by a second enzyme, biliverdin reductase, to bilirubin. As bilirubin is a potentially toxic waste product, hepatic handling is designed to eliminate it from the body through the biliary tract. Transfer of bilirubin from blood to bile involves four inter-related steps

1. hepatocellular uptake
2. intracellular binding
3. conjugation
4. biliary excretion.

Bilirubin enters the hepatocyte by both a facilitated transport mechanism (predominant) and by passive diffusion. OATP2 (also called SLC21A60) is thought to mediate high-affinity bilirubin uptake from albumin-containing media. Inside the cell-bilirubin partitions between the lipid environment of intracellular membranes and the aqueous cytosol. Glucuronidation renders the bilrubin water soluble. Bilirubin glucuronidation is catalyzed by a specific UDP-glucuronosyltransferase of UGT1 family. Normal bile typically contains less than 5% unconjugated bilirubin, 7% bilirubin monoconjugates, and 90% bilirubin diconjugates. The proportion of mono-conjugates increases in the presence of either an increased bilirubin load (hemolysis) or a reduced bilirubin-conjugating capacity. Bilirubin mono- and diglucuronides are transported across the canalicular plasma membrane into the canaliculus by an ATP-dependent transport process mediated by a canalicular membrane protein called multidrug resistance-associated protein 2 (MRP2). Multidrug resistance-associated protein 2 is a member of the MRP gene family, other members of which are involved in the transport of drug conjugates and anti-cancer drugs. Following biliary excretion, conjugated bilirubin reaches the duodenum and passes down the gastrointestinal tract without reabsorption by the intestinal mucosa. An appreciable fraction of bilirubin is converted to urobilinogen and related compounds by bacterial metabolism within the ileum and colon. Urobilinogen undergoes entero-hepatic circulation, and the portion of urobilinogen not taken up by the liver is cleared by the kidneys.

Unconjugated bilirubin is not excreted in urine as it is tightly bound to albumin for effective glomerular filtration, and there is no tubular mechanism for its renal excretion. Numerous diseases occur because of hereditary or acquired defects in bilirubin metabolism. A discussion of these conditions is beyond the scope of this chapter.

Bile metabolism

Bile is a lipid-rich secretion that originates from secretion of the hepatocytes into biliary canaliculi. Four main ATP-driven pumps have been identified that generate the solutes that are actively transported into bile. The solutes that are actively secreted are known as primary solutes. The osmotic action of primary solutes pulls water and filterable solutes through the paracellular junctions. Canalicular bile is modified in the biliary ductules with absorption of some secondary solutes, secretion of bicarbonate, and hydrolysis of glutathione by gamma-glutamyl transpeptidase. The gallbladder concentrates bile by removing electrolytes and also acidifies it. In humans gallbladder bile obtained after overnight fasting is about three times as concentrated as hepatic bile. There is a very efficient enterohepatic circulation for conserving bile acids. The normal bile acid pool size is approximately 2 to 4 grams. During digestion of a meal, the bile acid pool undergoes at least one or more enterohepatic cycles depending on the size and composition of the meal. Normally, the bile acid pool circulates approximately five to ten times daily. Intestinal absorption of the pool is about 95% efficient, so fecal loss is in the range of 0.3 to 0.6 g/day. The fecal loss is compensated by an equal daily synthesis of bile acids by the liver, and thus the bile salt pool is maintained. It is of note that the bile salts returning to the liver suppress *de novo* hepatic synthesis of primary bile acids from cholesterol by limiting the rate-limiting enzyme 7 alpha hydroxyls. While the loss of bile salts in stool is generally matched by increased hepatic synthesis, the maximum rate of synthesis is approximately 5 g/day, which may be insufficient to replete the bile acid pool when there is pronounced impairment of intestinal bile salt reabsorption.

The primary bile acids, cholic and chenodeoxycholic acid, are synthesized from cholesterol in the liver, conjugated with glycine or taurine, and excreted into the bile. Secondary bile acids, deoxycholate and lithocholate, are formed in the colon as bacterial metabolites of the primary bile acids.

Lithocholic acid is much less efficiently absorbed from the colon than deoxycholic acid. In normal bile, the ratio of glycine to taurine conjugates is about 3:1, while in patients with cholestasis, increased concentrations of sulfate and glucuronide conjugates of bile acids are found.

The four major primary solutes include conjugated bile acids, phospholipids, cholesterol, and bilirubin diglucuronide. The conjugated bile acids are the major driving force for bile flow. They also detach biliary phospholipids from the luminal face of the canalicular membrane. The major function of conjugated bile acids is to solubilize cholesterol in the biliary tract and to promote lipid absorption in the small intestine. The phospholipids in bile are mostly phosphatidylcholine. A phospholipids flippase flips phosphatidylcholine into the luminal face of the canalicular membrane. The phospholipids solubilize the cholesterol in bile, keeping it in solution. In addition, the association of phospholipids and conjugated bile acids occurs at a relatively low concentration. This keeps the molecular concentration of bile acids low and prevents damage to the bile duct epithelium. Cholesterol in bile is functionless and biliary excretion of cholesterol promotes its elimination from the body. Increased concentration of cholesterol in bile explains the high prevalence of cholesterol gallstone disease. In addition, bilirubin diglucuronide is also excreted through the bile. Some metals such as copper are also secreted into bile via a canalicular transporter. There are numerous hepatocyte pumps and transporters which orchestrate the complex process of bile formation. The canalicular pumps include the bile salt export pump (BSEP, ABC 11), phospholipids flippases (mdr2, mdr3), multiple organic anion transporter (mrp2), multidrug resistance protein (mdr1) and polyvalent cation transporters. Bile salt export pumps transport conjugated bile salts uphill, thereby establishing an osmotic gradient that generates bile flow. Lack of this transporter results in primary infantile cholestasis II, which is characterized by severe cholestasis and death. As the defect is at the canalicular level, bile acids do not enter bile and there is no ductular damage. Because gamma glutamyl transpeptidase (GGT) is a ductular enzyme, its levels are not elevated in this rare inborn error of metabolism. The phospholipids flippases flip phosphatidylcholine across the canalicular membrane. The flipped molecules form blebs on the luminal surface of the canalicular membrane, and these are washed by the conjugated bile acids to form mixed micelles. Deficiency of flippases is associated with neonatal and adult cholestatic disease, and possibly biliary microlithia-

sis. MDR1 exports many anti-cancer drugs into bile and is a transporter for cationic drugs. The major carriers of the basolateral membrane that are related to bile production are those involved in bile-acid transport. A sodium-coupled bile-acid transporter (NTCP, natrium taurocholate transporter) appears to be the major player in the uptake of conjugated bile acids. A second family of transporters which are sodium independent belong to the OATP family. These transport a bile acid in, and an anion out. MRP3 is a recently identified basolateral transporter that is ATP energized and is upregulated in chronic liver disease.

Hepatic biochemical tests

Hepatic biochemical tests – often referred to as liver function tests – are useful in the evaluation and management of liver disease. They provide a non-invasive method of screening for the presence of liver dysfunction. In addition, the pattern of abnormalities help in recognizing the general type of liver disorder. They also help to assess the severity of liver dysfunction and evaluate response to therapy.

In general there are three different groups of liver function tests

1. tests that detect injury to hepatocytes (liver-injury tests)
2. tests of hepatic biosynthetic capacity
3. tests to detect chronic inflammation in liver, altered immune regulation, and viral hepatitis.

Tests that detect injury to hepatocytes (liver-injury tests)

Aminotransferases

The serum aminotransferases are sensitive indicators of hepatic injury. Alanine aminotransferase (ALT, also known as serum glutamic-pyruvic transaminase or SGPT) and aspartate aminotransferase (AST, also known as serum glutamic-oxaloacetic transaminase or SGOT) are the most frequently used indicators of hepatocyte dysfunction. These enzymes catalyze the transfer of the alpha-amino groups of alanine and aspartic acid, respectively, to the alpha-keto group of ketoglutaric acid. Both require pyridoxal 5'-phosphate as cofactor. In tissues ALT is found in the cytosol, whereas AST occurs in both cytosol and mitochondria. Both aminotransferases are normally present in serum in low concentrations (less than 30 to 40 IU/L). Aspartate aminotransferase is found in the liver, cardiac muscle, skeletal muscle, the kidneys, the brain, the pancreas, the lungs, leukocytes, and erythrocytes, in decreasing order of concentration. Alanine aminotransferase is present in the highest concentration in the liver and is a more sensitive as well as specific test of acute hepatocellular damage. Aspartate aminotransferase is cleared more rapidly than ALT. Most of the aminotransferases are cleared by the reticuloendothelial system. Neither ALT nor AST has isoenzymes that are tissue specific.

Aminotransferases are elevated in all types of acute and chronic hepatitis, cirrhosis, infectious mononucleosis, heart failure, malignancy, and alcoholic liver disease. The highest increases occur in disorders associated with extensive hepatocellular injury (for example injuries caused by viral infections and drugs), acute heart failure, and following exposure to hepatotoxins such as carbon tetrachloride. They are usually less than 300 IU in alcoholic liver disease and seldom more than 500 IU in obstructive jaundice or cirrhosis. A single exception is acute common-duct obstruction due to common bile duct stone where aminotransferases reach the thousands within 24 to 48 hours and then rapidly decline to lower levels. There is a poor correlation between the extent of hepatocellular damage and elevation of serum aminotransferases. The AST:ALT ratio is of value in the recognition of alcoholic liver disease where a value greater than 3 is highly suggestive of the same. This is because of the low serum activity of ALT. Alcoholic liver disease results in a deficiency of pyridoxal 5′-phosphate and ALT synthesis in liver requires more of this factor than AST synthesis. A second, much less common disorder characterized by a disproportionate elevation of AST relative to ALT is acute Wilson's disease. A ratio above 4 in the appropriate clinical setting, especially with a low alkaline phosphatase, is suggestive of fulminant Wilsonian hepatitis. Elevations in aminotransferases may herald acute viral hepatitis and serum bilirubin elevation may lag behind by 1 week. Drugs such as para-aminosalicylic acid and erythromycin in addition to diabetic ketoacidosis and high-sucrose diets may result in falsely elevated aminotransferase values if older calorimetric tests are used. Rarely, AST may exist as a macroenzyme complex with albumin in serum, resulting in persistent elevation of the serum enzyme activity. Low AST values may be seen in patients with uremia. These low values increase after dialysis, suggesting that a dialyzable inhibitor is present in uremic serum.

Other tests of hepatocellular necrosis, which are seldom used, include glutamate dehydrogenase, isocitrate dehydrogenase, lactate dehydrogenase and sorbitol dehydrogenase. Lactate dehydrogenase has a wide tissue distribution and transient, massive elevations of this enzyme may occur in ischemic hepatitis. Sustained lactate dehydrogenase elevations when accompanied by alkaline phosphatase elevation suggest malignant infiltration of the liver.

Alkaline phosphatase

Alkaline phosphatase (AP) comprises a group of enzymes present in a wide variety of tissues including liver, bone, intestine, kidney, placenta, leukocytes, and various neoplasms. Alkaline phosphatase catalyzes the hydrolysis of a large number of organic phosphate esters, optimally at an alkaline pH, and inorganic phosphates and the organic radical are generated by this reaction. It tends to increase in tissues undergoing metabolic stimulation, hence the increase in alkaline phosphatase during adolescence and pregnancy. Liver and bone are the major sources of serum alkaline phosphatase. Individuals with blood groups O and B may have a significant serum alkaline phosphatase level derived from the small intestine, particularly after a fatty meal, providing the rationale for obtaining a fasting measurement. Hepatic AP is present on the apical domain of the hepatocyte plasma membrane and in the luminal domain of bile-duct epithelium. Increases of AP in liver disease are from increased synthesis and release into serum rather than from impaired biliary secretion. As serum elevation of AP requires synthesis of new enzyme, AP may not become elevated for 24 to 48 hours after acute biliary obstruction. In addition, because the half-life of serum AP is approximately 1 week, the level in serum may remain elevated for weeks after resolution of biliary obstruction.

Levels of AP up to three times normal are relatively non-specific and occur in different liver diseases. However, remarkable increases in serum AP are seen in both intra- and extrahepatic biliary obstruction and in infiltrative hepatic diseases. The level of AP does not differentiate between intra- and extrahepatic obstruction. Rarely, AP is normal despite extensive hepatic metastasis or common bile duct obstruction. Regan isoenzyme is biochemically distinct from liver AP and has been identified in different cancers including lung neoplasms. Elevations of AP in the setting of Hodgkin's lymphoma and renal cell cancer may be due to a non-specific hepatitis. In addition, certain families may have increased serum AP that is genetic in origin. Extremely low levels of AP can be seen in patients with fulminant Wilson's disease complicated by hemolysis.

Gamma glutamyl transpeptidase

Gamma glutamyl transpeptidase is found in many tissues including the liver, kidney, spleen, pancreas, heart, lung, and brain. It is not found in appreciable quantities in bone, and it is thus helpful in confirming the hepatic origin of an elevated AP. Gamma glutamyl transpeptidase is a microsomal enzyme, and as such is inducible by alcohol and several drugs such as warfarin and anticonvulsants. A GGT:AP ratio greater than 2.5 has been reported to be suggestive of alcohol abuse, although the enzyme level does not rise during alcohol binges. In rare conditions such as Byler disease and benign recurrent intrahepatic cholestasis, the alkaline phosphatase is elevated without an elevation in GGT.

5'-nucleotidase

5'-nucleotidase (5'NT) is found in many tissues including the liver, cardiac muscle, brain, blood vessels, and the pancreas. It catalyzes the hydrolysis of nucleotides such as adenosine 5'-phosphate and inosine 5'-phosphate, in which the phosphate is attached to the 5 position of the pentose moiety. In spite of this widespread tissue distribution, significant elevations of 5'NT are found almost exclusively in the setting of liver disease. It is located in both the hepatocyte sinusoidal and the canalicular plasma membranes. Its physiologic function is unknown. An increased serum 5' NT level in a non-pregnant person suggests that a concomitantly increased serum AP is of hepatic origin. However, a normal 5'NT in the presence of an elevated serum AP does not rule out the liver as the source of AP.

Leucine aminopeptidase

Leucine aminopeptidase is present in a variety of different tissues but is most abundant in biliary epithelium. It hydrolyzes tissue amino acids from the N-terminal of proteins and polypeptides. It is most active when leucine is the N-terminal residue, hence the name. Unlike 5'NT it is elevated during pregnancy. Leucine aminopeptidase is as sensitive as AP and 5'NT in detecting obstructive, infiltrative, or space-occupying lesions of the liver. The highest values of leucine aminopeptidase are found in biliary obstruction.

Bilirubin

Bilirubin normally present in serum represents a balance between input from production and hepatic removal of pigment. Causes of hyperbilirubinemia include overproduction of bilirubin, impaired uptake, conjugation, or excretion of bilirubin, and regurgitation from damaged hepatocytes or bile ducts. The major value of fractionating total serum bilirubin into unconjugated and direct-reacting moieties is in the detection of conditions characterized by unconjugated hyperbilirubinemia. Such a diagnosis is needed when the serum indirect-reacting bilirubin is in excess of 1.2 mg/dL and the direct reacting fraction is less than 20% of the total serum bilirubin. When the serum bilirubin is minimally elevated it is difficult to distinguish the nature of bilirubin elevation because of the inaccuracy of the diazo reaction. Total serum bilirubin is not a sensitive indicator of hepatic dysfunction and may not always accurately reflect the degree of liver damage. In a steady state, the serum bilirubin usually reflects the intensity of jaundice and the increase in total body bile pigment. The height of total serum bilirubin does not specify the cause of jaundice in the individual patient. In acute alcoholic hepatitis, hyperbilirubinemia in excess of 5 mg/dL indicates a poor prognosis. However, uncomplicated hemolysis seldom causes a serum bilirubin value in excess of 5 mg/dL. Fractionation of serum bilirubin in jaundiced patients does not allow a distinction to be made between parenchymal and cholestatic jaundice. Newer high performance liquid chromatography methods for measuring serum bilirubin demonstrate that conjugated and unconjugated bilirubins are both increased in hepatobiliary disease. Urinary bilirubin is always conjugated as the unconjugated form is bound to albumin and is not filtered by a normal glomerulus. A fraction of circulating conjugated bilirubin found in the setting of prolonged cholestasis, the delta fraction, is tightly bound to albumin and contributes to the tendency of hyperbilirubinemia to resolve more slowly.

Tests of hepatic biosynthetic capacity

Prothrombin time and serum albumin are the most commonly used tests of hepatic biosynthetic capacity. Prothrombin time measures the activity of several of the coagulation factors involved in the extrinsic coagulation pathway including factors I, II, V, VII, and X. The causes of an elevated prothrombin time include vitamin K deficiency, warfarin use, disseminated intravascular coagulation, and liver disease. Levels of factor VIII are low in disseminated intravascular coagulation but are normal in liver disease. Parenteral vitamin K (10 mg SQ) should reduce a prolonged prothrombin time secondary to vitamin K deficiency by at least 30% within 24 hours. Because of the short life of some of the coagulation factors measured by prothrombin time, changes in prothrombin time are extremely useful in monitoring hepatic synthetic function in patients with acute hepatic failure. The prothrombin time is not a sensitive test of liver disease because even cirrhotics can have a normal prothrombin time.

Serum albumin, which is quantitatively the most important plasma protein, is synthesized exclusively in the liver. Approximately 10 grams of albumin are synthesized and secreted by hepatocytes each day. With progressive hepatocellular injury, hepatic synthetic capacity decreases and albumin levels fall. As the serum half-life of albumin is approximately 20 days, its measurements are less useful than prothrombin time in acute liver failure. Heavy alcohol abuse and chronic inflammation inhibit albumin synthesis. Hypoalbuminemia is not specific for liver disease and may occur in protein malnutrition of any cause. Hence, serum albumin should not be used for screening in patients with no suspicion of liver disease.

Hepatocellular and cholestatic diseases have characteristic patterns of abnormal biochemical tests as illustrated in Table 1.1.

Tests to detect chronic inflammation in the liver, altered immune regulation, and viral hepatitis

Serum immunoglobulins are produced by stimulated B lymphocytes and are elevated in chronic liver disease. Elevation of immunoglobulins in chronic liver disease is due to impaired function of reticuloendothelial cells in the sinusoids or shunting of portal venous blood around the liver. Profound increases in serum immunoglobulins are found in autoimmune hepatitis. Diffuse polyclonal increases in immunoglobulins G and M are found in most types of cirrhosis and are non-specific. Increases in immunoglobulin A are seen in alcoholic cirrhosis, and immunoglobulin M in primary biliary cirrhosis. Hypergammaglobulinemia, with or without hypoalbuminemia, is not specific for liver disease and may be found in other chronic inflammatory and malignant diseases.

A detailed description of tests for viral hepatitis can be found in other chapters in this text book.

Dynamic liver function tests

Also known as quantitative liver function tests, these tests were considered superior to conventional biochemical tests in establishing the presence of liver disease and predicting the prognosis. However, their use is currently limited to research centers as they are expensive, cumbersome, and labor intensive. Indocyanine green clearance, galactose elimination capacity, aminopyrine breath test, antipyrine clearance, monoethylglycinexylidide

Table 1.1 General patterns of biochemical liver tests

Type of disorder	Aminotransferases	Alkaline phosphatase	Bilirubin	Albumin	Prothrombin time
Hepatocellular disease					
Toxic/ischemic	50–100×	1–3×	1–3×	↓in chronic	↑↑ ↑[1]
Viral hepatitis	5–50×	1–3×	1–30×	↓in chronic	↑↑[1]
Alcoholic liver disease	2–5×	1–10×	1–30×	↓in chronic	↑↑[1]
Biliary obstruction					
Complete	1–5×	2–20×	1–30×	usually normal	↑↑ [2]
Partial	1–5×	2–10×	1–5×	usually normal	↑↑ [2]
Infiltrative disease					
	1–3×	1–20×	1–5×	usually normal	usually normal

[1] *unresponsive to parenteral vitamin K in severe disease.*
[2] *responsive to parenteral vitamin K.*

test, and caffeine clearance are some of the quantitative liver function tests.

In the indocyanine green test the concentration of dye which is taken up almost exclusively by hepatocytes and excreted unchanged in bile is measured photometrically in blood samples taken at regular intervals after a bolus intravenous injection of 0.5 mg/kg. Clearance of the dye decreases with loss of hepatocyte mass. It may predict death in patients with primary biliary cirrhosis and outcome after orthoptic liver transplantation. Rare cases of anaphylaxis have been reported with this dye. It provides a reasonable approximation of hepatic blood flow in healthy adults, but not in cirrhotics. In the caffeine clearance test caffeine metabolites are measured in saliva samples over 24 hours after oral administration of a 280 gram dose of caffeine. It is a safe and relatively easy test to perform, although drug interactions may influence the results.

History and physical examination

The paramount importance of a good history and physical examination in the evaluation of hepatic diseases was pointed out by the late Franz Ingelfinger who stated that the cause of jaundice could be identified in 85% of patients by these procedures together with standard laboratory data. Jaundice is the term used to describe yellow-appearing skin, which can be the presenting symptom in patients with liver and biliary tract disease (Box 1.1). Anorexia, fever, and chills are non-specific symptoms of early viral hepatitis. Right upper quadrant abdominal pain in addition to fever and chills may be seen in choledocholithiasis and ascending cholangitis. Pruritus suggests a cholestatic liver disorder. History of blood transfusions prior to 1990 and intravenous drug use are important modes of acquisition of hepatitis C. Tattoos, body piercing, intranasal cocaine use, and razor or tooth-brush sharing are also means of contracting viral hepatitis. Health care professionals, especially those in dialysis and trauma units, are at increased risk for contracting hepatitis C. Ingestion of raw shellfish, travel to endemic areas such as Mexico, and residents of mental institutions, are at risk for acquisition of hepatitis A. Use of both prescription and over-the-counter medications, can be potential causes of hepatic disease. Fever, arthritis, rash, and eosinophilia are suggestive of drug-induced liver disease. Occupational exposure to known hepato-

---

Box 1.1   Differential diagnosis of jaundice

Common causes
  viral hepatitis
  alcoholic liver disease
  drug-induced liver disease
  common bile duct stones
  metastatic liver disease

Rare causes
  Gilbert syndrome
  sickle cell anemia
  primary biliary cirrhosis
  primary sclerosing cholangitis

Causes and presumed sites of cholestasis
Hepatocellular causes
  viral hepatitis
  alcoholic liver disease
  alpha-1-antitrypsin deficiency

Hepatocanalicular causes
  drugs – androgens
  sepsis
  postoperative causes
  total parenteral nutrition
  amyloidosis

Ductular causes
  sarcoidosis
  primary biliary cirrhosis

Bile ducts
  primary sclerosing cholangitis
  cholangiocarcinoma
  Caroli's disease

Recurrent cholestasis
  Dubin–Johnson syndrome
  benign recurrent intrahepatic cholestasis

Modified from Schiff ER, Sorrell MF Maddrey WC. Schiff's Diseases of the Liver 8th edn. Philadelphia PA, Lippincott Williams and Wilkins, 1999.

---

toxins should be considered in industrial workers. Alcohol consumption, especially more than 30 g/day in women and 60 g/day in men, over a period of 5 to 10 years can cause hepatic damage. The CAGE criteria are reliable indicators of excessive alcohol use. The CAGE criteria relate to four questions.

1. Has the patient tried to *cut back* on alcohol use?
2. Does the patient become *angry* when asked about his or her alcohol intake?

3. Does the patient feel *guilty* about his or her alcohol use?
4. Does the patient need an *eye opener* in the morning?

Scleral icterus should ideally be determined in natural daylight. It can usually be detected if serum bilirubin is greater than 3.0 mg/dL. Wasting suggests neoplastic or chronic liver disease. Skin excoriations suggest chronic cholestasis. Needle tracts or evidence of skin popping suggest parenteral drug use. Ecchymosis or petechiae suggest clotting problems or thrombocytopenia. Grey Turner's sign – discoloration of the abdomen – is seen in severe acute pancreatitis and suggests an increased risk of mortality. Congestive heart failure, if chronic, can result in jaundice and rarely to signs of portosystemic encephalopathy. Spider angiomata are usually noted in the distribution of the superior vena cava, and if more than a dozen are found they suggest portal hypertension. The triad of gynecomastia, Dupuytren's contracture, and parotid enlargement suggests chronic alcoholism. Testicular atrophy is also common in chronic alcoholics.

Examination of the abdomen helps in determining the liver size as well as the presence of an enlarged spleen. Inspection, percussion, palpation, and auscultation are all necessary and complementary in evaluating the abdomen. Palpation should be done with warm hands and light palpation should precede deep palpation. The normal liver edge is sharp, smooth, and not hard. A rounded edge suggests liver disease. A pulsatile liver denotes tricuspid regurgitation. Liver span as assessed by liver dullness measures between 10 to 12 cm in men, and 8 to 11 cm in women. Normally the spleen is not palpable. Percussion over the spleen reveals an area of dullness extending from the tenth rib in the posterior midaxillary plane to the anterior chest. It may be a challenge to differentiate an enlarged spleen from a kidney (Table 1.2). An enlarged gallbladder can be palpated at the angle formed by the lateral border of the rectus abdominis and the right costal margin. The gallbladder is palpable in approximately 25% of cases of carcinoma of the head of pancreas (Courvoisier's law). Fluid wave and shifting dullness are two physical signs in ascites. The former is demonstrated by tapping the left flank sharply with the right hand while the left hand is placed against the opposite flank. A second examiner must place the ulnar surface of his or her hand in the midline of the abdomen. In a positive test an impulse on the opposite flank is felt after tapping the right flank. Percussion of the abdomen with the patient in a supine position will elicit tympany over the anterior abdomen and dullness in the flanks. If the patient turns to one side, the dullness shifts and it is tympanitic in the flanks. This sign is called shifting dullness. Both tests need at least 1000 cm^3 of fluid to become positive and have a sensitivity of 60% when compared to ultrasound examination. Right upper quadrant pain, aggravated by inspiration (Murphy's sign), is suggestive of acute cholecystitis. In addition there may be an area of hyperalgesia over the right subcapsular area in acute cholecystitis, this being known as the Boas' sign. While modest increases in liver size can occur in numerous conditions, marked enlargement is seen in malignancy, severe congestive heart failure, infiltrative diseases such as myelofibrosis and amyloidosis, and chronic myelogenous leukemia. Abdominal bruits are heard in alcoholic hepatitis, hepatoma, hepatic arteriovenous fistulae, splenic artery or aortic aneurysms, and in renal artery stenosis. Signs of decompensated liver disease in cirrhotics include jaundice, ascites, portal hypertension with bleeding esophageal or gastric varices, oliguria, and hepatic encephalopathy. Hypothermia, asterixis, and fetor hepaticus are seen in hepatic

Table 1.2 Differentiation of an enlarged spleen from a kidney

Spleen	Kidney
sharp edge	rounded edge
characteristic notch	no notch
angular poles	rounded poles
dull on percussion	vertical band of colonic resonance in front
bimanually not palpable	bimanually palpable
moves freely with respiration	movement on respiration not marked
tendency to bulge forward	tendency to bulge into loin

encephalopathy. Fetor hepaticus is a pungent odor of the breath caused by excretion of sulfur-containing amino acid by-products. Asterixis is the downward drift and abnormal recovery motion of the hand with the fingers either together or outstretched. It is not pathognomonic of hepatic encephalopathy and is seen in patients with renal, cardiac, or pulmonary failure. Documented chronic parenchymal liver disease, evidence of portosystemic shunting, behavioral alterations, and an abnormal electroencephalogram are suggestive of chronic portosystemic encephalopathy.

Imaging of the liver

Radionuclide scanning, ultrasound, computed tomography (CT), and magnetic resonance imaging (MRI) have replaced traditional techniques (oral cholecystogram) in imaging the liver.

Plain radiographs of the abdomen may identify hepatic or gallbladder calcifications, opaque gallstones, and air in the biliary tree. Oral cholecystogram is seldom used today. Radionuclide scanning involves the hepatic extraction of an injected radiopharmaceutic agent from blood, the most commonly used being technetium 99 m (^{99m}Tc). The liver–spleen scan uses a ^{99m}Tc sulfur colloid, which is rapidly extracted by the reticuloendothelial cells. Generally there is uniform distribution of radioactivity, and the position, size, and contour of the liver can be readily evaluated. Replacement of cells by a space-occupying lesion produces a *cold spot*. A ^{99m}Tc scan aids in differentiating focal nodular hyperplasia from adenoma – the former takes up radioactivity while the latter does not. These scans are also occasionally used in diagnosing hemangiomas. Cholescintigraphy uses ^{99m}Tc-imidoacetic acid derivatives to evaluate the hepatobiliary excretory system. A minimum 2-hour fast is necessary. A normal scan shows rapid, uniform liver uptake, prompt excretion into the bile ducts, and visibility of the gallbladder and duodenum by 1 hour. In acute cholecystitis the gallbladder will not be visible by 1 hour. Chronic cholecystitis is diagnosed when gallbladder visualization is delayed beyond 1 hour, sometimes until 24 hours. Cholescintigraphy can assess hepatobiliary integrity (bile leaks) and anatomy (choledochal cyst). After cholecystectomy, cholescintigraphy can quantitate biliary drainage and assist in diagnosing sphincter of Oddi dysfunction. Ultrasound depends on the reflection of sound waves at interfaces between tissues of different acoustic impedance. Real-time systems provide two-dimensional grayscale pictures providing the flexibility of dynamic organ imaging. Ultrasound is better at focal lesions (larger than 1 cm in diameter) than diffuse disease. The ability to localize focal lesions permits sonography-guided aspiration and biopsy. In general, cysts are echo free, solid lesions are echogenic. Ultrasound is the least expensive, safest, and most sensitive modality in evaluation of hepatobiliary disease. Gallstones cast intense echoes with distal shadowing and move with gravity. Criteria for acute cholecystitis include a thickened gallbladder wall, pericholecystic fluid, and sonographic Murphy's sign. Ultrasound is the test of choice to evaluate cholestasis, and to differentiate extrahepatic from intrahepatic causes of jaundice. A dilated common bile duct is virtually pathognomonic for extrahepatic obstruction, but a normal common duct does not exclude this because the obstruction may be recent or intermittent. Doppler ultrasound measures the frequency change of an ultrasound wave reflected from moving red blood cells and is used to evaluate the patency of hepatic vessels and direction of flow.

Computed tomography is becoming the preferred technique for imaging the hepatobiliary system, with perhaps the exception of the gallbladder which is better imaged with ultrasound. Computed tomography allows for a more thorough evaluation of the liver and other abdominal structures than ultrasound, and is less dependent upon operator skills. A CT scan is created by passing fine X-ray beams through the patient, with rotating detectors located on the opposite side of the body to record the amount of radiation not attenuated by the tissues being imaged. This information is then processed by a computer which calculates the attenuation values with reference to a standard water value of 0 (Hounsfield units). Intravenous iodinated contrast material is used to opacify vessels, and to determine the vascularity of lesions relative to that of normal liver parenchyma. The timing of image acquisition is crucial in hepatic imaging; images should be obtained during an interval of sustained hepatic enhancement before the equilibrium phase is reached. At equilibrium, lesions may become isodense with the liver parenchyma and therefore not visible. Images are acquired during the vascular phase to document tumor vascularity, arterial patency, and blood supply; this is most useful to identify lesions such as hepatocellular carcinoma. Images are acquired during the redistribution phase when portal opacification has reached a maximal level; this is most useful to identify lesions such as colorectal cancer metastases. In contrast to ultrasound, successful CT of the liver can be obtained despite obesity, overlying bowel gas, or ascites. The latest generation of CT scanners use a technology called helical or spiral CT scanning. This technique was developed to optimize detection and characterization of lesions that may be missed by conventional incremental contrast-enhanced CT. Helical technology also permits single-level multiscan or continuous data acquisition at a single anatomical level. In the liver this is used for lesion characterization and plays a diagnostic role in identifying hemangiomas and vascular metastases. Thus, helical CT is superior to conventional CT in detecting and characterizing the vascularity of liver tumors.

Computed tomography arterial portography (CTAP) is currently considered to be the most sensitive technique for the detection of intrahepatic tumors and portal vein obstruction. It involves portal enhancement of the liver by infusion of contrast material via an angiographically placed catheter in the superior mesenteric artery, providing good delineation of intrahepatic vessels and the hepatic parenchyma. Since most liver tumors receive an arterial blood supply, this technique enhances differences between the normal parenchyma and most liver lesions. Magnetic resonance imaging has rapidly become an important tool in the investigation of patients with hepatobiliary disease, particularly for the characterization and staging of liver lesions seen on other imaging tests. It is also having an increasing role as a non-invasive means of imaging the biliary tree. Magnetic resonance imaging uses a strong magnetic field to align rotating hydrogen protons within the tissue being imaged. During realignment of the protons, energy is released and sampled at different time intervals. The measured signal intensity from this energy depends upon the degree and rate of realignment within a very specific time period, which in turn depends upon the water and fat content of the different tissues. These signals are then converted into gray-scale cross-sectional images, which can be depicted in multiple planes or in three dimensions. The advantages of MRI include excellent contrast resolution, multiplanar imaging, reproducibility, lack of the need for iodinated contrast agents in patients with renal failure, and safety, since the patient is not exposed to radiation. The major disadvantages of MRI are motion artifacts, high cost, availability, and claustrophobia, which is experienced by some patients.

Liver biopsy

A liver biopsy is usually performed only after a thorough non-invasive clinical evaluation. The biopsy tissue can provide information that is otherwise unavailable regarding the structural integrity of the liver, and the type or degree of injury. There are several methods of obtaining liver tissue: percutaneous, transjugular, laparoscopic, or ultrasound or CT-guided fine needle aspiration. The percutaneous liver biopsy is the simplest and most commonly performed approach in modern medical practice, and is very safe in experienced hands. Fine needle aspiration provides a small number of cells for cytological examination and is often used when a specific lesion needs to be sampled. Laparoscopic liver biopsy is likely to have a higher diagnostic yield in patients with cirrhosis compared to percutaneous liver biopsy and is excellent for staging the extent of disease in patients with various intraabdominal malignancies. The transjugular technique is more invasive than the percutaneous approach, but is useful in patients with a bleeding diathesis or in whom the percutaneous technique is otherwise contraindicated.

Conclusion

The liver is a complex organ which plays a critical role in maintaining the overall well being of the human body. A thorough understanding of the structure and function of the liver is indispensable for successful practice of medicine. Dysfunction of the liver manifests most commonly as jaundice and its evaluation can be challenging. Biochemical tests, radiological imaging, and liver biopsy aid in appropriate diagnosis and therapy of hepatic diseases.

Further reading

Arias IM, Boyer JL, Fausto N, *et al. The Liver: Biology and Pathobiology* 3rd edn. New York, Raven Press, 1994.

Berk PD, Noyer C (eds). Bilirubin metabolism and the hereditary hyperbilirubinemias. *Semin Liver Dis* 1994; 14(4): 321–322.

Couinaud C. *Surgical Anatomy of Liver Revisited*. Paris, Couinaud, 1989.

Feldman M, Scharschmidt BF, Sleisenger MH (eds). *Sleisenger and Fordtran's Gastrointestinal and liver disease* 6th edn. Philadelphia PA, W.B. Saunders, 1998.

Gollan JL (ed.). The molecular basis of hepatic transport. *Semin Liver Dis* 1997; 16(2):

Nathanson MH, Boyer JL. Mechanisms and regulation of bile regulation. *Hepatology* 1991; 14: 551–566.

Schiff ER, Sorrell MF, Maddrey WC. *Schiff's Diseases of the Liver* 8th edn. Lippincott Williams and Wilkins, Philadelphia PA, 1999.

Chapter 2

Liver Pathology

Emma E. Furth

The normal liver

Overview

The liver in the postnatal period is composed of vascular (portal veins, hepatic veins, hepatic arteries, sinusoids, lymphatics), biliary, parynchemal (hepatocytes), mesenchymal, and hematopoetic systems organized in a relatively repetitive, yet complex, fashion. This organization optimizes the many functions of the liver that can be broadly divided into two groups – synthetic activities and clearing activities.

Embryology

The liver is derived from the hepatic diverticulum, an out pouching from the duodenum, and is of mesodermal origin. Perhaps this embryology explains the not unusual finding of ectopic pancreas in the hilum of the adult liver. Hepatoblasts are present by the seventh week of gestation. By the eighth week of gestation these stem cells, that give rise to the hepatocytes and the bile ducts, start to yield differentiated cells. Specifically, the cells destined to become the bile ducts surround the portal vein forming a complete ring. Later, this ring develops a lumen, which continues to completely encircle the portal vein; these primitive biliary cells express high molecular weight cytokeratins while the stem cells and hepatocytes do not (Figure 2.1). With the activation of apoptosis in a specific subset of the circle of biliary cells at the twelfth week of gestation, part of the circle dies leaving an eccentric lumen which abuts the portal vessels. This structure is now a mature bile duct. This process is complex involving numerous factors including important epithelial–mesynchymal contact interactions. One of these important factors is the Jagged/Notch signaling pathway that is disrupted in Alagille's syndrome. The hepatocytes also grow and differentiate so that by the twelfth week of gestation some maturity such as bile cannilicular formation has occurred. Extramedullary hematopoiesis (Figure 2.2) is an important function for the liver during embryology but discontinues at about week 36 of gestation. However, the postnatal and adult livers have the capability to support extramedullary hematopoiesis under specific conditions.

The postnatal and adult liver

As the liver grows both in fetal and postnatal life, the bile ducts and portal structures must also continue to grow. This growth is outward away from the hilum. Thus, the liver closer to the capsule is "younger" than the liver closer to the hilum (Figure 2.3). Processes that affect the liver in the late fetal or postnatal state may therefore have their

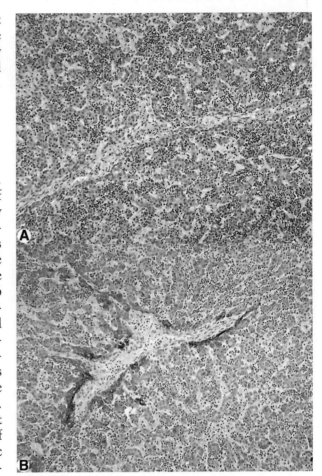

Figure 2.1 A. The beginning bile ducts are seen in the fetal liver as a band of cells adjacent to the portal vein and can be seen on routine sections. B. These cells express high molecular weight cytokeratin, which is shown by immunohistochemistry (*see plate section for color*).

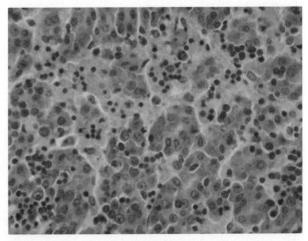

Figure 2.2 Extramedullary hematopoiesis occurs in the sinusoids of the fetal liver (x400) (*see plate section for color*).

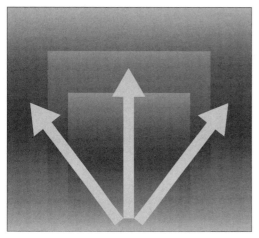

Figure 2.3 The liver continues to grow outwardly postnatally and as such bile ducts continue to develop as well.

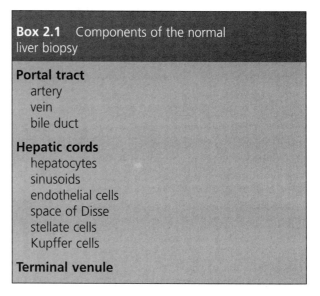

Box 2.1 Components of the normal liver biopsy

Portal tract
   artery
   vein
   bile duct

Hepatic cords
   hepatocytes
   sinusoids
   endothelial cells
   space of Disse
   stellate cells
   Kupffer cells

Terminal venule

largest effect on this outer segment. This explanation is invoked to help explain the geographic heterogeneity of the absence of bile ducts in Allagille's syndrome.

The normal liver in the adult weighs approximately 1500 grams and has a smooth surface. On cross sectioning, the liver is brown and homogeneous with visible vessels and bile ducts (Figure 2.4). The vascular system of the liver is composed of the portal vein and hepatic artery. These structures enter the liver at the hilum while the confluence of the right and left hepatic ducts forms the common bile duct, which exits at the hilum. The bile duct, artery, and vein travel together as they branch in the liver down to the microscopi-

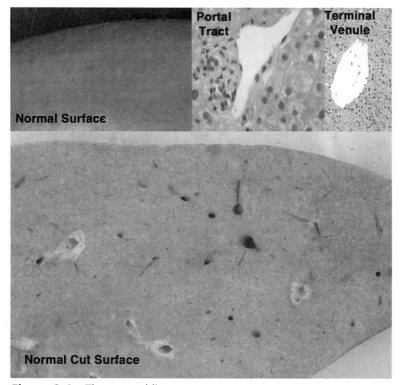

Figure 2.4 The normal liver.

cally defined portal triad. The portal triad, composed of a bile duct, artery, and vein (Figure 2.4), is embedded in a collagen matrix containing types I and II collagen, which is stained by the trichrome stain (Figure 2.5). The terminal venule may have a slight amount of collagen if it is a large vessel (Figure 2.5); for small terminal venules, little to no collagen-supporting framework is seen on trichrome stain. While most portal tracts have all three structures, it is acceptable to have occasional portal tracts without all three elements. Additionally, sole bile-duct structures may be found in the liver without much in the way of a surrounding matrix.

The arterial and venous blood mix as they enter the sinusoids of the liver. Fenestrated endothelial cells line the sinusoids. The space of Disse is a space in between the endothelial cells and the hepatocytes. This "space" actually contains several matrix elements including laminin without their forming a structural basement membrane. Thus, the reticulin (Figure 2.6) but not trichrome stain will highlight the space of Disse. Additionally, the stellate cells reside in the space of Disse. These cells store vitamin A and when stimulated

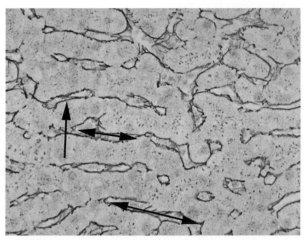

Figure 2.6 Reticulin stain of normal liver. Red arrows show sinusoidal spaces, which are bounded by the endothelial cells, and space of Disse (blue arrow). (*see plate section for color*).

by a variety of signals transform into myofibroblasts and are responsible for the fibrosis as they make collagen types I and II. These cells are normally not seen on a routine liver biopsy. When these cells accumulate vitamin A to an abnormal level, they are visible with routine light microscopy as cleared out cells with a "spider web" cytoplasm and a nucleus with a scalloped contour (Figure 2.7).

The hepatic cords are composed of the hepatocytes bounded by the endothelium. The hepato-

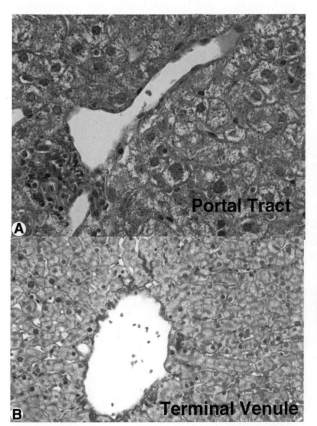

Portal Tract

Terminal Venule

Figure 2.5 Trichrome staining of normal liver (*see plate section for color*).

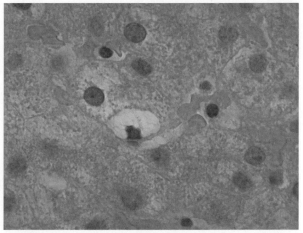

Figure 2.7 The hepatic stellate cells reside in the space of Disse and are normally not visible in a routine liver biopsy. When they become engulfed with Vitamin A they are evident. These cells may transform to myofibroblasts, which leads to liver fibrosis (x1000) (*see plate section for color*).

cytes couple to each of their adjacent neighbors and form in the center of this coupling the bile caniliculus. In adults the hepatic cords are one cell thick, but in infants and regenerative states the cords may become two layers thick. The hepatocytes take up the water-insoluble unconjugated bilirubin and congutate it with glucuronide to form a water-soluble molecule. This conjugated bilirubin is transported out of the hepatocyte into the bile caniliculus through active transport mechanisms. The bile caniliculi eventually empty into the bile ducts. Normally, the bile caniliculi are not seen on routine light microscopy. They may become dilated and visible in cholestatic conditions (Figure 2.8).

The nuclei of the hepatocytes are fairly uniform. However, with age and certain drugs such as methotrexate, nuclear variability may be increased (Figure 2.9). This variability is shown by variation in nuclear size and hyperchromaticity. With diabetes and/or obesity, glycogenation of the hepatocyte nuclei may occur leading to "clearing" on routine sections. This clearing should not be mistaken for a viral inclusion (Figure 2.10).

Handling and processing liver biopsies

General principles

As with all medical specialties, communication is a key element in achieving optimal care for the patient. For the patient undergoing a liver biopsy, communication with the pathologists is important, even before the biopsy is done, to ensure proper handling of the tissue. While many special studies

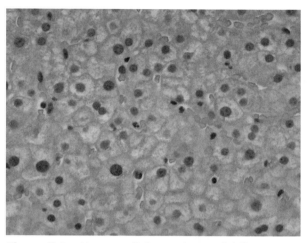

Figure 2.9 Hepatocellular nuclear variability may be found with increasing age and methotrexate use (x400).

may be performed on fixed and processed tissue, there are certain tests that require fresh tissue, e.g. frozen sectioning, electron microscopy, and enzyme analysis. Additionally, the turn around time for diagnosis may vary and special processing may be needed to ensure a same-day analysis, the results of which may be important in the care of the liver transplant patient. The hepatologists, surgeons, interventional radiologists, and pathologists form a team whose goal is good patient care. The method of handling the liver biopsy is driven by the clinical presentation, questions to be answered, and time period in which the evaluation must be done (Figure 2.11).

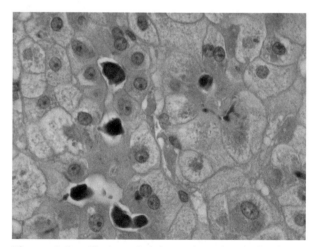

Figure 2.8 Cholestatic injury. There is canillicular plugging by bile (x630) (*see plate section for color*).

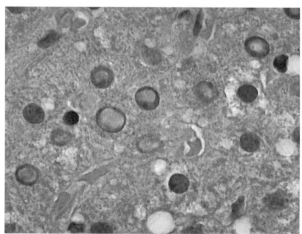

Figure 2.10 Glycogenated hepatocellular nuclei are associated with diabetes and obesity. These nuclear inclusions should not be mistaken for a viral infection (x1000) (*see plate section for color*).

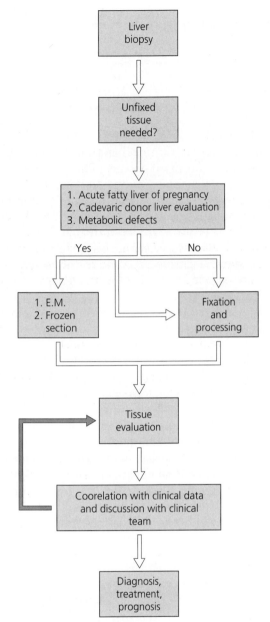

Figure 2.11 General analysis.

Standard processing

Most liver biopsies are handled in a standard manner in terms of fixation, processing, sectioning, and staining. There are essentially three methods used to obtain a liver biopsy: 1) percutaneous biopsy, 2) surgically obtained biopsy, 3) interventional radiology biopsy, either guided or unguided. Regardless of the approach, the tissue, if standard processing is chosen, should be placed in formalin immediately. Most needle liver biopsies require 2 hours of fixation prior to the 4 hours of tissue processing. During the processing, the tissue undergoes a series of dehydration and hydration steps with solvents that always remove neutral lipids and variably remove glycogen. Therefore, the pathologist evaluates steatosis by observing spaces in hepatocytes that were presumptively filled with lipid. There are no stains to "see" these lipids after this processing. Standard tissue fixation and processing, however, will not remove metals such as copper and iron and thus their semi and quantitative evaluation may be performed on processed tissue. However, if an acidic fixative such as Bouin's is used, iron may be leached from the tissue leading to an erroneously low quantitative measurement. Most laboratories use formalin fixation for the liver biopsies. After the processing, the tissue is embedded in paraffin wax and cut into a series of 5-micrometer sections and placed on a slide for subsequent staining.

Standard stains

Most laboratories do a standard panel of stains on all non-transplant liver biopsies. These include

- hematoxylin and eosin to show the histology
- trichrome stain to show the degree of fibrosis
- reticulin stain to show the fine hepatic-cord architecture
- PAS after diastase reaction to show Kupffer-cell hyperplasia and intrahepatocellular globules such as alpha-1-antitrypsin
- Gomori's iron stain to show hemosiderin deposition.

Box 2.2 Normal liver biopsy caveats

1. Not all portal tracts have all three structures.
2. The caliber of the terminal venule determines the presence and extent of normal collagen matrix.
3. Occasional megakaryocytes in the sinusoids is a normal finding and should not be mistaken for a malignant process.
4. Lipofuschin may be confused with intrahepatocellular bile.
5. Transjugular liver biopsies may have zone three dilatation which occurs during the course of the biopsy and should not be mistaken for venous outflow obstruction or nodular regenerative hyperplasia.

Special techniques

The vast majority of liver biopsy evaluation may be accomplished with the above standard practice. There are certain situations, however, which require either immediate evaluation of a frozen section, same-day evaluation requiring early receipt and special processing in the pathology laboratory, and/or special evaluation methods.

Frozen sections

Frozen section evaluation is done with fresh tissue only. Thus, if immediate evaluation is needed, fresh tissue is invaluable. Frozen sections are made by embedding and freezing the tissue in a matrix and then sectioning it with a microtome into 10-micrometer sections, which are placed on a slide and then fixed in methanol for 1 minute. Hematoxylin and eosin staining is performed immediately after this brief fixation. The frozen section can be evaluated about 15 minutes after receipt in the pathology laboratory. For the evaluation of microvesicular steatosis, which may be warranted in the work-up of acute fatty liver of pregnancy, frozen sections are cut and placed briefly in formalin instead of methanol which would leach out the lipid. An Oil Red O stain is done which stains the neutral lipids red. This fat stain requires an additional hour and is performed by a special histotechnologist.

While the rapidity of the frozen section is impressive, the limitations of its evaluation make this technique useful only under certain restricted circumstances. The frozen section is limited in that the fine histology is often lost with frozen section artifacts, and the liver panel of stains requires additional time. In general, frozen section analysis is needed for the following circumstances

- intraoperative consultation where the diagnosis will alter the surgical management
- cadaver donor liver biopsy evaluation
- work-up for fatty liver of pregnancy
- other suspected microvesicular steatotic disorders.

Electron microscopy

If electron microscopy is warranted, the tissue should be placed in a special gluteraldehyde fixative in extremely small pieces. The pathologist is the best person to do such handling. Electron microscopy requires several days of processing for evaluation and has extremely limited use for liver biopsy analysis. It is useful, however, for the evaluation of mitochondrial disorders and research purposes.

Quantitative metal analysis

As stated above, a Gomori's iron stain is used to show hemosiderin deposition. For the work-up of hemochromatosis, it is important to send the tissue for a histological evaluation first before sending it for metal analysis. All metal analysis may be done on standard processed tissue. This approach is important for several reasons, one of the most important being that histological evaluation ensures that adequate and appropriate tissue is sent for evaluation. For example, although it happens rarely, occasionally percutaneuos liver biopsies hit the liver and other organs, such as the kidney and lung, are biopsied instead. Also, if a fibrous area of the liver is sent for evaluation, a false negative result may be given. The pathologist can first evaluate the tissue and then choose, if appropriate, the piece to be sent for quantitative analysis.

In the case of hemochromatosis, there is a relatively linear relationship between the grading of intrahepatocellular hemosiderin and the quantitative iron analysis. Thus, if there is no staining with the iron stain in a 50-year-old man presenting with increased transferrin saturation, the quantitative iron analysis would inevitably yield a negative result for hemochromatisis. The pathologists can also determine the cellular compartment in which the hemosiderin resides. If the hemosiderin is deposited primarily in the Kupffer cells, while the quantitative iron analysis may yield a "high" result, the interpretation of that result must be made in light of the non-hepatocellular deposition. Thus, in this case, hemochromatosis would not be a consideration and causes of increased red cell turnover should be considered.

For Wilson's disease, the stains used for copper are notoriously insensitive in contrast to the iron stain. If clinically indicated, a processed portion of the biopsy can be sent for copper analysis regardless of the stains. However, as discussed later, the interpretation of the result must be made in light of the pathology, as chronic cholestatic liver conditions will lead to increased copper deposition and thus increased quantitative copper tissue measurement.

Quantitative metal analysis is a very specialized type of analysis requiring ashing (i.e. burning and destroying) the tissue for analysis. This test is done by a few reference laboratories such as the Mayo Clinic in Rochester Minnesota. The results are usually available in 2 weeks.

Immunohistochemistry

Immunohistochemistry is a technique used to specifically identify molecules with an antibody. Most immunohistochemistry may be done with standard processed tissue. For medical liver biopsy evaluation, immunohistochemistry may be used as an adjunct for the evaluation of hepatitis B infection and alpha-1-antitrypsin globules. While antibodies have been developed against hepatitis C, their role in liver biopsy analysis is little to none. In most circumstances, immunohistochemistry plays a minor role in evaluation. However, for the evaluation of tumors, this technique is often key in determining the histogenesis of the tumor cells.

In situ hybridization

In situ hybridization is a technique used to determine the presence of specific nucleotide sequences in tissue specimens. A "probe" which consists of a short (approximately 25 base pair) sequence with a biotinylated tail (used for colorimetric detection) is applied to the tissue. With subsequent steps, a colorimetric reaction occurs where there is specific binding. Thus, the pathologists can detect the presence and also the cellular localization of specific agents. For research purposes this technique has been developed to detect the hepatitis C virus, while clinically it is used to detect the Epstein–Barr virus in the work-up of post-transplant lymphoproliferative disorders. This technique requires special technologists and reagents and, again, has limited clinical use.

Patterns of liver injury

The pathologist should assess the liver biopsy in a consistent and systematic fashion (see Figures 2.11, 2.12) and determine its adequacy. The criteria for this assessment will vary depending on the questions to be answered. For example, at least four portal tracts are needed to evaluate for acute cellular rejection in the liver allograft, while over twenty portal areas may be needed to evaluate for chronic rejection. On the other hand, the diagnosis of a neoplasia may require a very small amount of material. After concluding that the biopsy is large enough, the pathologist must decide if the tissue is normal or abnormal, and if abnormal, then whether the disease process is neoplastic or non-neoplastic. If dealing with a non-neoplastic process, i.e. a medical liver biopsy,

then the pattern of injury present must be determined and one may begin to elucidate the etiology of the process. The determination of the patterns of injury will affect the prognosis and therapy of the disease.

Broadly speaking, the patterns of liver injury may be divided into six categories

- hepatitic injuries
- cholestatic injuries
- infiltrative injuries (e.g. amyloidosis, granulomatas storage diseases)
- steatotic injuries
- vascular injuries
- metabolic injuries.

There may be overlap among these categories leading to an admixed picture. Each of these categories may encompass both acute and chronic processes, and numerous etiologies of injury with widely disparate prognoses and treatments. Therefore, while general statements about each category of injury may be made, complete generalization must be avoided.

To categorize the patterns of injury, one must determine the presence and type of inflammation in the liver. Also, one must determine the form of hepatocellular reactions and mode of cell death. For example, hepatitic injuries are characterized by hepatocyte apoptosis (Councilman bodies) (Figure 2.13) and an inflammatory infiltrate composed of lymphocytes and plasma cells. Ballooning, feathery hepatocellular degeneration, is the hallmark feature of cholestatic injury. Also present in this form of injury maybe bile-ductule proliferation, inflammation of the portal tracts composed of neutrophils and eosinophils, and cannilicular bile plugging.

Infiltrative processes span a wide array of diseases. Amyloidosis can manifest as arterial thickening and/or space of Disse expansion by an amorphous substance. On the other hand, granulomas, another infiltrative process, are scattered in the liver with variable degrees of chronic inflammation (Figure 2.14) and possible bile-duct loss. Hepatocytes filled with neutral lipid characterize steatosis, while progression to ballooning degeneration with the steatotic hepatocyte is the hallmark of steatohepatitis (Figure 2.15). With steatohepatitis, variable amounts of neutrophils and Mallory's hyaline (ubiquinated intermediate filaments) may involve the liver (Figure 2.16). The pattern of vascular injuries is dependent on the degree of inflow versus outflow injuries. With acute outflow injury, zone three congestion is typical. With mild inflow abnor-

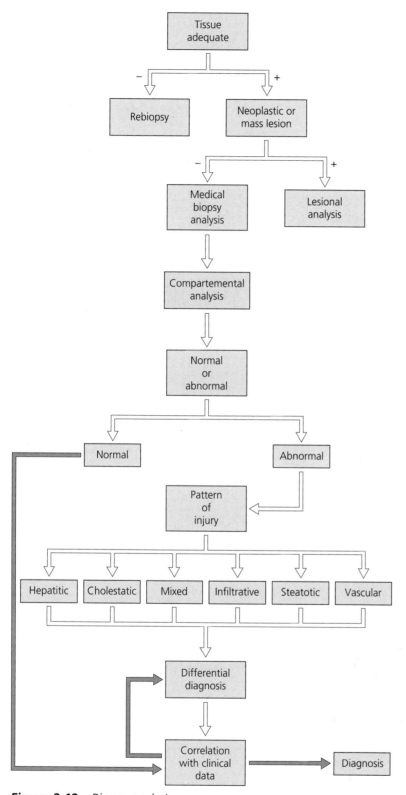

Figure 2.12 Biopsy analysis.

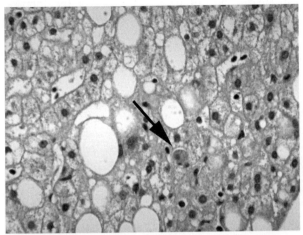

Figure 2.13 Apoptotic hepatocytes (arrow) are seen in a variety of hepatitic injuries (x630) (*see plate section for color*).

malities, nodular regenerative hyperplasia may be seen. The metabolic diseases affecting the liver are incredibly vast and may manifest themselves as many forms of injury. However, there are specific diseases for which specific phenotypes are present. For example, hemochromatosis is characterized by hemosiderin in the heptocytes (Figure 2.17) with little inflammation. Alpha-1-antitrypsin deficiency may appear as a cholestatic form of injury, however, the presence of intrahepatic, PAS diastase resistant, eosinophilic globules (Figure 2.20) is not typical of other cholestatic etiologies.

The pattern of fibrosis is also helpful in determining the class of liver injury. Most hepatitic injuries lead to portal-to-portal fibrosis with thin bridges. In contrast, cholestatic injuries may give thick bands of

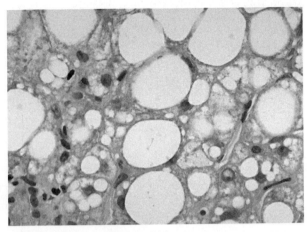

Figure 2.15 Steatohepatitis.

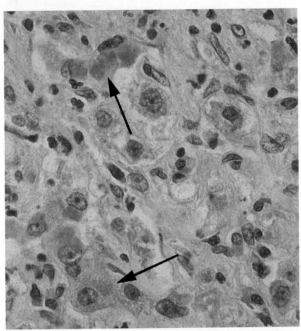

Figure 2.16 Mallory's hyaline in steatohepatitis (x400) (*see plate section for color*).

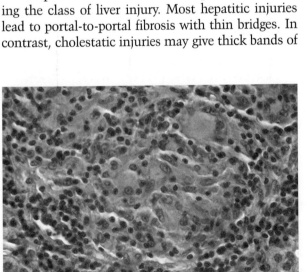

Figure 2.14 Hepatic granuloma (x400).

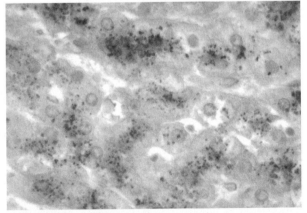

Figure 2.17 Prussian Blue iron stain showing intrahepatocellular hemosiderin (x630) (*see plate section for color*).

Portal to portal
   viral hepatitis
   autoimmune disease
   biliary etiologies

Central to portal
   cardiac disease
   Budd–Chiari syndrome
   alcohol injury
   chronic allograft rejection

portal-to-portal fibrosis. Amyloidosis, one form of infiltrative disease, may appear as "fibrosis" of the space of Disse. However, the trichrome stain shows this deposition to be a light-blue color rather than the rich, dark-blue color of mature collagen. Collagenization of the space of Disse and perivenular fibrosis is typical of steatohepatitis.

Acute hepatitis

Definition

In contrast to chronic hepatitis, acute hepatitis is a time-limited injury to the liver, which, for the most part, does not lead to fibrosis. With the advent of sensitive and specific serologic testing for viral hepatitis and autoimmune markers, the hepatologist rarely performs a biopsy for the clinical presentation of "acute hepatitis." Thus, currently, the pathologist is usually faced with evaluating a subset of very difficult biopsies from patients for whom the etiology of their "acute" injury is unknown.

Histology and etiologies

The morphology of acute hepatitis may span the full spectrum of liver injuries. As with chronic hepatitis, a lympho-plasmacytic inflammatory infiltrate may involve the portal tracts and lobules with accompanying apoptotic hepatocytes. While overlapping histological features exist, there are specific patterns of injury that may help to identify the process as an acute hepatitis. Specifically, panlobular/panacinar hepatitis is a pattern of acute injury. In panlobular/panacinar hepatitis the lympho-plasmacytic infiltrate is distributed roughly equally

among the portal tracts, all zones of the lobules, and terminal venules. This distribution differs from that in chronic hepatitis where the inflammatory infiltrate is most dense in the portal tracts. However, not all acute inflammatory hepatitides have a panlobular pattern. If significant fibrosis is present, then one should consider a chronic process. However, even in acute, self-limited injuries, a small degree of fibrosis may be present.

In contrast, cytomegalovirus, herpes simplex virus, and Epstein–Barr virus infections have characteristic features, with cytomegalovirus and herpes simplex virus producing characteristic cellular inclusions. For cytomegalovirus, the virus may infect the hepatocyte, the biliary epithelium, and/or the endothelium. Regardless of the cell infected, the cell becomes enlarged with nuclear and cytoplasmic inclusions, and neutrophils surround the infected hepatocyte giving rise to "micro-abscesses." Herpes simplex virus infects the hepatocyte with coagulatively necrotic hepatocellular foci scattered in the liver with no zonal predilection. The typical nuclear inclusions are best seen along the perimeter of the necrotic foci. Immunohistochemical stains are available to highlight these viruses although the histology itself is sufficient for identification.

In contrast, the Epstein–Barr virus does not yield characteristic nuclear inclusions. Epstein–Barr virus hepatitis may present as lymphocytic "beading" in the sinusoids. Specifically, the lymphocytes line up in the sinusoids. Care must be taken to exclude hairy-cell leukemia, which may also give rise to sinusoidal "beading." *In situ* hybridization studies may help to show the presence of Epstein–Barr virus.

Ischemic injury may lead to markedly elevated transaminases into the several hundreds to thousands. The liver biopsy will show zone three necrosis and scattered apoptotic hepatocytes.

Patients with viral hepatitis B and A (rarely C) may present with acute hepatitis but, as previously stated, rarely require liver biopsy analysis. The most common etiology of acute hepatitis seen in the liver biopsy consultation is drug-induced injury. Additionally, one must keep in mind that autoimmune hepatitis may present as an acute episode with a liver biopsy showing panlobular/panacinar hepatitis. In addition, metabolic disorders such as Wilson's disease may present as acute liver failure with acute hepatitis. Thus, the diagnosis of "acute hepatitis" is not a diagnosis rendered on the basis of the liver biopsy alone.

The liver biopsy for acute fatty liver of pregnancy may have an inflammatory infiltrate of lymphocytes.

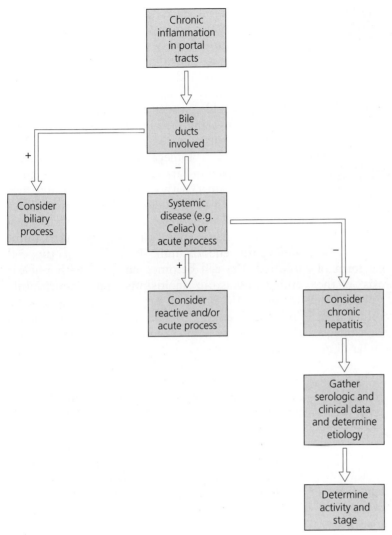

Figure 2.18 Hepatitis.

The microvesicular steatosis, however, is seen only with a frozen section and fat stain. Thus, fresh tissue is needed to make this diagnosis.

Chronic hepatitis

Definition

Chronic hepatitis is an inflammatory state of the liver with propensity to cause fibrosis. The histological hallmark of this process is an influx of chronic inflammatory cells, lymphocytes, and plasma cells. While this definition may seem straightforward, in practice it may be difficult to apply. The prior definition requiring elevation of liver function tests for more than 6 months has been abandoned with the discovery and understanding of the biology of hepatitis C, whose insidious behavior may defy this old criteria. The pathologist is obliged to correlate the histological findings with the clinical data to avoid the over diagnosis and misclassification of conditions which may at first glance appear to be "chronic hepatitis."

Caveat The finding of chronic inflammation in the liver is not a sine qua non with chronic hepatitis. Additionally, a diagnosis of chronic hepatitis does not connote a specific etiology to the liver disease. Further histological evaluation and the gathering of clinical data are imperative to render a useful and correct diagnosis. A general approach is highlighted in Figures 2.18 and 2.19.

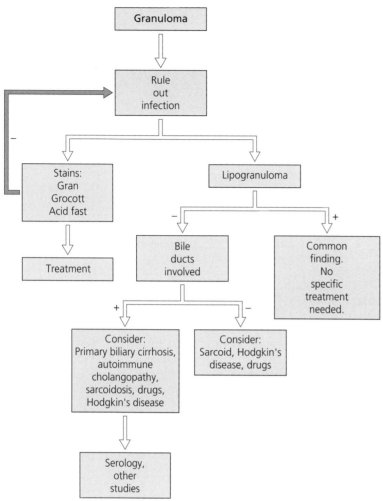

Figure 2.19 Granuloma.

Specific caveats

Chronic inflammation in the liver a chronic hepatitis does not make! For example, patients with celiac disease may present with mildly increased liver function tests and a liver biopsy showing a chronic inflammatory infiltrate. However, this picture may be part of a "reactive hepatopathy" associated with a systemic disease. As the viral serologies are invariably negative, the possibility of autoimmune hepatitis is often considered and over use of immunosuppressive agents may ensue. In addition, at autopsy, it is not uncommon to find a portal tract infiltrate with no definable etiology for a hepatitic process.

Patients presenting with acute viral hepatitis A may have a portal lymphoplasmacytic infiltrate; these patients, of course, do not go on to develop a chronic liver disease. Patients presenting with an acute drug reaction may also present with a histological picture of "chronic" hepatitis. Thus, the pathologist must be extremely careful before rendering a diagnosis of chronic hepatitis.

The term "chronic" may be misleading as the term may be applied either to a temporal feature or to the composition of the inflammatory infiltrate. As such, neutrophils are not part of the composition of the inflammation in chronic hepatitis. The term "surgical hepatitis" is an unfortunate term but it signifies that with surgical manipulation of the liver, neutrophils may migrate into the liver. Thus, a biopsy during and/or after this manipulation may show an impressive influx of these inflammatory cells throughout the lobules and portal tracts. However, the neutrophils should not involve the bile ducts and, if found, should raise the possibility of an acute cholangitis. The liver recovers quickly from this mechanical insult with no long-term consequences. Similar histological findings may be found in liver segments taken out for acute trauma on the same biologic principle. However, there are important forms of chronic liver injury which are manifested by a neutrophilic response such as steatohepatitis and cytomegaloviral infection. From a pathologic standpoint the term "surgical hepatitis" is not used.

It is equally important not to misclassify chronic inflammatory disorders such as primary biliary cirrhosis as chronic hepatitis. *Caveat* Primary biliary cirrhosis may initially appear histologically as a chronic hepatitis. On further inspection, subtle features of bile-duct damage may emerge (Figure 2.20).

Similarly, mechanical obstruction such as that seen with biliary stricures and intrahepatic cholelithiasis may lead to a chronic inflammatory infiltrate into the portal tracts. Further analysis usually reveals that the inflammation is surrounding the ducts and is thus "ductocentric." Loss of bile ducts may follow (Figure 2.21).

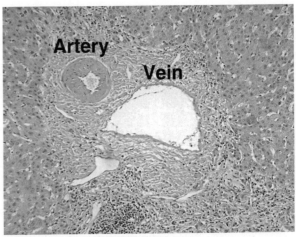

Figure 2.21 Ductopenia (*see plate section for color*).

In addition, granulomatous diseases such as sarcoidosis may involve the liver with an accompanying lymphocytic infiltrate. It would not be correct to render a diagnosis of chronic hepatitis in this setting even though chronic inflammation is part of the process.

Specific terms

Chronic hepatitis of numerous etiologies shares certain common histological patterns. The lymphocytes infiltrating the portal tract are mostly composed of B cells while parenchymal lymphocytes are rich in T cells. The behavior of the lymphocytes in the portal tracts with regard to the limiting plate (Figure 2.22), the juncture of the portal tract with the lobules, is an important feature, which is used in grading the activity of the inflammatory process (Figure 2.23). The more the lymphocytes breach this limiting plate with so-called interface hepatitis, the higher the activity is scored. The grade is determined in part by how extensively, and over what percentage of the perimeter of the portal tract interface hepatitis is occurring. Usually accompanying this interface activity is a lobular component to the inflammatory process. The lymphocytes travel into the hepatic cords and may kill the hepatocytes. This killing may in part be mediated by the apoptotic cell death pathway through a Fas-mediated process. As a result apoptotic (or the older term Councilman) bodies are seen as small pink-to-red spherules. Experienced pathologists have arbitrarily integrated the features of the interface hepati-

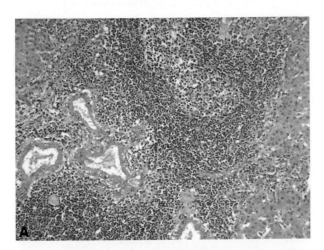

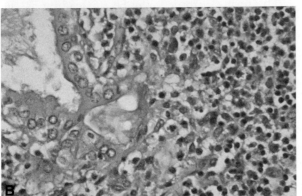

Figure 2.20 Alpha-1-antitrypsin globules (PAS after Diastase, x630).

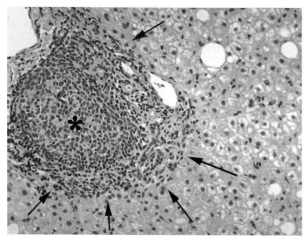

Figure 2.22 Hepatitis C with interface activity. Hepatitis C is characterized by a dense, chronic inflammatory infiltrate in the portal tracts. At times, germinal centers are formed (asterisk). The level of activity of a chronic hepatitis is dictated in part by the amount of interface hepatitis. Interface hepatitis is present when the lymphocytes breach the limiting plate (arrows) (x20).

tis and the lobular component to arrive at an overall grade for the process. Studies have shown that hepatopatholgists place about two thirds of the activity score based upon interface hepatitis and the other one third based upon the lobular component when using the global grade approach.

Grading and staging schemes

There are several schemes by which to evaluate and report liver injury. One must use caution, however, because the clinical relevance of these schemes is applicable only in the right clinical context. Specifically, the use of the Knodell system was developed for hepatitis B while the METAVIR and modified Scheurer systems are more generalized to both hepatitis B and C viral infections. Additionally, while each of these schemes may use a numerical system of reporting various histological features, one should not overestimate the accuracy and precision of these numbers. Specifically, in evaluating for progression in liver disease, direct slide-to-slide comparison is the best method by which to compare, rather than assuming that a numerical difference or non-difference is significant.

The Knodell system was based on an extremely limited number of patients with liver biopsies for hepatitis B. Numbers are assigned to four histological features, and are then summed to arrive at a total score. This system is problematic in that it groups activity features (e.g. inflammation) with staging (i.e. fibrosis). In addition, the numerical system is non-linear. For example, the category of "periportal bridging necrosis" has numerical choices of 0, 1, 3, 4, 5, 6, and 10. Additionally, the numerical scoring across features is not equivalent and thus an arbitrary bias to certain features is given; for example, the feature of "intralobular degeneration and focal necrosis" has numerical score choices of 0, 1, 3, and 4. For these reasons, the Knodell scoring system is not widely used because of the evolution of more meaningful and user friendly systems.

The stage of a disease refers to the degree of fibrosis. Most, but not all, chronic liver diseases result in portal fibrosis with progression to septae, bridging, and cirrhosis. Septae are strands of fibrosis that emanate from the portal tract with beginning

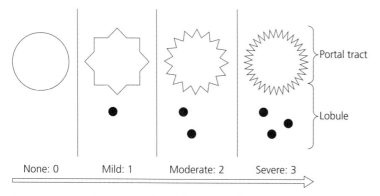

Figure 2.23 Diagram of activity scores for chronic hepatitis. While various schemes have been devised for grading activity, the system presented utilizes the extent of both interface (circle and polygons) and lobular (filled circles) hepatitis to arrive at a single activity score. However, not all cases show concordance with the portal and lobular components. In such cases, an integration of the differing levels is done.

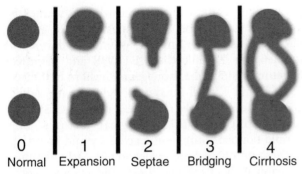

0	1	2	3	4
Normal	Expansion	Septae	Bridging	Cirrhosis

Figure 2.24 Diagram of staging. The differing stages of fibrosis may be given numbers as shown. The blue color represents fibrosis. The circles show portal tracts.

<table>
<tr><td colspan="2">Box 2.4   Staging of fibrosis</td></tr>
<tr><td>0. None
1. Portal expansion
2. Septae
3. Bridging
4. Cirrhosis</td></tr>
</table>

architectural distortion. Bridging occurs when fibrosis connects two structures. The most common form of bridging is portal to portal. However, with alcohol, steatohepatitis, and venous outflow obstruction, central to portal bridging may occur. The end stage of fibrosis, cirrhosis, is defined as disruption of hepatocellular architecture by fibrosis and regenerative nodules. As with activity, numerical scores from 0 to 4 may be assigned to this progression of fibrosis (Figures 2.24, 2.25).

Specific etiologies

There are histological features that are typical, and often diagnostic, for many of the etiologies of chronic hepatitis. However, there is still no substitute for serologic testing. Hepatitis C may have a dense, tight, lymphoid infiltrate in the portal tracts, termed a Poulsen lesion (Figure 2.22). Plasma cells and eosinophils are not a common component of the inflammatory infiltrate in hepatitis C. In contrast hepatitis B and autoimmune hepatitis have inflammatory infiltrates rich in plasma cells but relatively devoid of eosinophils. Ground glass hepatocytes, composed of hepatitis B surface antigen, are diagnostic of hepatitis B. One must be careful to exclude pseudo-ground glass hepatocytes which may be seen in patients who use seizure medication, and which result in smooth endoplasmic reticulum proliferation. A significant number of eosinophils may be present as part of the inflammatory response to drug reactions.

Steatohepatitis may or may not have an inflammatory component. The hallmark of steatohepatitis is ballooning hepatocellular degeneration and steatotic hepatocytes. If there is no ballooning degeneration but there are hepatocytes filled with fat, the term steatosis is applied. Apoptotic hepatocytes are not a common feature of steatohepatitis.

Metabolic and congenital abnormalities

Overview

There are numerous inherited disorders with varying pathologic and clinical presentations that may result in liver damage. These conditions are arbitrarily divided into structural and metabolic categories. The purpose of this section is to highlight

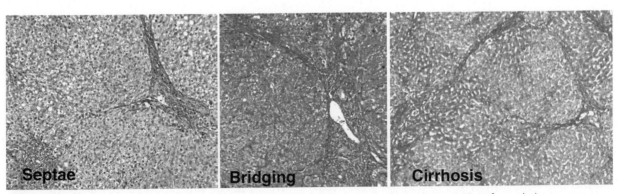

Figure 2.25 Trichrome staining of differing stages of fibrosis (x10) (*see plate section for color*).

the key histological features typical of these processes.

Structural abnormalities

While congenital abnormalities of the vascular supply to liver may occur, these abnormalities are usually not detected on a liver biopsy. In contrast, abnormalities in bile-duct development may be readily apparent on a biopsy. As previously stated, the development of the intrahepatic bile ducts is a complex process of differentiation and remodeling. This process begins in early fetal life and continues in infancy with continued liver growth. Abnormalities in the ductal-plate development may result in numerous intrahepatic biliary disorders such as congenital hepatic fibrosis, polycystic liver disease, Caroli's disease, von Meyenburg complexes, and Alagille's syndrome.

The absence of bile ducts in a biopsy for neonatal jaundice may indicate the condition of Alagille's syndrome, which is due to a defect in the Jagged/Notch signaling pathway. Specifically this condition is due to haploinsufficiency of the Jagged 1 gene (JAG1). This autosomal disorder affects the liver, heart, skeleton (butterfly vertebrae), eye (posterior embryotoxon), face (triangular facies), and the kidney. Of course, the absence of bile ducts alone is not sufficient to make this specific diagnosis, as there are other conditions in which there is a paucity of bile ducts.

Congenital hepatic fibrosis (Figure 2.26) is a conglomeration of ectatic ducts with fibrosis throughout the liver giving the appearance of "puzzle pieces" with intervening hepatocytes. While there is fibrosis associated with this the portal tract abnormality, there are no regenerative nodules and hence the term "cirrhosis" is not applied. This condition may result in portal hypertension. Also, in contrast to cirrhosis, the risk of hepatocellular carcinomas is not appreciably increased in this condition.

In contrast, polycystic liver disease has marked dilatation of the bile ducts resulting in diffuse, macroscopically visible cysts (Figure 2.27). This condition does not necessarily result in hepatic dysfunction, as the hepatocytes are unaffected.

Metabolic abnormalities

The numerous inborn errors of metabolism may affect the liver with a huge array of injury patterns. The most common genetic metabolic abnormality is hemochromatosis. In this genetic disease, the absorption of iron is unregulated at the level of the small bowel. With enteral absorption, the excess iron is deposited in organs such as the heart, pancreas, and liver. In the liver, the iron is deposited

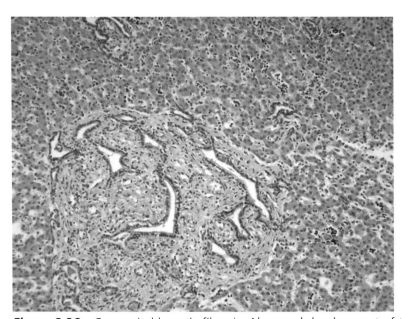

Figure 2.26 Congenital hepatic fibrosis. Abnormal development of the bile duct plate may lead to congenital hepatic fibrosis in which almost every portal tract has abnormal bile duct with surrounding increased fibrous matrix. In isolation, this same pictured lesion resembles a bile duct hamartoma. (x100)

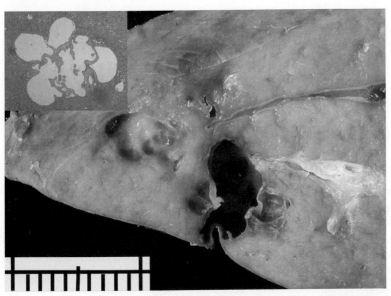

Figure 2.27 Polycystic liver disease. These diseases are also due to abnormal bile duct plate development. The gross pathology is shown with the insert showing the histology of the cystic area. The cysts are lined by unremarkable biliary epithelium.

first in zone one hepatocytes paralleling the blood flow gradient along the three zones. The iron is converted to hemosiderin, which is seen on routine sectioning as a brown pigment. A Prussian blue stain highlights the hemosiderin. The amount of hemosiderin in the hepatocytes is graded on a semi-quantitative scale from 0 to 4 by visual inspection of the biopsy after Prussian blue staining. This visual assessment is correlated with the quantitative iron measurement. If applicable, the pathologist may elect to send the liver tissue for quantitative iron measurement for calculation of the hepatic iron index. An index greater than 1.9 is considered indicative of genetic hemochromatosis rather than an iron over load secondary to a primary liver disease such as viral hepatitis. The hepatic iron index is valid only if underlying hematologic disorders such as thalassemia have been excluded. It is imperative that the pathologist examines the biopsy for full validation of the numbers. Specifically, if the iron is deposited primarily in the Kupffer cells, then the hepatic iron index is not valid. In such a case, the patient has most likely had prior blood transfusions.

In contrast, in Wilson's disease, a rare genetic disorder resulting in a defect in copper exportation from the hepatocyte into the bile, the excess copper is not visualized by standard means. While special stains exist to highlight copper, these stains are very insensitive. Thus, if clinically indicated, quantitative measurement of copper in liver tissue is a very good test to evaluate for Wilson's disease. Histolog-ically, Wilson's disease may present as a chronic hepatitis, steatosis, steatohepatitis, and/or fulminant hepatic necrosis.

Alpha-1-antitrypsin deficiency is a recessive disease usually caused by a point mutation in the gene resulting in abnormal folding of the protein impeding its export from the hepatocyte. Patients may present with neonatal jaundice. Over time, especially for those patients who had neonatal jaundice, approximately 10% of individuals will develop chronic liver damage. When liver damage does occur, it may take the form of a chronic biliary cholestatic pattern. Finding the alpha-1-antitrypsin globules in the periportal hepatocytes, however, does not make the diagnosis of an underlying homozygous genetic disorder, because other diseases such as alcohol use and viral hepatitis may secondarily result in the formation of the globules particularly in homozygous individuals. Thus, Pi phenotyping and measurement of the serum levels of the protein are needed to establish the diagnosis.

Vascular injury

Overview

The liver is a highly vascular organ with several different anatomic and biologic vascular components. While the endothelial cells, which line all vascular spaces, at first appear to be a homogeneous cell population, in reality they are incredibly diverse in structure, function, and biochemistry. As such, it follows that each of these compartments differs in its susceptibilities and reactions to varying insults. Considering the etiologies of disruption to mechanical inflow and outflow of the liver, toxic and metabolic injury, and thrombotic and embolic processes may cause vascular damage to the liver. Anatomically three compartments may be considered

- inflow compartments – hepatic artery, portal vein
- intrahepatic compartments – branches of the portal vein and hepatic artery, sinusoids, and terminal venules
- outflow compartments – hepatic veins.

Normal vasculature

Blood is supplied to the liver by the hepatic artery and portal vein; both vessels enter into the hilum of the liver and then branch into the parenchyma. During fetal life, the umbilical vein is the major blood source of the liver carrying enriched blood from the placenta. The two vitelline veins, which later fuse to become the portal vein, are a minor source of blood in fetal life. Postnatally, the umbilical vein regresses through active constricting mechanisms and becomes the falciform ligament.

The hepatic artery and portal vein branches travel together in the liver in the portal tracts. The venous and arterial blood systems jointly enter the sinusoidal spaces and this mixed blood travels to the terminal venules. The terminal venules drain into the hepatic veins, which enter into the inferior vena cava. However, the caudate lobe has an additional direct venous drainage into the inferior vena cava which may bypass the hepatic veins. This independent drainage is the reason why the caudate lobe may hypertrophy in the setting of hepatic vein thrombosis (Budd–Chiari syndrome).

Endothelial cells line the vascular spaces. Particularly in the sinusoids, these cells vary with respect to their microanatomy and physiology. For example, in the sinusoids the endothelial cells are fenestrated leaving spaces for exchange of large particles with the hepatocytes. In contrast, the other endothelial cells form a tight, continuous sheet of cells. Different endothelial cells may express different proteins. For example, the endothelial cells in zone one express CD34 while the other sinusoidal endothelial cells do not. The significance of this particular finding is unknown but serves to highlight differences among this cell population.

Pathology

Inflow

The dual blood supply makes the normally functioning liver relatively resistant to damage by vascular occlusion. Ischemia is damage caused when there is compromise of oxygen delivery. When ischemia does occur, the pattern and location of the damage is dictated by the caliber of vascular compromise. Hepatic infarction is one consequence of ischemic damage. The gross appearance of a hepatic infarct is similar to that seen in other organ systems. There is a central area of pallor surrounded by a hyperemic border. Because of hemodynamics, the subcapsular region is the most common site for these infarctions. Histologically, the central area is composed of sheets of hepatocytes with coagulative-type necrosis.

Table 2.1 Vascular pathologies	
Entity	Histological findings
Ischemia	Zone three necrosis.
Portal tract venopathy	Decreased size and fragmentation of portal veins.
Nodular regenerative hyperplasia	Thin zone three and thick zone one cords.
Focal nodular hyperplasia	Localized fibrosis with feeding vessel and variable central scar.
Portal vein thrombosis	"Non-cirrhotic portal hypertension" may be "normal" or have portal tract venopathy and/or nodular regenerative hyperplasia.
Veno-occlusive disease	Loose, fibrous occlusion of venules.
Budd–Chiari syndrome	Zone three congestion and fibrosis/thrombosis of terminal venules.
Cardiac-type fibrosis	Central venular, radiating fibrosis.

Coagulative necrosis is a form of cell death, which is passive unlike the active process of apoptosis. The cells maintain their size and shape but loose color on staining. Surrounding this area of coagulative necrosis in infarctions is usually a perimeter of apoptotic hepatocytes, which are characterized by a shrunken, very pink (on hematoxylin and eosin staining) appearance. Interestingly, hepatic infarction does not incite a brisk inflammatory reaction.

In contrast, a state of hypotension leads to global liver ischemia. With this type of ischemic injury, the zone three hepatocytes are the most affected as their oxygen supply is the least of all the zones to begin with. These hepatocytes may undergo coagulative and apoptotic-type necrosis yielding zonal necrosis with surrounding hemorrhage (ie. small infarctions) in zone three throughout the liver. In the case of the cirrhotic liver, hypotension may lead to infarction of individual nodules in a somewhat random pattern. The gross appearance of these infarcted nodules may raise the differential diagnosis of hepatocellular carcinoma as the color of the infarcted nodules is very distinctive from the surrounding viable nodules.

Unlike the dual blood supply to the hepatocytes, the bile duct is dependent solely on hepatic arterial blood. This tenuous association may lead to serious problems with hepatic arterial compromise. For example, acute thrombosis of the hepatic artery in the post-liver transplant patient may lead to necrosis of the intrahepatic bile ducts with subsequent formation of bilomas. Bilomas are very prone to superimposed infection. Bile duct strictures may form over time in both post-liver transplant and non-transplant patient populations with diminished arterial flow. Additionally, in the liver transplantation patient, decreased hepatic artery blood flow due to vascular-type rejection is postulated to be one of the etiologies of ductopenic-type late chronic rejection.

Obstruction of the main portal vein in the otherwise uncompromised liver may not necessarily lead to liver dysfunction or changes on liver biopsy. Of course such a situation may lead to portal hypertension and thus is one of several causes of so-called "non-cirrhotic portal hypertension."

While such thrombosis may lead to no discernable change in the liver biopsy, there are some cases where changes extend into the liver proper. A portal vein thrombus may lead to propagation of thrombi, and/or emboli, into the smaller portal venous branches. When these thrombi or emboli are organized by the endothelium lining the veins, the caliber of the vein may

not necessarily be restored to its original state. The portal vein branch may thus become smaller than its original size. The liver biopsy will show this change and warrant a diagnosis of portal tract venopathy (Figures 2.28, 2.29). However, portal tract venopathy may have other etiologies apart from portal vein thrombosis. The decreased size of the portal vein branch leads to increased resistance to the blood flow and thus increased pressure within the portal venous system. Because this form of portal vein injury may not affect all the portal veins equally, the less affected branches will have an increased portal vein flow as their resistance is less than the smaller-sized branches. With this increased flow and altered hemodynamics in these branches, they may become dilated with projections into the adjacent space of Disse. Thus, the key pathologic features of portal tract venopathy are

- decreased size of the portal venous branches
- fragmentation and/or protrusion into the sinusoids of other branches.

Other embolic and prothrombotic conditions have been associated with portal venopathy. For example, prior appendicitis has been linked to this entity.

The fibrosis in portal tract venopathy remains confined to the portal tract and does not lead to cirrhosis and is thus one of several features compatible with non-cirrhotic portal hypertension. While thrombotic and embolic etiologies may lead to portal tract venopathy, other etiologies may do the same, for example toxic injury from radiation or chemotherapeutic agents. Unfortunately, portal tract venopathy is also represented in the literature as "portal sclerosis." Additionally, portal tract venopathy may be a secondary event to chronic venous outflow obstruction as may be seen with Budd–Chiari syndrome and congestive heart failure. The increased hepatic venous pressure is transmitted back to the portal venous branches. This increased pressure alone may incite a fibrotic response in these vascular compartments.

In some instances, nodular regenerative hyperplasia may occur as a secondary consequence of the alteration in portal blood flow through the liver in portal tract venopathy. This entity will be discussed in detail below.

Sinusoids

The endothelium lining the sinusoids is fenestrated leading to gaps that allow the passage of plasma as small particles such as lipoproteins

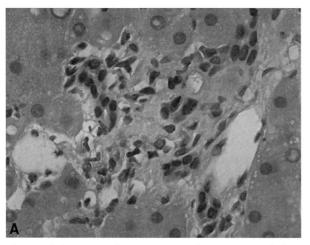
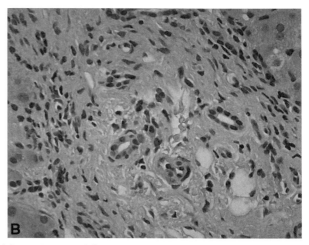

Figure 2.28 Portal tract venopathy. Decreased size, obliteration, and fragmentation are all features of this entity whose etiologies are varied. Portal tract venopathy may lead to portal hypertension without cirrhosis and hence is one of several etiologies of `non-cirrhotic portal hypertension' (x400) (*see plate section for color*).

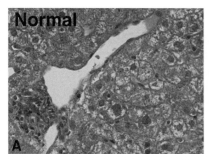
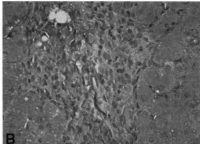
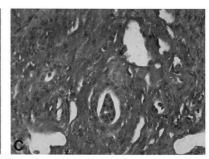

Figure 2.29 Trichrome stain of portal tracts in portal tract venopathy. The fibrosis does not extend very far out from the portal tracts. A. Normal portal tract for comparison (*see plate section for color*).

into the space of Disse. Interestingly, the endothelium in zone one expresses the antigen CD34 while the other sinusoidal endothelia do not express CD34 even in the cirrhotic state. The endothelia of the arteries and portal veins also express CD34. While the true biologic significance of this expression is unknown, this pattern has proved helpful as an additional feature in diagnosing hepatocellular carcinoma. Specifically, the endothelium lining a hepatocellular carcinoma expresses CD34 while that of a hepatic adenoma does not. As with any test, there are exceptions to the rule and this pattern of CD34 is not 100% sensitive or specific for making a diagnosis of hepatocellular carcinoma.

Toxins, such as arsenic, may injure the endothelium of the sinusoids. While vitamin A does not directly injure these cells, it may lead to fibrosis in the space of Disse with so-called "capiliraization." This fibrosis may increase the resistance in the sinusoids leading to portal hypertension.

Outflow

Blocking the outflow of the liver may occur at the level of the lungs, heart, superior vena cava, hepatic veins, and terminal venules. The etiologies affecting these vascular beds differ tremendously. However, the effects on the liver have remarkable similarities. In general, obstruction of the outflow initially causes sinusoidal dilatation in zone three. Over time, with continuation of the obstruction, fibrosis in the terminal venular area with extension into the space of Disse along zone three ensues. The pattern of long-term injury may be central to portal bridging fibrosis. In the setting of cardiac disease with resultant right-sided heart failure and "back up" of blood flow to the liver, the term "cardiac cirrhosis" may used by hepatologists. However, the pathologist should not use this term because, technically speaking, there is no cirrhosis and instead "cardiac-type fibrosis" is the appropriate term. Cirrhosis is defined by the disruption of the hepatic architecture by fibrosis and regenerative nodules of hepatocytes. In the setting of cardiac failure, while the fibrosis may be very impressive, there is often little in the way of hepatic regeneration and nodule formation. The liver grossly, as well, does not have the typical nodular surface associated with cirrhosis; the surface is usually very smooth and only by inspecting the tissue with one's fingers can one appreciate that fibrosis exists before viewing the tissue microscopically. The finding of cardiac-type fibrosis in a liver biopsy may be the first evidence for an underlying cardiac etiology of a presumptive primary liver disease. One must keep in mind that there are numerous non-liver diseases which may present as primary liver issues. Such a presentation and the finding of true liver pathology do not always equate to a primary liver disease. Cardiac failure is merely one of many examples of this point.

Thrombosis of the hepatic veins results in the clinical entity known as Budd–Chiari syndrome (Figure 2.30). In the acute phase, the patient presents with hepatomegaly and ascites. The liver biopsy shows zone three sinusoidal dilatation usually to a much greater degree than that seen in car-

diac failure. At low power, the terminal venules are obliterated by hemorrhage. Because of the sudden increased pressure, the red cells may be extravasated into the space of Disse. As with cardiac failure, the heptocytes do not undergo necrosis or apoptosis, nor is there an inflammatory reaction to this insult. Somewhat counter-intuitively, the hemorrhage does not result in Kupffer cell hemosiderin deposition. Over time fibrosis will ensue. The caudate lobe is relatively spared and actually hypertrophies because, unlike cardiac causes, it escapes the increased pressure with its independent outflow directly to the inferior vena cava bypassing the hepatic veins.

Nodular regenerative hyperplasia

Nodular regenerative hyperplasia is defined as thin hepatocellular cords in zone three with relatively hypertrophied (i.e. thick) cords in zone one throughout the liver (Figure 2.30A). This alteration in the cord thicknesses gives rise to the "nodular" appearance of the liver seen particularly with imaging studies. The thinness of the cords in zone three leads to apparent sinusoidal dilatation, which is not due to outflow obstruction. The trichrome stain shows no increased fibrosis; this finding helps to distinguish the sinusoidal dilatation in nodular regenerative hyperplasia from that seen in outflow obstruction. Thus, the nodularity in nodular regenerative hyperplasia is not due to fibrosis. Because imaging studies detect the nodularity of nodular regenerative hyperplasia, these patients may be

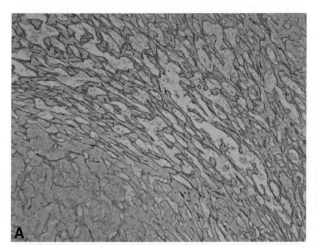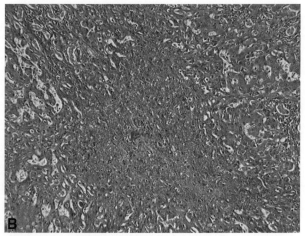

Figure 2.30 Vascular injury. Nodular regenerative hyperplasia. A. Highlighted by a reticulin stain. Nodular regenerative hyperplasia (NRH) has atrophic hepatic cords juxtaposed thicker, regenerative cords. NRH may cause non-cirrhotic portal hypertension. It may be caused by abnormalities of blood inflow but is also associated with a wide variety of etiologies. B. In contrast, venous outflow obstruction will lead to perivenular fibrosis as shown by the trichrome stain (x100) (*see plate section for color*).

erroneously given a diagnosis of cirrhosis. The diffuse nodularity may also be misinterpreted as metastatic malignancy.

Alteration in blood flow in the liver is one potential cause of nodular regenerative hyperplasia. Thus, a nodular regenerative hyperplasia pattern may be seen as a secondary consequence of other primary vascular injuries such as portal tract venopathy. Pure nodular regenerative hyperplasia may be associated with underlying connective tissue disorders caused by unknown mechanisms. It may lead to portal hypertension and is thus another cause of non-cirrhotic portal hypertension. The liver maintains its synthetic function; however, the size of the liver may decrease, remain unchanged, or increase.

Transplantation pathology

Donor liver biopsy analysis

The evaluation of the donor liver biopsy often aids surgeons in deciding whether or not to use the organ. The published criteria for rejection of the organ pertain to cadaveric organs with only emerging data for living related donors. The evaluation of the cadaveric liver is done quickly by frozen sectioning, as fixation and processing take many hours. The finding of a malignancy automatically and universally precludes the use of the organ. The pathologist must evaluate the liver biopsy for steatosis based upon the frozen section; an Oil Red O stain is not needed for the evaluation of fat in this setting and in fact the use of this stain may lead to an overestimate of the most important form of the steatosis. The pathologist must determine the extent based upon percentage of hepatocellular involvement by macrovesicular steatosis. Care must be taken not to evaluate microvesicular steatosis. Unfortunately, steatosis is usually a mixture of these types. Individual institutions may vary in their cut off for steatosis, however, 60% macrovesicular steatosis should preclude the use of the liver. The significance of chronic inflammation in the liver must be taken in light of the serologic data of the donor.

Harvest injury

When the liver is placed in the recipient and the blood flow is established, many changes in the liver allograft occur immediately and over time as a result of reperfusion injury. Apoptotic hepatocytes are seen early and distributed among all zones of the liver. This form of cell death abates quickly in approximately 1 week or longer. Cholestasis may follow and may take several weeks to resolve.

Rejection

Definition

Rejection is broadly defined as an immnunologic attack on the foreign organ. Rejection may take the form of an acute injury and/or a chronic injury. As such, rejection is categorized as acute and chronic. Such a designation is based upon the biology of the process and not the time period of the finding. Underlying this designation is the driving biology of rejection whereby acute rejection is manifested by a mixed inflammatory infiltrate with activated lymphocytes and occasional eosinophils and neutrophils, which injure structures such as the endothelium and bile ducts. It therefore follows that if this acute injury persists and is sufficient to cause "irreversible" injury to those targeted structures, then the morphologic features of "chronic" rejection follow. We thus may view chronic rejection as a consequence of prior acute rejection injury. The distinction between acute and chronic rejection is based purely on histopathologic analysis as, despite the terminology, both acute and chronic rejection may occur both very early and very late post-transplantation. However, as with the concept that chronic rejection is a result of acute cellular rejection, chronic rejection usually temporarily follows, although not inevitably, episodes of acute cellular rejection.

Diagnosis

Acute cellular rejection   The histological diagnosis of acute cellular rejection is made difficult in the setting of recurrent inflammatory disorders such as viral hepatitis C. However, the diagnosis of acute cellular rejection is made by the presence of a lymphocytic attack on endothelial cells, portal and/or terminal veins, and bile ducts (Figure 2.31). Interestingly, hepatocytes are not a primary target of this form of immunologic destruction. Therefore, while apoptotic hepatocytes may be seen in severe rejection, they are not the hallmark of cellular rejection and their presence should lead to the investigation of other injury etiologies such as viral hepatitis. Endotheliitis is seen when lymphocytes undermine, and at times lift off, the endothelium. However, in the case of the terminal/central venular area, the structure of the endothelium is not the same as it is in the portal vein. Thus, the histopathology of cellular rejection in the terminal venular area ("central venulitis") is shown by a lymphocytic infiltrate with hepatocyte drop-out and hemorrhage (Figure 2.31B). In the case of the bile-duct compartment, lymphocytes infiltrate and damage the epithelial cells. This damage is shown by cytoplasmic vacuolization and nuclear irregularities. Most likely secondary to this bile-duct damage, eosinophils are often a component of the rejection-type inflammatory infiltrate but are not viewed as the primary immunologic component of injury. Arteritis is an extremely rare feature of rejection in the allograft biopsy.

Which of these compartments and to what extent they must be involved to diagnose rejection is a matter of discussion. The original diagnosis of rejection was based on portal tract-type rejection. Even with that, one is left with the same quantitative issue. The "rejection activity index" is an attempt to solve this problem. Specifically, this index is based on assigning a score from 0 to 3 for rejection-type damage for the bile duct and endothelium and for the amount of portal tract inflammation. The scores are summed for a possible maximal score of 9. The assignment of the rejection to grades of none, mild, moderate, severe may then be based on this score. Unfortunately, this scoring system presumes a rejection-type infiltrate. Particularly in the case of portal tract inflam-

Box 2.5 Grading of acute cellular rejection

1. None
2. Indeterminate
3. Mild
4. Moderate
5. Severe

mation, this score is problematic in that recurrent hepatitis may as well yield portal tract inflammation. Therefore, the pathologists must determine the extent of inflammation due to rejection versus hepatitis. Such a distinction is extremely difficult. In contrast, the global assessment method of diagnosing rejection has been adapted by many. Fortunately, this method is comparable to that of the scoring system although it does not itself deal with the issue of recurrent hepatitis. As with so much in liver pathology, experience and active discussions with the rest of the transplant team are key factors that enable the pathologist to render a correct and useful diagnosis.

The histological features indicative of hepatitis versus rejection include interface and lobular hepatitis. The inflammatory component of viral hepatitis does not usually involve and injure the bile ducts, endothelium and especially the terminal vein. However, one must be careful as vigorous hepatitis may have lymphocytic infiltration, but not extensive damage, into the endothelium and bile ducts. As hepatocytes are not the target of cellular rejection, apoptotic hepatocytes with an associated

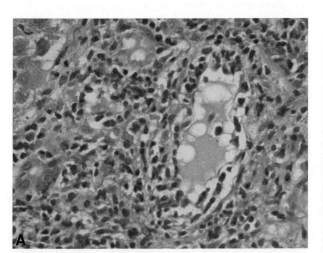 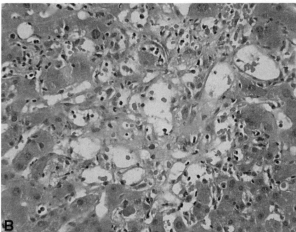

Figure 2.31 Acute cellular rejection. In acute cellular rejection, the lymphocytes target, infiltrate, and injure bile ducts and vessels. A. ductitis and endothelietitis in a portal tract. B. terminal venule involvement by cellular rejection ('central venulitis') (*see plate section for color*).

lymphocytic infiltrate (i.e. lobular hepatitis) are usually a feature of viral hepatitis rather than rejection. Interestingly, lobular hepatitis may precede the typical portal tract-type hepatitis with recurrence of viral hepatitis in the allograft.

The terminal venule is an interesting structure whose involvement by acute cellular rejection has gained recent attention. Given portal tract-type rejection, the finding of a central venular rejection infiltrate may bump the grade of rejection up to severe. An interesting dilemma arises, however, when the biopsy shows only terminal venular involvement, or so-called isolated central venulitis. While debate in the transplant community continues, there is a general consensus that isolated central venulitis is a form of acute cellular rejection.

While transaminase, gamma-glutamyl transpeptidase, and bilirubin elevations are indicative of liver injury, neither the extent nor pattern of elevation can distinguish rejection from other forms of injury. Also, attempts to distinguish acute cellular rejection from other inflammatory processes by ancillary tools such as immunophenotyping of the inflammatory infiltrate and flow cytometry of circulating mononuclear cells have failed. Thus, histological examination of the liver biopsy remains the gold standard by which a diagnosis of rejection is made.

Chronic rejection Chronic rejection as well is a diagnosis made by histopathogic analysis of the liver biopsy. The pathogenesis of chronic rejection is somewhat enigmatic although we believe it to be the result of an acute cellular rejection injury. Given the compartments involved in acute cellular injury, it follows that the compartments involved with chronic rejection are the bile duct and vascular structures. Going along with the thought that chronic rejection is a result of prior acute rejection, the first year post-transplantation is the most likely period when chronic rejection occurs. Previously, chronic rejection was diagnosed when there was ductopenia (loss of at least 50% of bile ducts). However, practitioners have begun to recognize that structures other than the bile duct may be chronically damaged. In addition, the "all or nothing" concept of chronic rejection has been questioned. Specifically, the terminal venule may acquire fibrosis, presumably as a result of prior inflammation (i.e. central venulitis). Thus, the finding of this fibrosis is now part of a component of chronic rejection. Also, disruption of the bile-duct architecture is viewed as a component of chronic rejection. However, we do not know the plasticity of this feature; specifically, we do not know if the architecture

may be restored with increased immunosupression or if this feature heralds the true loss of the duct. Thus, the concept of "early chronic rejection" has emerged and therefore chronic rejection is broken up into "early" and "late" forms.

Tumors

Overview

Broadly speaking, a tumor is a mass lesion and therefore technically the term implies a malignant or even a neoplastic process. Additionally, what may seemingly be a lesion on an imaging study such as an MRI may not be a lesion at all but simply a reflection of abnormal blood flow and/or hepatic architecture. Thus, given the finding of a "lesion" or "mass", one must determine the reality of the lesion and then classify it in terms of its biologic potential. For malignant tumors, one must determine if the lesion is metastatic or a primary hepatic tumor.

Non-neoplastic lesions

Inflammatory processes may lead to a localized mass in the liver. At times, these lesions may be confused initially as a potential malignant process. Inflammatory "pseudotumors" are masses formed of mostly chronic inflammatory cells and may

---

Box 2.6 Primary hepatic lesions

Benign
focal nodular hyperplasia
hepatic adenoma
bile-duct adenoma
bile-duct hamartoma
biliary cyst
hemangioma
focal fat

Neoplastic
hepatocellular carcinoma
hepatoblastoma
cholangiocarcinoma
angiosarcoma
biliary cystadenoma and/or carcinoma
sarcoma

occur in many organs. While an infectious etiology has been postulated for this rare lesion, no infectious agent has been identified. However, there are reports that the Epstein–Barr virus has been identified in the inflammatory cell component in a small percentage of these lesions. Inflammatory pseudotumors are rare accounting for 0.4% of localized liver lesions and are often worrisome on imaging studies for a malignant tumor. These lesions are composed of often dense chronic inflammatory cells admixed with variable degrees of fibrosis and liver parenchyma. Most liver inflammatory psuedotumors are single lesions with no association with their development in other organs despite rare reports of multiple lesions. The term "inflammatory psuedotumor" has encompassed a wide range of lesions in the literature. In other organ systems, this term has encompassed a potentially true neoplastic lesion – the myofibroblastic tumor. This tumor expresses the anaplastic lymphoma kinase protein while true liver inflammatory pseudotumors do not express this protein.

These tumors may present as incidental masses and patients may complain of vague pain and fevers. The age range of presentation is large and includes pediatric and elderly populations. Most of these tumors are resected surgically, partly because they are often mistaken for malignancies.

In contrast, hepatic abscesses may form a mass but are clearly related to an infectious etiology (e.g. bacterial or fungal organisms). Echinococcal cysts may present as liver masses with characteristic radiologic findings. Histlogically, these lesions are composed of an inner membrane composed of a homogeneous eosinophilic substance and, if nonsterile, scolices and/or their hooklets may be found (Figure 2.32). Fine-needle aspiration may identify these components.

There are a number of primary liver lesions which have no malignant potential. For example, bile-duct hamartomas are embryologic abnormalities in bile-duct formation which may present as single or multiple small, i.e. 1 to 2 mm, white lesions on the surface of the liver discovered at the time of surgery. These lesions are composed of ectatic multiple ducts in a portal area usually with intraluminal bile. Especially when inflamed, bile-duct hamartomas may mimic metastatic adenocarcinoma. Bile-duct hamartomas may be multiple. While not a tumor, congenital hepatic fibrosis is the confluence of numerous bile-duct hamaromatous lesions.

In contrast to bile-duct hamartomas, the less common bile-duct adenomas do not communicate with the biliary system and thus do not contain intraluminal bile, although they are composed of a localized proliferation of bile-duct-type glands. These lesions are usually small, i.e. several millimeters in size, although larger lesions on the order of 1 to 2 cm have been reported. Lymphocytes usu-

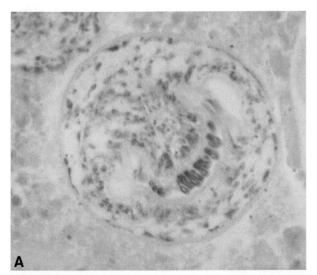
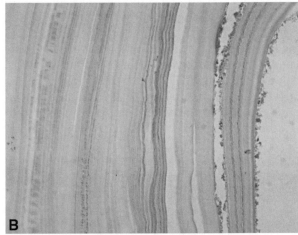

Figure 2.32 Echinococcal cyst. The hooklets stain red with acid-fast stain. A. The membrane of the cyst contains a layered, acellular material, which is pink with hemaotyxylin and eosin stain (x630) (*see plate section for color*).

ally infiltrate the lesion peripherally. Histologically, these lesions may mimic a small cholangiocarcinoma. Bile-duct adenomas are not considered a precursor for cholangiocarcinoma.

Hemangiomas are composed of benign blood vessels (Figure 2.33). Their size may range from a few millimeters to large so-called "giant cavernous hemangiomas". Grossly, these lesions may appear on cross sectioning similar to a hemorrhagic sponge, as they are composed of small spaces filled with blood. Over time, these lesions may undergo involution and may appear white and firm to touch reflecting the abundant fibrosis; these sclerosed lesions are termed sclerosed hemangiomas. The solid, white, often gritty appearance of scelerosed hemangiomas may be confused for a malignant process such as a metastatic carcinoma by imaging studies and intraoperatively.

Focal nodular hyperplasia

Focal nodular hyperplasia is a benign liver mass composed of hepatocytes, bile ductules, and abnormal arterial branches. Fundamentally, this lesion develops because of abnormal arterial blood flow, usually from a defined "feeding" artery. The original term of "localized cirrhosis" is not technically correct, as the histogenesis of this lesion is actually not one of cirrhosis. While rare case reports of hepatocellular carcinoma arising within this lesion exist, this lesion is not considered premalignant. Most focal nodular hyperplasia lesions occur in women, while they occur infrequently in children. Despite the female predominance, there is little association between focal nodular hyperplasia and oral contraceptives or pregnancy. These lesions are often found incidentally during imaging studies for unrelated reasons.

The gross appearance of focal nodular hyperplasia may vary as not all lesions contain the typical central scar (Figure 2.34). Usually, these lesions are single and appear slightly undulating but relatively well circumscribed with surrounding normal liver. While the contour of these lesions is not smooth, it is not nodular in the same manner as cirrhosis. The color of focal nodular hyperplasia is light brown with no evidence of a green color to suggest bile staining. If cholestasis were a feature of the lesion, then consideration for fibrolamellar carcinoma should be given. Additionally, the rare telangiectatic form of focal nodular hyperplasia appears grossly as a blood-filled area and may be confused with a hemangioma.

Histologically, abnormal arteries within the portal tract-type areas typify the mass. However, on a needle biopsy, there may be great difficulty in diagnosing this lesion and also distinguishing focal nodular hyperplasia from a liver adenoma. For example, a needle biopsy of focal nodular hyperplasia may yield a large fragment of hepatocytes without portal structures if the biopsy hits a hepatocyte-rich area. Additionally, because the bile ducts may not be well formed, the pathologist may misinterpret the localized changes as reflective of a systemic liver disease and consider causes of

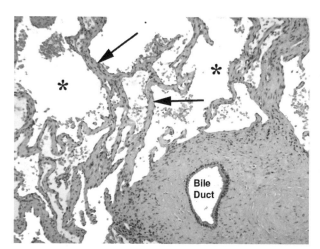

Figure 2.33 Hemangioma. These benign tumors are composed of vessels with blood filled spaces (*) bounded by endothelial cells (arrows) (x100).

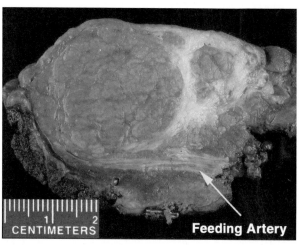

Figure 2.34 Focal nodular hyperplasia (FNH). These lesions are localized and may or may have a central scar. As FNH is a result of abnormal blood flow, a feeding artery usually is found at the periphery of the lesion. The lobular contour of FNH contrasts to the smooth surface of the adjoining normal liver.

biliary damage. In typical focal nodular hyperplasia, there is a variable degree of fibrosis and bile-duct proliferation. In the telangiectatic form, there is little fibrosis but abnormal portal structures with sinusoidal dilatation.

Hepatic adenomas

Hepatic adenomas are benign liver tumors formed by a clonal expansion of hepatocytes mostly under the influence of hormones. As such, 73% of these tumors express estrogen and progesterone receptors. Thirty percent of cases express the androgen receptors. While activation of the Wnt signaling pathway is evident in 46% of cases as shown by nuclear beta catenin staining, mutations in the adenomatous polyposis coli gene (APC), or beta catenin itself, are not present unlike the situation in hepatocellular carcinomas.

Hepatocellular carcinoma

Hepatacellular carcinomas are the most common primary malignant tumor of the liver. The vast majority arise in a chronically injured liver. The gross appearance of these tumors may vary and distinguishing hepatocellular carcinoma nodules from benign, macroregenerative nodules may be difficult (Figures 2.35, 2.36). In general, livers with cirrhosis have a higher probability of having a hepatocellular carcinoma than liver with a lower stage of fibrosis. Interestingly, the etiology of the liver disease may play a role in determining the probability of developing hepatocellular carcinoma. For example, cirrhosis due to hemochromatosis has a higher probability of developing hepatocellular carcinoma compared to cirrhotic liver due to primary biliary cirrhosis. In contrast, the important variant fibrolamellar hepatocellular carcinoma is not associated with underlying liver disease.

As with all tumors, hepatocellular carcinoma may display varying degrees of differentiation (well, moderate, and poor). The level of differentiation is based upon architectural and cytological features (Figures 2.39–2.40). Making the diagnosis of a well-differentiated hepatocellular carcinoma by needle biopsy may be a challenge as the distinction from a benign regenerative process and/or a hepatic adenoma must be made. The feature of macrotrabecular architecture is a very useful finding to help diagnose hepatocellular carcinoma. For this fea-

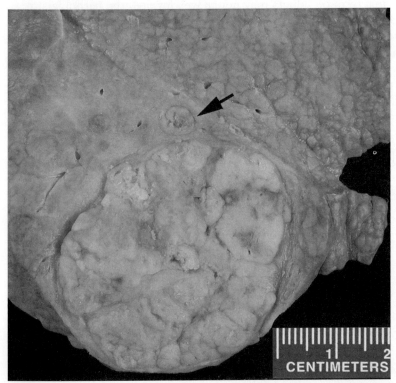

Figure 2.35 Hepatocellular carcinoma. Hepatocellular carcinomas (HCC) usually arise in a chronically damaged liver. The HCC shown arose in a cirrhotic liver. The arrow shows a satellite lesion of the tumor (*see plate section for color*).

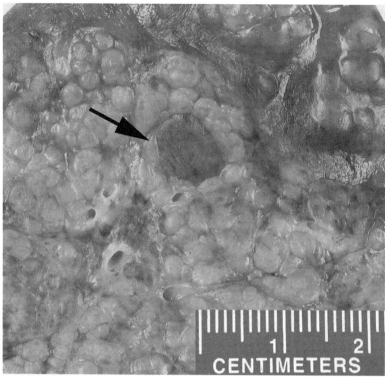

Figure 2.36 Macroregenerative nodule. These lesions may be difficult to distinguish from hepatocellular carcinoma. Microscopic examination of this lesion is needed for diagnosis (*see plate section for color*).

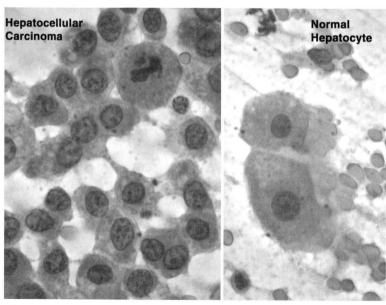

Figure 2.37 Cytology of hepatocellular carcinoma and normal hepatocytes (x630) (*see plate section for color*).

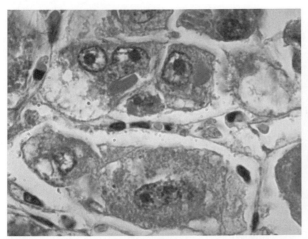

Figure 2.38 Poorly differentiated hepatocellular carcinoma (x630) (*see plate section for color*).

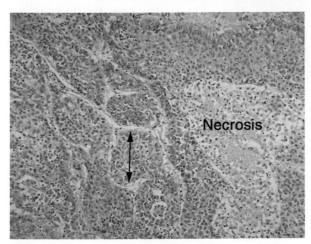

Figure 2.39 Macrotrabecular architecture of hepatocellular carcinoma (reticulin stain, x100) (*see plate section for color*).

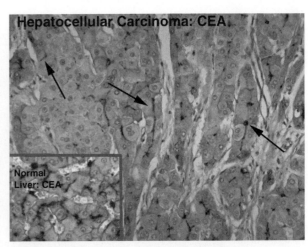

Figure 2.40 Immunohistochemistry using a polyclonal antibody to CEA. Hepatocellular carcinomas show cannilicular staining pattern (arrows) similar to that of normal hepatocytes (insert) (x200) (*see plate section for color*).

ture, the malignant hepatocytes are grouped into at least three cell layers thick by benign endothelial cells. A reticulin stain helps define this grouping. In addition, the endothelial cells that surround these malignant hepatocytes diffusely express CD34, which is normally expressed only in the periportal endothelial cells. Thus, the pattern of CD34 expression may further aid in diagnosing an extremely well-differentiated hepatocellular carcinoma. However, the staining pattern of CD34 is not 100% specific for a diagnosis of hepatocellular carcinoma as focal nodular hyperplasia may at times display a similar pattern.

The putative "precursor" of hepatocellular carcinoma is the dysplastic nodule. Dysplastic nodules are vaguely defined as 1 to 2 cm lesions which are not regenerative nodules but which do not yet have sufficient histological criteria to be diagnosed as hepatocellular carcinoma. The natural history of a dysplastic nodule is difficult to define; however, studies have shown that many of these lesions may regress and/or remain static. The feature of small cell dysplasia in the hepatocytes of these nodules is a predictor of progression to hepatocellular carcinoma.

The important pathologic prognostic parameters for hepatocellular carcinoma in a liver resection specimen include the presence or absence of vascular invasion, differentiation, size, number of lesions, and status of the margins of resection.

The variant fibrolamellar carcinoma has a very distinctive pattern of growth with intervening fibrotic plates among the neoplastic hepatocytes with prominent nucleoli (Figure 2.41).

Fibrolamellar carcinoma

Fibrolammellar hepatocellular carcinoma is a rare form of hepatocellular carcinoma (7% of all primary liver cancers) that occurs, in sharp contrast to usual hepatocellular carcinoma, in a completely normal liver with equal male and female distribution. As such, there are no known etiologic factors for its development as there are for usual hepatocellular carcinoma. However, as with hepatocellular carcinoma, this tumor is malignant and has the capability to metastatsize although the biologic behavior of fibrolamellar may be less malignant than hepatocellular carcinoma. Fibrolamellar carcinomas, unlike hepatocellular carcinoma's, have little genomic instability, a characteristic that has been postulated to explain their potentially more indolent nature.

Grossly, fibrolamellar hepatocellular carcinomas are seemingly localized lesions often with a central scar. However, unlike focal nodular hyperplasia, these tumors are essentially always green from the bilirubin produced by the tumor cells (Figure 2.41). The surrounding liver is unremarkable with no evidence of fibrosis. Interestingly, when these tumors metastasize, their gross morphology including the greenish color and central scar is preserved.

Histologically, fibrolamellar carcinomas derive their name from the alternating sheets of fibrosis that interdigitate among the malignant hepatocytes. The malignant hepatocytes are very distinctive with a prominent nucleus and nucleolus. The cytoplasm contains pale bodies, which are collections of material representing abnormal fibrinogen. Eosinophilic globules are common. Care must be taken in classifying a hepatocellular carcinoma as fibrolamellar, since usual hepatocellular carcinoma may have foci resembling this distinct and separate entity.

In contrast to hepatocellular carcinomas, fibrolamellar carcinomas do not have elevated alpha fetoprotein but may have elevated serum vitamin B_{12} binding globulin and neurotensin. Also, unlike hepatocellular carcinomas, fibrolamellar carcinomas are not associated with any known underlying liver disease. As such, they usually in occur in adolescents and young adults. Surgical resection is the treatment of choice.

Cholangiocarcinoma

Cholangiocarcinoma (Figures 2.42, 2.43) is a malignant tumor derived from neoplastic transformation of the biliary epithelium. As with most epithelial neoplasias, the dysplasia–carcinoma sequence usually prevails. As these tumors are glandular derived, cholangiocarcinomas may form true glands and may produce a scant amount of mucin. These tumors are notorious for inciting a desmoplastic response, although the epithelial variant induces less of this response. Cholangiocarcinomas may arise from the extrahepatic or intrahepatic bile ducts. Peripheral cholangiocarcinomas are tumors which are derived from the small ducts and are, as the name states, located in the periphery of the liver. In contrast, the nonperipheral tumors are derived from the large ducts and arise in the hilum or extrahepatic bile ducts. In contrast to hepatocellular carcinoma, cirrhosis alone is not a strong risk factor for the development of cholangiocarcinoma. Instead, chronic injury states of the biliary system are risk factors for the development of cholangiocarcinoma. For example, liver flukes, which live in the biliary tract, may predispose to the development of these

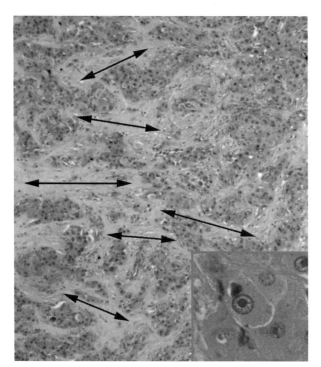

Figure 2.41 Fibrolamellar carcinoma. This specific type of hepatocellular carcinoma occurs in the background of normal liver and is characterized by intervening plates of fibrosis. The insert shows the cytology of this tumor (x50, x630) (*see plate section for color*).

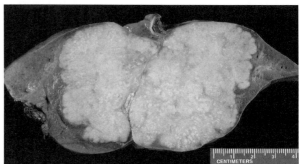

Figure 2.42 Cholangiocarcinoma. This malignant tumor derives from the biliary epithelium and may present as an isolated white mass. Cholangiocarcinomas usually arise in non-cirrhotic livers.

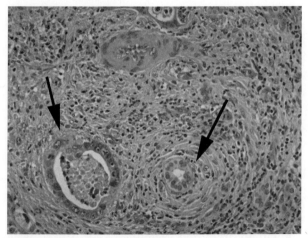

Figure 2.43 Cholangiocarcinoma. Cholangiocarcinomas form glands (red arrow) recapitulating the formation of the bile duct (blue arrow) (x200) (*see plate section for color*).

tumors. As well, choledochal cysts, perhaps due to chronic bile stasis, are at risk for the development of cholangiocarcinomas. While primary sclerosing cholangitis is associated with the development of cholangiocarcinoma, most of these tumors occur in the extrahepatic biliary tract.

As cholangiocarcinomas are true adenocarcinomas and do not necessarily develop in a cirrhotic liver, distinction of this tumor from a metastatic colon cancer may pose a diagnostic challenge (Figure 2.44). Often the morphology alone is adequate

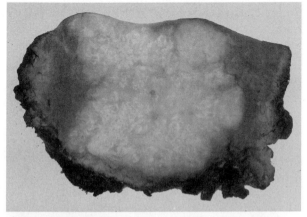

Figure 2.44 Metastaic carcinoma. The gross appearance of metastatic carcinomas may mimic that of cholangiocarcinomas. As well, metastatic malignant tumors are the most common malignancy in the non-cirrhotic liver.

to distinguish between these possibilities. However, the immunohistochemistry for cytokeratins 7 and 20 may also be helpful. In general, colon cancers do not express cytokeratin 7 but strongly express 20. Peripheral and non-peripheral cholangiocarcinomas both strongly express cytokeratin 7. However, the non-peripheral tumors may also express cytokeratin 20 while the peripheral tumors do not.

Further reading

Abraham S, Furth EE. Quantitative evaluation of histologic features in "Time Zero" liver allograft biopsies as predictors of rejection and/or graft failure: Receiver operator characteristic analysis application. *Human Pathol* 1996; 27(10):1077–1084.

Abraham S, Furth EE. Receiver operator characteristic analysis of serum chemical parameters as tests of rejection and correlation with histology. *Transplantation* 1995; 5(59):740–746.

Abraham S, Furth EE. Receiver operator characteristic analysis of glycogenated nuclei in liver biopsies: Quantitative evaluation of their relationship with diabetes and obesity. *Human Pathol* 1994; 25(10):1063–1068.

Argani P, Furth EE. Intrahepatic iron variation may greatly affect the hepatic iron index. *Intl J Surg Path* 1996; 3(4):263–266.

Bedossa P, Poynard T. An algorithm for the grading of activity in chronic hepatitis C. The METAVIR Cooperative Study Group. *Hepatol* 1996; 24(2):289–293.

Bioulac-Sage P, Balabaud C, Wanless IR. Diagnosis of focal nodular hyperplasia: not so easy. *Am J Surg Pathol* 2001; 25(10):1322–1325.

Chan JK, Cheuk W, Shimizu M. Anaplastic lymphoma kinase expression in inflammatory pseudotumors. *Am J Surg Pathol* 2001; 25(6):761–768.

de Boer WB, Segal A, Frost FA, Sterrett GF. Can CD34 discriminate between benign and malignant hepatocytic lesions in fine-needle aspirates and thin core biopsies? *Cancer* 2000; 90(5):273–8.

Desmet VJ. Ludwig symposium on biliary disorders– part I. Pathogenesis of ductal plate abnormalities Mayo Clinic Proceedings 1998; 73(1):80–9.

Epstein BE, Pajak TF, Haulk TL, Herpst JM, Order SE, Abrams RA. Metastatic nonresectable fibrolamellar hepatoma: prognostic features and natural history. Am J Clin Oncol. 1999 Feb;22(1):22–8.

Esnaola NF, Lauwers GY, Mirza NQ, *et al.* Predictors of microvascular invasion in patients with hepatocellular carcinoma who are candidates for orthotopic liver transplantation. *J Gastrointest Surg* 2002; 6(2): 224–232.

Fabre A, Audet P, Vilgrain V, Nguyen BN, Valla D, Belghiti J, Degott C. Histologic scoring of liver biopsy in focal nodular hyperplasia with atypical presentation. Hepatology. 2002 Feb;35(2):414–20.

Hillaire S, Bonte E, Denninger MH, *et al.* Idiopathic intrahepatic portal hypertension in the West: a reevaluation in 28 patients. *Gut* 2002; 51(2):275–80.

Jarnagin WR, Weber S, Tickoo SK, *et al*. Combined hepatocellular and cholangiocarcinoma: demographic, clinical, and prognostic factors. *Cancer* 2002; 94(7):2040–6.

Kajiyama K, Maeda T, Takenaka K, Sugimachi K, Tsuneyoshi M. The significance of stromal desmoplasia in intrahepatic cholangiocarcinoma: a special reference of 'scirrhous-type' and 'nonscirrhous-type' growth. *Am J Surg Pathol* 1999; 23(8):892–902.

Chapter 3

Acute and Chronic Viral Hepatitis

Barbara Piasecki, Lisa Forman and Kyong-Mi Chang

CHAPTER OUTLINE

General introduction to viral hepatitis

Before the advent of molecular and serologic methods, viral hepatitis was classified as either infectious hepatitis (A) or serum hepatitis (B), based on the mode of transmission identified in observational studies. The first major breakthrough in the field of viral hepatitis came in 1965 with Dr Blumberg's description of the Australia antigen, a protein first identified in the blood of an Australian aborigine and subsequently shown to be the envelope or surface antigen for the hepatitis B virus. The identification of hepatitis B virus was followed by the isolation of hepatitis A virus from stools of infected volunteers in 1973 by the workers at the National Institutes of Health. These discoveries then led to the development of highly effective vaccines that are in wide use today for both viruses. In 1980, Rizzetto and colleagues described the hepatitis D or the Delta agent that infects the liver with help from the hepatitis B virus. Following the sero-epidemiologic characterization of hepatitis A and B, a third type of hepatitis following blood transfusions was recognized and was named the non-A, non-B hepatitis. Although it was felt to be a distinct type of hepatitis, an agent was not easily identified. Finally, in 1989 using the latest molecular cloning technology, the hepatitis C virus was identified and determined to be the causative agent of the previously described parenterally transmitted non-A, non-B hepatitis. Both hepatitis E and G were also identified in the 1980s and 1990s. The identification and characterization of the hepatitis E virus, has primarily been in developing countries and has had a significant impact on the health of many people in certain areas of the world. The pathogenetic role of hepatitis G virus in causing acute and chronic liver diseases is less clear. The following sections describe the main clinically relevant hepatitis viruses that infect humans, including their overall virological characteristics, epidemiology (e.g. transmission, natural history, diagnosis), clinical features, complications, treatment, and prevention.

HEPATITIS A

Hepatitis A virus was the first recognized cause of infectious jaundice. It is an enterically transmitted virus, usually causing self-limited acute hepatitis without chronic sequelae. Importantly, effective vaccines against hepatitis A virus are available.

The virus

Hepatitis A virus is a 27 nanometer, non-enveloped, icosahedral, positive-stranded RNA virus, classified in the hepatovirus genus of the Picornaviridae family. The hepatitis A virus genome is of approximately 7.5 kilobases in length and encodes a single polyprotein. Four distinct genotypes of the virus exist but they have not been shown to demonstrate significant biologic or clinical differences.

Epidemiology

Hepatitis A virus causes infections worldwide and is estimated to affect 1.4 million people each year (Figure 3.1). According to the Sentinel County Study on Viral Hepatitis, 63% of acute viral hepatitis in the US is attributed to hepatitis A virus. Based on serologic evidence of hepatitis A virus exposure (i.e. anti-hepatitis A virus antibody), the prevalence of hepatitis A virus infection is more than 30% among adults, with greater prevalence among Mexican Americans followed by African Americans and white persons according to the Third National Health and Nutrition Examination Survey (NHANES III). Hepatitis A virus infection may be endemic, or at least far more common in the western states (e.g. California, Nevada, New Mexico, Arizona, Washington) and in Alaska, than elsewhere. The incidence of hepatitis A virus infection in the US has a cyclical pattern with increased rates occurring every decade or so.

Transmission

The hepatitis A virus is spread via the fecal–oral route by person-to-person contact or by ingestion of contaminated food. It is rarely associated with blood exposure such as injecting drug use or transfusion. The prevalence of hepatitis A virus infection is related to the sanitation conditions and hygienic practices of individuals. Hepatitis A virus can be acquired from contaminated water, food (especially shellfish), or sporadically. As living conditions improve in less developed countries, the global burden of hepatitis A virus infection is decreasing. However, with fewer individuals being exposed to hepatitis A virus, this could also reduce the overall immunity in the population as a whole and result in a greater proportion of individuals being at risk for acquiring the disease during epidemic outbreaks.

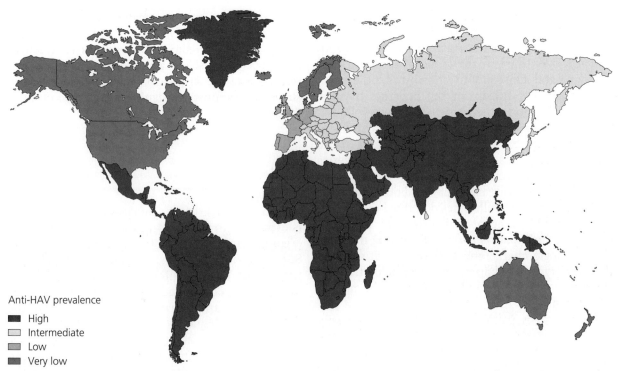

Figure 3.1 Geographic distribution of hepatitis A virus (HAV) infection. From Centers for Disease Control and Prevention (www.cdc.gov).

Natural history

Hepatitis A virus infection presents as an acute hepatitis without chronic evolution. Most often, particularly in areas where it is endemic, the infection is subclinical. The active damage is believed to be immune-mediated as the virus replicates within the infected hepatocytes. Acute hepatitis A can progress to fulminant liver failure in rare cases. The risk for fulminant hepatitis A is greater among patients with other underlying liver disease (e.g. hepatitis C) and advanced age. Hepatitis A virus infection may also trigger autoimmune hepatitis (a form of chronic liver disease).

Diagnosis

Serologic tests

The diagnosis of hepatitis A virus infection or exposure is based on serologic tests that detect anti-hepatitis A virus antibodies. The hallmark for acute hepatitis A virus infection is the detection of anti-hepatitis A virus immunoglobulin M (anti-HAV IgM) which remains positive for approximately 4 to 6 months following exposure. This is then followed

by anti-HAV IgG which remains detectable for decades. Thus, in the setting of acute hepatitis, anti-HAV IgM indicates acute hepatitis A whereas anti-HAV IgG signifies past exposure and immunity (Figure 3.2).

Liver-associated laboratory tests

In symptomatic patients who present with acute hepatitis A, the transaminases, alanine amino-

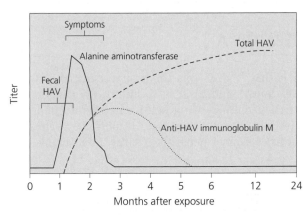

Figure 3.2 Typical serologic course of hepatitis A virus (HAV) infection. From Centers for Disease Control and Prevention (www.cdc.gov).

transferase (ALT) and aspartate aminotransferase (AST), are usually greater than 1000 IU/dL with ALT typically higher than AST. The total and direct bilirubin levels may be elevated with total bilirubin exceeding 10 mg/dL. The transaminases usually peak earlier than the bilirubin levels.

Clinical picture

Acute hepatitis A infection may be subclinical or it may present with symptoms typical of hepatitis including jaundice, fatigue, anorexia, nausea, fever, and abdominal pain. Children under the age of 2 years are usually asymptomatic whereas children over the age of 5 years and adults tend to be symptomatic. Usually, there is an incubation period of approximately 30 days (range 15 to 50 days) before the symptoms develop. Once symptoms begin, jaundice generally develops within 1 week. The incidence of jaundice is strongly related to the age of the infected individual, occurring in less than 10% of children below 6 years of age, and in 70% to 80% of people above 14 years. On physical examination, the most common findings are jaundice and hepatomegaly. Less common findings include splenomegaly, cervical lymphadenopathy, an evanescent rash, arthritis, and rarely a vasculitis. In most cases, acute hepatitis A is self-limited with complete recovery without any chronic complications and life-long immunity. In 5% to 10% of patients, a relapsing form of acute hepatitis A may occur weeks to months after an apparent initial resolution. Rarely, patients may develop cholestatic hepatitis with jaundice and pruritus that can persist for many months to a year. However, both variants of acute hepatitis A result in complete recovery. The hepatitis A virus has also been identified as a trigger for autoimmune hepatitis in certain individuals.

Complications

Although most cases of acute hepatitis A virus resolve without clinical sequelae, 1% to 5% may develop fulminant hepatic failure or aplastic anemia. According to Centers for Disease Control estimates, the overall case fatality for hepatitis A virus infection is low (0.3%) but may be higher among persons over 50 years of age (1.8%). The risk of fulminant hepatitis A is also higher among individuals with underlying chronic liver disease.

Extrahepatic manifestations

The extrahepatic manifestations associated with hepatitis A virus infection include vasculitis, arthritis, aplastic anemia, red cell aplasia, optic neuritis, transverse myelitis, and thrombocytopenia.

Treatment

Acute hepatitis A is usually self-limited and most patients recover fully within a few months. Thus, treatment is merely supportive in most cases. However, it has a significant economic impact in that approximately 11% to 20% of affected persons will require hospitalization. In the rare cases of fulminant hepatitis A, this includes monitoring in the intensive care unit as well as liver transplantation.

Prevention

Prevention of hepatitis A virus infection is readily available through effective vaccination and anti-HAV Ig. In addition, improvement in sanitation and sociohygenic conditions can effectively decrease the spread of the virus.

Hepatitis A virus vaccination

The hepatitis A virus vaccine is an inactivated vaccine prepared from hepatitis A virus grown in cell culture. Two types of hepatitis A virus vaccinations are currently available: HAVRIX (Glaxo Smith Kline) and VAQTA (Merck Sharp Dohme). Although they differ in the strain of hepatitis A virus used, both are considered safe and effective. The most commonly reported adverse side-effect of hepatitis A virus vaccination is local pain at the injection site, attributed to the aluminum hydroxide that is used as an adjuvant. There has been no evidence for inducible hypersensitivity. Vaccination of an already immune person does not increase the risk for adverse events. Recently, hepatitis A virus and hepatitis B virus vaccines have been combined into one preparation for simultaneous immunization that appears to be well-tolerated and highly immunogenic.

Since humans are the only known reservoir for hepatitis A virus, effective vaccination campaigns could theoretically eradicate the virus completely. However, universal immunization is not currently recommended. According to the guidelines from the Advisory Committee on Immunization Practices of the Centers for Disease Control, vaccination is recommended only for individuals at high risk for hepatitis A virus exposure including international travelers, military personnel, people living in areas where hepatitis A virus is endemic, and certain populations known to have a high-prevalence of hepatitis A virus such as Alaskan natives, Native Americans, and homosexual men (Box 3.1). Other high-risk groups that may qualify for vaccination include illicit drug users, employees of day-care centers and institutions, laboratory workers, persons with chronic liver disease, and handlers of primate animals.

Pre-exposure prophylaxis

Pre-exposure prophylaxis can be achieved by administering polyclonal immune globulin prior to exposure to hepatitis A virus. Given within 2 weeks of exposure, this provides effective passive immunity for up to 6 months. However, since the development of effective hepatitis A virus vaccine, the utility of immune globulin for pre-exposure prophylaxis has

been minimal. There are also significant drawbacks to using immune globulin, these include injection-site pain, considerable expense, non-permanent immunity, and the potential risk of transmitting other viruses in these pooled blood products. Furthermore, the antibody concentration achieved after hepatitis A virus vaccination is much greater than that after the administration of immune globulin. Therefore, it appears that the vaccine is superior to the immune globulin in efficacy, safety, and cost in most cases. However, the use of immune globulin rather than vaccination is recommended in persons with a known allergy to the vaccine or an impaired immune system that cannot mount an effective response to the vaccine. Finally, immune globulin offers immediate protection whereas there is a lag period in the development of protective antibody after vaccination.

Post-exposure prophylaxis

Post-exposure prophlyaxis is appropriate for individuals with recent exposure to hepatitis A virus but without previous hepatitis A virus vaccination. Post-exposure prophylaxis includes the administration of immune globulin as a single intramuscular dose of 0.02 mL/kg as soon as possible after the exposure – ideally within 2 weeks of the exposure. Notably, persons who have received at least one dose of the hepatitis A virus vaccine at least 1 month before the exposure do not need the immune globulin since a single dose of vaccine confers significant protective immunity while the second vaccine dose lengthens the duration of immunity.

Persons considered at risk for hepatitis A virus exposure include unvaccinated household and sexual contacts of the index patient, persons who have shared illicit drugs with the index patient, unvaccinated staff and attendees of day-care centers or institutions, and food handlers exposed to the index patient. An index case is identified by positive serologic evidence for acute hepatitis A infection (positive HAV IgM). A lack of immunity to hepatitis A virus need not be demonstrated before giving the prophylaxis to the exposed or at-risk individuals since this will only delay the immunization. In the case of unclear immune status based on history, post-exposure prophylaxis should be administered in the form of immune globulin. If the exposed individual is at risk for repeated exposure to hepatitis A virus, a concurrent administration of hepatitis A virus vaccination is also recommended as post-exposure prophylaxis,

> **Box 3.1** Advisory Committee on Immunization Practices of the Centers for Disease Control recommendations of persons at increased risk for hepatitis A virus infection who should be routinely vaccinated
>
> Persons traveling to or working in countries that have high or intermediate endemicity of infection.
> Men who have sex with men.
> Illegal drug users.
> Persons who have occupational risk for exposure – persons working with hepatitis A virus-infected primates or hepatitis A virus in a research laboratory.
> Persons who have clotting-factor disorders and are administered clotting-factor concentrates, especially solvent-detergent-treated preparations.
> Persons with chronic liver disease.

conferring both passive and active immunization. The hepatitis A virus vaccine is still efficacious when administered in this fashion, although the overall antibody titers may be somewhat lower. For individuals with an exposure, but no risk for repeated exposure, immune globulin should be provided as soon as possible, but without vaccine.

Further reading – hepatitis A virus

Feinstone SM, Kapikian AZ, Purcell RH. Hepatitis A: detection by immune electron microscopy of a viruslike antigen associated with acute illness. *Science* 1973; 182(116): 1026–1028.

Kemmer NM, Miskovsky EP. Hepatitis A. *Infect Dis Clin North Am* 2000; 14(3): 605–615.

Koff, RS. Hepatitis vaccines. *Infect Dis Clin North Am* 2001; 15(1): 83–95.

Prevention of hepatitis A through active or passive immunization: recommendations of the Advisory Committee on Immunization Practices (ACIP). *Morbidity and Mortality Weekly Report* 1999; 48(12): 1–37.

HEPATITIS B

Hepatitis B virus is a hepatotrophic DNA virus that causes acute and chronic hepatitis in people throughout the world. More than 300 million people worldwide are chronically infected with hepatitis B virus and are at risk for the development of cirrhosis and hepatocellular carcinoma. However, hepatitis B virus infection is readily preventable because of an effective vaccine that has been available for nearly 20 years. Therefore, the challenge in hepatitis B virus infection includes not only the treatment of currently infected patients, but also the primary prevention of hepatitis B virus infection including proper vaccination and public health measures to decrease the overall worldwide prevalence of hepatitis B virus.

The virus

The hepatitis B virus is a 3.2 kilobases long partially double-stranded DNA virus belonging to the Hepadnaviridae family. It codes for a number of viral proteins (envelope, core/precore, polymerase and X) in overlapping open reading frames. The complete infectious virion (also called the Dane particle) is 42 nanometers in diameter with the hepatitis B virus envelope antigens on its surface and with a nucleocapsid core. Hepatitis B virus envelope or surface antigen (HBsAg) can be visualized in electron microscopy as non-infectious subviral particles circulating in the blood of infected patients. The hepatitis Be antigen (HBeAg) is a readily secreted viral antigen derived from the precore region of hepatitis B virus, with overlap of the hepatitis B virus core region. Presence of HBeAg is usually associated with a high replicative state of hepatitis B virus. Hepatitis B virus nucleocapsid or core antigen contains the infectious hepatitis B virus genome and the viral polymerase within the Dane particle. Unlike the s or e antigens, hepatitis B core antigen (HBcAg) is not secreted into the blood. The role of the hepatitis B virus X protein is not well established, although it is a transcriptional transactivator with an important role in the hepatitis B virus life cycle.

Seven genotypes of hepatitis B virus (A–G) with unique geographic distributions have been identified based on the viral sequences. The predominant geographic distributions are as follows

- genotype A in northwest Europe, North America, and Central Africa
- genotypes B and C mainly in southeast Asia and Japan
- genotype D in the Mediterranean area, the Middle East and India
- genotype E in Africa
- genotype F in Native American and Polynesian populations.
- genotype G, a new genotype, has been reported in the US and France.

There is increasing evidence that hepatitis B virus genotypes may influence HBeAg seroconversion rates, mutational patterns in the precore and core promoter regions, and the severity of liver disease, although further research is needed to fully characterize the clinical impact.

Although hepatitis B virus is a DNA virus, it has an RNA intermediate that is reverse transcribed to DNA in its life cycle, similar to a retrovirus. As a result, its mutation rate is as high as that of an RNA virus. A number of clinically relevant hepatitis B virus variants and mutants have been described. These include the precore stop codon mutation and core promoter mutations associated with the loss of HBeAg but resolution of the disease and viral replication as well as the glycine-145-arginine substitution in the S gene associated with the vaccine escape variants. These have been implicated in worsening severity of liver disease because of altered hepatitis B virus replication or the expression of immunogenic epitopes. Recently, the therapeutic inhibition of hepatitis B virus polymerase with antiviral compounds such as lamivudine or famciclovir has resulted in selection of polymerase gene mutants.

Epidemiology

Infection with hepatitis B is a global health problem. The prevalence of hepatitis B virus carriers is estimated to be more than 300 million in the world and 1.25 million in the US. Each year 250 000 people die from hepatitis B virus-associated liver disease. The carrier state is defined by the presence of detectable HBsAg in the serum. The prevalence of hepatitis B virus infection shows significant geographical variation based primarily on the mode of transmission and the age at the time of infection (Figure 3.3). The highest prevalence of hepatitis B virus carriers is observed in parts of the world where hepatitis B virus is transmitted in the perinatal period. These areas include southeast Asia and sub-Saharan Africa where the prevalence may reach 10% to 20%. In intermediate-prevalence areas (e.g. Mediterranean countries, Japan, India, and Singapore), exposure to hepatitis B virus occurs mostly in early childhood and the prevalence is 3%

to 5%. In contrast, in low-prevalence areas (e.g. the US, western Europe, Australia, and New Zealand), most infections are acquired in early adult life through sexual contact or intravenous drug use and the prevalence of hepatitis B virus carrier state is 0.1% to 2%. The prevalence of hepatitis B virus infection also tends to increase with age.

The epidemiology of hepatitis B virus infection has been quite dynamic, with a dramatic decline in hepatitis B virus cases in some regions of the world but not in others. In the US, the rate of acute hepatitis B infections has decreased by almost 76% over the last 20 years presumably because of widespread hepatitis B virus vaccination and the implementation of public health measures for high-risk groups. Interestingly, the greatest decline has been in cases associated with injection drug use.

Transmission

Hepatitis B virus is transmitted mainly by perinatal, sexual, and parenteral exposure. In parts of the world where hepatitis B virus is highly endemic (e.g. China) the rate of perinatal transmission may be as high as 90% in infants born to mothers who are HBeAg or hepatitis B virus DNA positive. In the US,

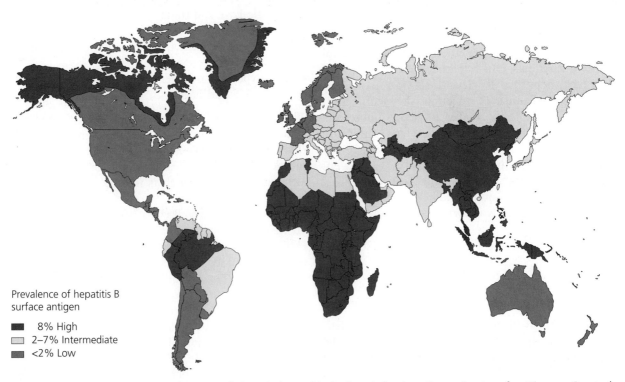

Prevalence of hepatitis B surface antigen

- ■ 8% High
- ▢ 2–7% Intermediate
- ■ <2% Low

Figure 3.3 Geographic distribution of chronic hepatitis B virus infection. From Centers for Disease Control and Prevention (www.cdc.gov).

perinatal transmission plays a much smaller role and the main mode of transmission is through sexual contact. In this setting, the risk of sexual transmission of the hepatitis B virus may be related to the number of lifetime sexual partners, education level, contact with prostitutes, and history of sexually transmitted diseases. Hepatitis B virus is also transmitted through parenteral or direct routes such as blood transfusion, hepatitis B virus-contaminated needle exposure during illicit intravenous drug use, and solid-organ transplantation from infected persons. Importantly, hepatitis B virus transmission through blood transfusion has been dramatically reduced since the 1960s in many countries because of the careful screening of blood donors for the presence of HBsAg and hepatitis B core antibody (anti-HBc). Thus, the current estimated risk of hepatitis B virus infection from a blood transfusion in the US is approximately 1 in 63 000.

Working in a health care field also poses a risk for hepatitis B virus infection. Although the risk is greatest with a percutaneous injury in this setting, hepatitis B virus transmission is possible by direct contact between infected instruments and skin surfaces with lesions (e.g. scratches, abrasions, burns) that disrupt the skin barrier. Indeed, it has been shown that the hepatitis B virus can survive in dried blood at room temperature on environmental surfaces for up to 1 week. Furthermore, hepatitis B virus has been detected in many types of body fluids including breast milk, bile, cerebrospinal fluid, feces, nasopharyngeal washings, saliva, semen, sweat, and synovial fluid (Table 3.1), although they are less efficient in hepatitis B virus transmission than the blood which has a higher concentration of infectious particles.

Natural history

Hepatitis B virus infection has both an acute and a chronic phase. Patients may present during the acute phase of infection or they may present many years thereafter either in spontaneous resolution or with long-term chronic infection. Acute hepatitis B virus infection may present in varying levels of acute liver injury including asymptomatic, icteric or fulminant hepatitis. Chronic hepatitis B virus infection can progress to cirrhosis and hepatocellular carcinoma after many years of infection. The specific clinical features are described below.

Diagnosis of hepatitis B virus infection

Various diagnostic markers provide clinically relevant information in the setting of hepatitis B virus infection. There are serologic assays for various hepatitis B virus antigens (HBsAg and HBeAg) as well as antibodies to these and other viral antigens (anti-HBs, anti-HBe, anti-HBc). Hepatitis B virus DNA can be directly measured in the serum through both hybridization and polymerase chain reaction (PCR)-based assays. The pattern of serologic markers will change over time and will depend on whether the infection is acute and self-limited or if the infection becomes chronic (Table 3.2). In the case of an acute infection with spontaneous recovery, HBsAg is initially detectable but eventually lost with resolution of hepatitis B virus infection (Figure 3.4). In contrast, HBsAg persists in the setting of acute hepatitis B that evolves into a chronic infection (Figure 3.5).

Serologic tests

Hepatitis B surface antigen and antibody

Hepatitis B surface antigen is an important marker of active hepatitis B virus infection. Detectable by enzyme immunoassays (EIA) or radioimmunoassay, it appears in the serum within 1 to 10 weeks of acute infection (Figures 3.4 and 3.5), and it is lost within 6 months thereafter in self-limited hepatitis B virus infection. Loss of HBsAg is followed by a rise in antibody to the HBsAg (anti-HBs), a neutralizing antibody that binds and removes the circulating viral particles. The presence of anti-HBs confers protective immunity that is life long in most cases. There may be a window period between the loss of HBsAg and the appearance of anti-HBs during which time neither marker is detectable. This window period can last for several weeks to months. During this time the presence of IgM antibody to hepatitis B core antigen (anti-HBc IgM) indicates acute hepatitis B virus infection. In con-

Table 3.1 Concentration of hepatitis B virus in various body fluids		
High	**Moderate**	**Low or not detectable**
blood	semen	urine
serum	vaginal fluid	feces
wound exudates	saliva	sweat
		tears
		breast milk

Table 3.2 Patterns of serologic markers

HBsAG[1]	HBeAg[2]	Anti-HBc IgM[3]	Anti-HBc IgG[4]	Anti-HBs[5]	Anti-HBe[6]	HBV DNA[7]	Interpretation
+	+	+	–	–	–	+	Early acute infection
–	–	+	–	–	–	+/–	Window phase
–	–	–	+	+	+	–	Recovery phase
			+	–			
+	+	–	+	–	–	+	Replicative chronic phase
+	–	–	+	–	+	+/–	Low nonreplicative chronic phase
+	+/–	+/–	+	–	+/–	+	Flare of chronic HBV
+	–	–	+	–	+/–	+	Precore/core mutants
–	–	–	–	+	–	–	Immunity due to vaccine or prior recovery

[1] *hepatitis B surface antigen.*
[2] *hepatitis Be antigen.*
[3] *immunoglobulin M antibody to hepatitis B core antigen.*
[4] *immunoglobulin G antibody to hepatitis B core antigen.*
[5] *antibody to hepatitis B surface antigen.*
[6] *antibody to hepatitis Be antigen.*
[7] *hepatitis B virus DNA. These results may depend on the types of assay used. For example, low level HBV viremia (e.g. during the window phase or low replicative phase of chronic infection) may not be detected unless highly sensitive PCR-based arrays are used with detection limit of 100–1000 copies/ml.*

trast, the presence of anti-HBc IgG without HBsAg or anti-HBs suggests a prior rather than an acute hepatitis B virus infection. Approximately 0.5% of patients with chronic hepatitis B infection may spontaneously develop anti-HBs and lose HBsAg each year. Both HBsAg and anti-HBs can coexist in a subset of patients, presumably because of the failure of the antibody to neutralize the antigen. In

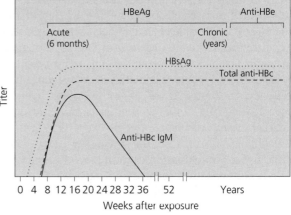

HbeAg = hepatitis Be antigen
anti-HBe = antibody to hepatitis Be antigen
anti-HBc = antibody to hepatitis B core antigen
HbsAg = hepatitis B surface antigen
anti-HBc IgM = Immunoglobolin M antibody to hepatitis B core antigen
anti-HBs = antibody to Hepatitis B surface antigen

Figure 3.5 Typical serologic course of the progression to a chronic hepatitis B virus infection. From Centers for Disease Control and Prevention (www.cdc.gov).

these cases there is chronic infection rather than recovery despite the presence of anti-HBs.

Hepatitis B core antigen and antibody

Hepatitis B core antigen resides within the infected hepatocytes but is not secreted. Therefore, it is detectable by immunohistochemical staining of

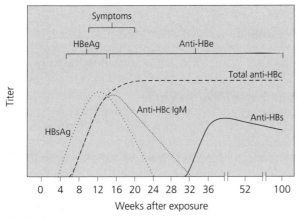

HbeAg = hepatitis Be antigen
anti-HBe = antibody to hepatitis Be antigen
anti-HBc = antibody to hepatitis B core antigen
HbsAg = hepatitis B surface antigen
anti-HBc IgM = Immunoglobolin M antibody to hepatitis B core antigen
anti-HBs = antibody to hepatitis B surface antigen

Figure 3.4 Typical serologic course of an acute hepatitis B virus infection with recovery. From Centers for Disease Control and Prevention (www.cdc.gov).

infected liver tissue but not in the serum. The antibody against the core antigen (anti-HBc) is detectable in the serum throughout hepatitis B virus infection starting with anti-HBc IgM during the acute phase and anti-HBc IgG thereafter. The anti-HBc IgM response usually lasts for several months, although it can be as long as 2 years. Unlike anti-HBs, presence of anti-HBc is associated with neither hepatitis B virus clearance nor protective immunity. However, exacerbations of chronic hepatitis B can be associated with a resurgence of anti-HBc IgM, thus leading to a diagnostic confusion since anti-HBc IgM is typically associated with new infection and not a flare in an existing chronic infection.

Isolated hepatitis B core antibody

Occasionally, patients will display the serologic pattern of an isolated anti-HBc IgG without concurrent HBsAg or anti-HBs. While anti-HBc IgM, in the setting of acute hepatitis, is diagnostic for acute hepatitis B, the presence of anti-HBc IgG without clinical hepatitis may reflect a previous infection with clearance followed by loss of anti-HBs but not anti-HBc. Alternatively, it may occur in the setting of long-term chronic hepatitis B virus infection with a decrease in HBsAg level below the limit of detection. Isolated anti-HBc has been reported in 0.4% to 1.7% of blood donors in low-prevalence areas and in 10% to 20% of persons in higher prevalence areas where hepatitis B virus is endemic. The overall clinical significance of isolated anti-HBc is not clear. However, based on the appropriate clinical scenario, a consideration should be given to test for acute hepatitis B with anti-HBc IgM, ongoing low-level chronic hepatitis B virus infection by hepatitis B virus DNA and to repeat the testing of HBsAg, anti-HBs, and anti-HBc by radioimmunoassay.

Hepatitis Be antigen and antibody

The e antigen of the hepatitis B virus is processed from the precore region of the viral genome which overlaps with the core region. However, unlike HBcAg, it is readily secreted from the hepatocytes into the circulation. The detection of serum HBeAg is a marker for active hepatitis B virus replication and infectivity. The loss of HBeAg with the development of anti-HBe is termed HBeAg seroconversion. This seroconversion is usually associated with decreased serum hepatitis B virus DNA titer and remission of liver inflammation as well as an improved overall liver-related prognosis. An exception to this rule is the emergence of hep-

atitis B virus variants with a stop codon mutation in the precore region that blocks proper HBeAg production but not hepatitis B virus replication. These individuals may demonstrate ongoing liver injury and hepatitis B virus viremia despite loss of HBeAg. Thus, identification of these precore mutants with loss of HBeAg but not hepatitis B virus DNA is clinically relevant.

Hepatitis B virus DNA

The measurement of hepatitis B virus DNA assesses the replicative state of the hepatitis B virus infection as well as the antiviral treatment candidacy and efficacy in various clinical settings. The serum titer of hepatitis B virus DNA can be detected by both qualitative and quantitative assays with varying lower limits of detection and accuracy. These assays include hybridization assays, signal amplification branched DNA assays, and PCR assays. In the past, a lack of standardization of these assays between laboratories made interpretation of their results confusing and potentially unreliable. However, there has been a movement to standardize the measurements in recent years, as proposed by the World Health Organization. The hybridization and branched DNA assays that are currently used have a detection threshold of around 10^5 to 10^6 genome equivalents/mL. Although these assays are not particularly sensitive compared to the PCR-based methods (50 to 1000 genome equivalents/mL), the clinical signficance of low-level viremia (i.e. detectable by PCR but not by hybridization or branched DNA assays) is not yet clear. Thus, the utility of these more or less sensitive tests may depend on the clinical setting.

Liver histology in chronic hepatitis B virus infections

Liver biopsy plays an important role in patients with chronic hepatitis B virus infection by assessing the severity of liver injury and predicting the overall prognosis and response to antiviral treatment. Histological findings of chronic hepatitis B virus infection include primarily mononuclear inflammatory infiltrates in the portal tracts, and periportal necrosis as well as varying degrees of liver fibrosis. The degree of injury (grade) and amount of fibrosis (stage) can be assessed using the histology activity index or the Metavir score. Immunohistochemical staining may show hepatocytes staining for HBsAg and HBcAg, including the characteristic ground-glass hepatocytes which are full of HBsAg. However, the hepatitis B virus antigen-staining pattern does not correlate with disease severity.

Clinical picture

Acute hepatitis B

The clinical presentation of acute hepatitis B covers the entire spectrum from sub-clinical, anicteric, and icteric hepatitis to fulminant hepatic failure. The clinical features and outcome of acute hepatitis B virus infection is dependent on both host and viral factors. Age at the time of hepatitis B virus infection is a particularly important determinant in this regard. Indeed, most hepatitis B virus infection in the perinatal period or early childhood is asymptomatic but results in persistent infection. By contrast, acute hepatitis B virus infection in adulthood can result in symptomatic hepatitis (approximately 30%) but it does not go on to chronic infection in most cases. Thus, the rate of chronic hepatitis B virus infection is 90% for perinatal onset, 20% to 50% for onset between ages 1 to 5 years, and less than 5% for adult-onset infection. Rarely (0.1% to 0.5%), acute hepatitis B virus infection will result in fulminant hepatic failure, accounting for approximately 35% to 70% of all virally related cases of fulminant hepatitis.

The course of acute hepatitis B virus infection includes 1 to 4 months of incubation period, prodromal period, and the acute symptomatic phase followed by resolution or persistence. The prodromal period can be associated with a serum sickness-like syndrome followed by various constitutional symptoms such as malaise, anorexia, nausea, vomiting, low-grade fever, right upper quadrant pain, myalgia, fatigue, and a disordered sense of smell and taste. In cases of icteric hepatitis, jaundice may develop within 10 days of the onset of constitutional symptoms. The acute symptoms and jaundice may last up to 1 to 3 months while fatigue may persist in some patients even after normalization of transaminases. Physical examination may reveal icterus, low-grade temperature, and mildly tender hepatomegaly. Patients with fulminant hepatitis B will present with features typical of hepatic failure including encephalopathy and coagulopathy.

The laboratory findings in acute hepatitis B include marked elevations of the serum transaminases up to 1000 to 2000 IU/L, typically with ALT greater than AST. The rise in serum bilirubin levels tends to occur after the transaminase elevation, although it may remain normal in patients with anicteric hepatitis. The prothrombin time may also be elevated and is the best prognostic marker. In patients who resolve their infection, the acute clinical hepatitis is resolved with normalization of ALT levels usually within 1 to 4 months followed by normalization of bilirubin levels. If ALT remains elevated for more than 6 months, this suggests chronic liver injury due to chronic hepatitis B virus infection or some other cause.

Resolution of acute hepatitis and viral clearance is associated with loss of various serologic and viral markers of active hepatitis B virus replication and antigen synthesis (e.g. HBsAg, HBeAg, and hepatitis B virus DNA) and the appearance of anti-HBs that signals the development of antibody-mediated protective immunity to hepatitis B virus. This clinical and virological resolution is associated with a sustained vigorous host immune response directed against the virus. During acute fulminant hepatitis B, however, severe hepatic failure occurs as the result of an overwhelming antiviral immune response that destroys more infected hepatocytes than it protects. The replicative capacity of the infecting virus may also contribute to this, as suggested in several cases of fulminant hepatitis B associated with a viral variant with higher replicative capacity.

By contrast, the inability to clear hepatitis B virus is associated with an ineffective antiviral immune response, particularly the antiviral T-cell responses that are too weak or focused to clear the virus. Although it is not clear why this occurs in otherwise immune-competent adults, hepatitis B virus persistence during vertical transmission may be due to the immature immune system in neonates. It has also been suggested that the HBeAg may cross the placenta and function as a tolerogen, further blunting the antiviral immune response. Interestingly, in some patients with apparent "cure" from hepatitis B virus based on standard virological and serologic assays, traces of hepatitis B virus DNA may still be detected in serum, lymphocytes, or liver by highly sensitive PCR-based assays even decades after successful recovery. In fact, recurrent hepatitis B virus viremia with HBsAg and HBeAg has been observed in apparently recovered and immune individuals in the setting of profound immunosuppression (e.g. bone marrow or organ transplantation). Thus, the outcome of acute hepatitis B virus infection is a tight balance between the host immune system and the virus, and recovery from hepatitis B virus infection may indicate an immune-mediated control of the virus rather than complete eradication of the virus from the body.

Chronic hepatitis B

The clinical presentation of patients with chronic hepatitis B virus infection can vary from the asymptomatic carrier state to chronic hepatitis, cirrhosis, and hepatocellular carcinoma. The symptoms can range from none to vague constitutional symptoms (e.g. fatigue) as well as those associated with advanced liver failure. The physical examination may be unrevealing unless the person has stigmata of chronic liver disease. Laboratory tests may show mild to moderate elevation in serum AST and ALT (normal to several hundreds). During acute exacerbations of chronic hepatitis B, however, the ALT concentration may rise to as high as 50 times the upper limit of normal and alpha-fetoprotein levels may become very elevated up to 1000 ng/mL. Past history of acute hepatitis may be elicited in 30% to 50% of patients in low- to intermediate-prevalence areas (mostly adult onset) while such history is lacking in endemic areas with predominantly perinatal infection. The initial diagnosis of chronic hepatitis B virus infection can be made when serum HBsAg persists for more than 6 months after acute hepatitis or from its first detection during established chronic infection.

A number of factors may negatively influence survival in patients with chronic hepatitis B virus. These include a prolonged replicative phase of the virus, older age, hypoalbuminemia, thrombocytopenia, splenomegaly and hyperbilirubinemia, alcohol abuse, and co-infection with human immunodeficiency virus (HIV) or other hepatotrophic viruses. Notably, the presence of HBeAg is associated with active viral replication and more rapid progression of liver disease. In contrast, loss of HBeAg with detection of HBeAb (i.e. seroconversion) is associated with a more benign clinical outcome. It has been estimated that over 5 years, 12% to 20% of cases will progress from chronic hepatitis to cirrhosis, 20% to 23% will progress from compensated cirrhosis to hepatic decompensation, and 6% to 15% will progress from compensated cirrhosis to hepatocellular carcinoma.

The course of chronic hepatitis B virus infection may be considered in several phases

- the replicative phase with immune tolerance
- the replicative phase with immune clearance
- the low or non-replicative phase.

Replicative phase – immune tolerance

This phase is characterized by high levels of hepatitis B virus replications associated with the presence of HBeAg and high serum hepatitis B virus DNA titers without active liver disease (i.e. normal serum transaminases, few symptoms, and minimal changes on liver histology). This phase is typically seen in individuals with vertical or perinatal hepatitis B virus infection who display apparent immunological tolerance to hepatitis B virus (e.g. young Asian patients), with high levels of viral replication with little immune control and/or immune-mediated liver damage. This phase usually lasts approximately 10 to 30 years. Such patients are unlikely to clear HBeAg, either spontaneously or even with currently available antiviral therapy. However, rates of seroconversion may increase as the person ages and immune response becomes more activated.

Replicative phase – immune clearance

This phase of chronic infection may follow the replicative immune tolerance phase or it may occur sooner in cases acquired in adulthood. During this phase there is spontaneous loss of HBeAg associated with a drop in hepatitis B virus DNA to undetectable levels, at least by the conventional hybridization assays. This seroconversion from HBeAg-positive to HBeAb-positive state may be accompanied by an exacerbation of hepatitis with increased serum transaminase levels, suggesting an immune-mediated lysis of infected hepatocytes. There may also be a transient increase in serum hepatitis B virus DNA or a shift of HBcAg within the hepatocytes from nuclear to a predominantly cytoplasmic compartment. The precise mechanism of these changes is not well understood. Importantly, clinical exacerbation during spontaneous seroconversion may be misdiagnosed as an episode of acute hepatitis B in the absence of knowledge regarding pre-existing chronic hepatitis B virus infection. Indeed, such a flare may be accompanied by a rise in serum anti-HBc IgM titers, typically a marker of acute hepatitis B. Rarely such exacerbations may lead to hepatic decompensation, fulminant hepatic failure, and even death. In some cases, an individual may appear to enter the immune clearance phase but without clearing HBeAg or hepatitis B virus DNA from the serum. Such recurrent flares of hepatitis without seroconversion may promote progressive liver injury and increase the risk for cirrhosis and hepatocellular carcinoma.

Low or non-replicative phase

This phase is characterized by viral replication at either very low or undetectable levels in HBeAg-negative and HBeAb-positive individuals (i.e. after seroconversion). The ALT level is normal and active liver injury is not apparent. Some of these individuals may also be HBsAg negative. While the liver-related prognosis is generally excellent in these patients, hepatitis B virus infection can be reactivated if immunosuppression occurs.

Complications

Chronic hepatitis B virus infection can progress to cirrhosis, portal hypertension, hepatocellular carcinoma, and liver-related death. The rate of progression to these complications may be variable depending on the host's immune system, the host's age, the stage of infection, and geographic and genetic factors. Prolonged hepatitis B virus replication phase may be associated with a worse prognosis. Thus, HBeAg seroconversion is associated with a significantly better survival even in HBsAg-positive patients with cirrhosis.

Liver failure

Fulminant liver failure may occur in 1% of patients with acute hepatitis B. Chronic hepatitis B virus infection progesses to cirrhosis in 12% to 20% of cases. Of these cirrhotic cases, 20% to 23% may become decompensated, requiring consideration for liver transplantation.

Hepatocellular carcinoma

Infection with hepatitis B virus increases a person's risk for developing hepatocellular carcinoma. The rate of progression from compensated hepatitis B virus cirrhosis to hepatocellular carcinoma is estimated as being 6% to 15%. The currently available therapies for hepatocellular carcinoma are imperfect and prognosis depends on early detection and resection, ablation, or transplantation. Surveillance for hepatocellular carcinoma includes measurement of serum alpha-fetoprotein and abdominal ultrasound examination every 6 months. While early detection is clearly desirable for a better outcome, the true impact of such screening on mortality from hepatitis B virus infection is not yet clear.

Extrahepatic manifestations

Extrahepatic manifestations of hepatitis B virus infection occur in 10% to 20% of chronically infected individuals and are believed to be due to circulating immune complexes. They include polyarteritis nodosa and glomerular disease as well as a serum sickness-like syndrome during acute hepatitis B, mixed cryoglobulinemia, papular acrodermatitis (Gianotti's disease), and aplastic anemia. Treatment of the underlying hepatitis B virus infection as with interferon or lamivudine may help induce remission of these extrahepatic disorders. Immunosuppression as with steroids for polyarteritis nodosa may improve manifestations of the disorder but will perpetuate hepatitis B virus infection.

Treatment

Treatment of acute hepatitis B virus

Most acute hepatitis B infections are subclinical, and the treatment of acute symptomatic hepatitis B is mainly supportive. In patients with fulminant hepatitis B, however, close monitoring in the intensive care unit setting and even liver transplantation may be required. During the acute replicative phase of hepatitis B virus infection, patients should be educated about their risk for transmitting the virus to others. Patients should also be tested for other viral infections (e.g. HIV, hepatitis C virus, hepatitis delta virus) based on their risk factors. Barrier protection during intercourse should be used and contacts notified. Non-vaccinated individuals exposed to the person should be offered vaccination and post-exposure prophylaxis in the form of hepatitis B immunoglobulin. After the initial recovery of acute hepatitis B, patients should be monitored for loss of HBsAg and anti-HBs (self-limited course) or persistent HBsAg and HBeAg (chronic course).

Treatment of chronic hepatitis B virus

Patients with chronic hepatitis B virus infection should be assessed for the degree of their liver disease (e.g. liver function tests, alpha-fetoprotein, ultrasound to look for evidence of liver cirrhosis or mass and portal hypertension). They should also be counseled about their potential infectivity to others (i.e. test contacts and offer vaccine and/or immuno-prophylaxis) and educated about the disease, risk factors for further liver damage (e.g. alcohol, other viral hepatitis, drugs), and available treatment. The goals in the treatment of chronic hepatitis B virus are to suppress viral replication, to induce remission of liver disease, and ultimately to improve the clinical outcome and survival. A response to treatment can be measured in terms of biochemical response (normalization of transaminases), virological response (reduction in hepatitis B virus to less than 10^5 copies/mL and loss of HBeAg), and histological response (decrease in necroinflammation in the liver). Thus, it is important to consider the definition of response when assessing the efficacy of various treatment modalities.

Currently, the available therapies for chronic hepatitis B virus include interferon alpha and lamivudine. Notably, not everyone with chronic hepatitis B virus infection qualifies for interferon or lamivudine therapy based on their overall prognosis and likelihood of treatment response. Thus, treatment should be limited to those with established chronic infection (HBsAg positive for more than 6 months), active viral replication (hepatitis B virus DNA above 10^5 copies/mL) and who have active liver disease (ALT more than twice the normal level and chronic hepatitis on liver biopsy). However, with the advent of more antiviral agents and considerations for combination-rather than single-drug therapy, the field of hepatitis B virus therapeutics is evolving rapidly.

Interferon alpha

Interferons are endogenous antiviral factors with both immunomodulatory and antiviral effects, although their precise mechanism of action in hepatitis B virus infection remains unknown. Interferon alpha is a type-1 interferon. For patients with chronic hepatitis B, it is usually administered by subcutaneous injection at a dosage of 5 million units (MU) daily or 10 MU thrice weekly. Generally the treatment lasts for 4 months although it may be longer particularly in patients with HBeAg-negative hepatitis with precore variants. Positive predictive factors for a treatment response include

- high pretreatment ALT levels
- low pretreatment hepatitis B virus DNA levels
- adult onset of hepatitis B virus infection

- active liver histology
- female gender
- the absence of concomitant HIV or hepatitis delta virus infection.

The efficacy of longer acting pegylated interferon is not yet clear, although it is likely to be similar to the shorter acting interferons.

Lamivudine

Lamivudine blocks hepatitis B virus replication by inhibiting its reverse transcriptase. It is very effective in reducing hepatitis B virus DNA levels in patients with chronic hepatitis B virus infection and results in a similar rate of HBeAg seroconversion to interferon alpha with considerably fewer side effects. Remarkably, lamivudine treatment in some patients with end-stage liver disease was associated with a marked improvement in their liver synthetic function. However, there is no clear consensus about its treatment duration and patients are often placed on prolonged lamivudine therapy which can select resistant viral variants, including the so-called YMDD mutants involving the catalytic site of the hepatitis B virus polymerase. Such drug-resistant viral strains typically occur within 9 to 12 months of initiating therapy. Clinically, the development of a resistant strain may manifest itself as a flare of hepatitis and reappearance of hepatitis B virus DNA in the serum (after initial viral clearance). On the other hand, sudden withdrawal of lamivudine may also be associated with a more severe flare of liver disease and possibly liver failure. For this reason, abrupt withdrawal of lamivudine is recommended during a flare to a mutant strain during therapy. Although lamivudine is a highly effective medication for suppressing chronic hepatitis B virus replication, its main disadvantages remain the risk for the emergence of drug-resistant viral strains and the indefinite duration of therapy.

Novel therapies

There are numerous therapies under investigation for the treatment of chronic hepatitis B virus, including those effective against the YMDD mutants. These medications are currently undergoing clinical trials with significant promise. It is very likely that combination therapy including interferon, lamivudine, and other agents will become the most effective therapy for this highly mutable virus, similar to the treatment of HIV and hepatitis C virus.

Liver transplantation

In decompensated cirrhosis due to chronic hepatitis B, liver transplantation can now be considered. Although liver transplantation for hepatitis B virus infection was initially associated with high recurrence rates leading to graft failure and mortality, the current use of hepatitis B immunoglobulin and antiviral therapy such as lamivudine in the peritransplant period has had a dramatic effect in improving the outcomes for hepatitis B virus liver transplantation. However, the exact regimen of lamivudine and hepatitis B immunoglobulin and the duration of the different therapies is not yet standardized and varies between the individual transplant centers. Given the high cost of repeated hepatitis B immunoglobulin therapy, a more standardized approach is desirable in this setting.

Prevention

Active immunization

The available hepatitis B virus vaccine based on the HBsAg is highly effective and can induce long-term protective immunity in 95% of children and 90% of adults. The anti-HBs titers may remain above the "protective level" of 10 IU/mL in 50% of subjects for up to 15 years. Given the high efficacy of the vaccine, post-vaccination testing for immunity (i.e. anti-HBs titer) is recommended only in those persons whose medical management relies on hepatitis B virus immune status. Booster immunizations are recommended for immunosuppressed individuals or for those individuals with anti-HBs titers below 10 IU/mL with ongoing risk to hepatitis B virus infection. Cases of vaccine-escape mutants of hepatitis B virus have been reported, although this is uncommon and without significant clinical impact. Despite speculations regarding an association between hepatitis B virus vaccination and certain adverse reactions such as arthritis, autism, and demyelinating disease in the past, formal epidemiologic studies have failed to show any association.

Current recommendations include the routine vaccination of all infants as well as "catch-up" vaccination of children, adolescents, and adults in high-risk groups for hepatitis B virus exposure (Box 3.2). The ultimate goal is to eliminate hepatitis B virus transmission altogether, although it will take time for the majority of the population to become immune.

Passive immunization

For previously unvaccinated individuals who are exposed to hepatitis B virus, it is possible to provide passive immunization through the administration of immune globulin containing a high titer of anti-HBs or hepatitis B immune globulin. This is particularly recommended for babies born to HBsAg-positive mothers and for individuals with recent hepatitis B virus exposure (e.g. via percutaneous, mucosal membrane, or sexual contact) as well as for liver transplant patients with hepatitis B virus infection.

Further reading – hepatitis B virus

Bartholomeusz A, and Locarnini S. Hepatitis B virus mutants and fulminant hepatitis B: fitness plus phenotype. *Hepatology* 2001; 34(2): 432–435.

Blumberg BS, Gerstley BJ, Hungerford DA, London WT, Sutnick AI. A serum antigen (Australia antigen) in Down's syndrome, leukemia, and hepatitis. *Ann Intern Med* 1967; 66(5): 924–931.

Centers for Disease Control. Updated U.S. Public Health Service Guidelines for the management of occupational exposures to HBV, HCV, and HIV and recommendations for postexposure prophylaxis. *Morbidity and Mortality Weekly Report* 2001; 50(11): 1–42.

Chang KM, Chisari FV. Immune response in hepatitis B virus infection. *Liver Clin North Am.* 1999; 3(2): 221–240.

Chu CJ, Lok AS. Clinical significance of hepatitis B virus genotypes. *Hepatology* 2002; 35(5): 1274–1276.

Hunt CM, McGill JM, Allen MI, Condreay LD. Clinical relevance of hepatitis B viral mutations. *Hepatology* 2000; 315: 1037–1044.

Lok A, Heathcote EJ, Hoofnagle JH. Management of hepatitis B 2000 – summary of a workshop. *Gastroenterology* 2001; 120: 1828–1853.

Lok AS, McMahon BJ, for the Practice Guidelines Committee, American Association for the Study of Liver Diseases. Chronic Hepatitis B. *Hepatology* 2002; 34(6): 1225–1241.

Seeger C, Mason WS. Hepatitis B virus biology. *Microbiology and Molecular Biology Reviews* 2000; 64(1): 51–68.

HEPATITIS DELTA

The hepatitis delta virus (hepatitis D virus) is a defective RNA virus that requires the hepatitis B virus to provide its outer envelope (i.e. HBsAg). Since it cannot replicate in the absence HBsAg, hepatitis D virus infection occurs only in the setting of concurrent or pre-existing hepatitis B virus infection.

Box 3.2 Advisory Committee on Immunization Practices of the Centers for Disease Control recommendations of who should be routinely vaccinated against hepatitis B virus

Prevention of perinatal hepatitis B virus infection.
Test all pregnant women for hepatitis B surface antigen (HBsAg).
Infants born to mothers who are HBsAg-positive should receive the hepatitis B virus vaccine and hepatitis B immune globulin (HBIg) within 12 hours of birth. Both can be administered concurrently but at separate sites.
If the mother's HBsAg status is not known testing should be done at the time of delivery. The infant should receive hepatitis B virus vaccine within 12 hours of delivery. If the mother is found to be HBsAg-positive then hepatitis B immune globulin should be administered as soon as possible.
Household contacts and sex partners of HBsAg-positive women should receive the hepatitis B virus vaccine.

Universal vaccination of infants born to HBsAg-negative mothers.
Hepatitis B virus vaccination is recommended for all infants regardless of the HBsAg status of their mother.

Vaccination of adolescents.
All adolescents should be offered the vaccination if they have any risk of exposure to hepatitis B virus.

Vaccination of high-risk adults.
Adults with an occupational risk such as health care workers and workers who perform tasks involving contact with blood or blood-containing body fluids.
Clients and staff of institutions for the developmentally disabled.
Hemodialysis patients.
Recipients of certain blood products such as clotting-factor concentrates.
Household contacts and sex partners of hepatitis B virus carriers.
Adoptees from countries where hepatitis B virus is endemic.
International travelers who plan to spend more than 6 months in areas with high rates of hepatitis B virus.
Injecting drug users.
Sexually active homosexual and bisexual men.
Sexually active heterosexual men and women particularly if they have a history of a sexually transmitted disease, are prostitutes, or have more than one partner in 6 months.
Inmates of long-term correctional facilities.

The virus

Hepatitis D virus has a single strand RNA genome in a rod-like structure, and is classified in the Deltaviridae family. The hepatitis D virus virion consists of an outer lipoprotein envelope consisting of HBsAg and an inner ribonucleoprotein structure that contains the viral genome.

Epidemiology

The overall incidence of hepatitis D virus infection in developed countries has been decreasing concur-rently with the decreasing incidence of hepatitis B virus infection. It is estimated that approximately 5% of the world's HBsAg carriers are also infected with hepatitis D virus. Thus, with 300 million hepatitis B virus carriers worldwide, the number of individuals infected with hepatitis D virus is estimated to be 15 million. However, the geographical distribution of hepatitis D virus infection does not parallel that of hepatitis B virus because of their differences in relative efficiency of transmission. For example, hepatitis D virus prevalence is not particularly high in endemic areas where hepatitis B virus infection is acquired through vertical or perinatal transmission. The pattern of the distribution of hepatitis D virus infection has also been changing in recent years because of various public health measures aimed at better hygiene, hepatitis B virus vaccination, and control of HIV transmission which shares a similar route to hepatitis B virus (i.e. sexual, parenteral). Thus, hepatitis B virus and hepatitis D virus are now far less common in the developed countries compared to underdeveloped countries. Today, hepatitis D virus is not common in North America or northern Europe but can be found more commonly in several tropical and subtropical countries including India, Africa, and along the Mediterranean basin.

Transmission

The routes of transmission for hepatitis D virus are the same as those for hepatitis B virus although the relative efficiency of transmission by these different modes may differ for the two viruses. The important routes of transmission are sexual, parenteral, and household transmission.

Natural history

Hepatitis D virus infection always occurs in the setting of hepatitis B virus infection, either acquired together (co-infection) or in persons already chronically infected with hepatitis B virus (super-infection). Hepatitis D virus infection may be acute and self-limited or it may become chronic. Whether hepatitis D virus occurs as a co-infection or as a super-infection, influences the final outcome and the course of chronic disease. In hepatitis B virus/hepatitis D virus co-infection, the clinical presentation is similar to that in acute hepatitis B virus mono-infection. The rate of hepatitis D virus persistence is no greater than that of hepatitis B virus since the former virus relies on the latter to survive. Since hepatitis B virus infection is self-limited in most co-infections, hepatitis D virus infection is also self-limited and only an estimated 2% evolve to chronicity. Interestingly, acute hepatitis B virus/hepatitis D virus co-infection is associated with a higher rate of fulminant hepatitis (2% to 20%).

In hepatitis D virus super-infection of patients with pre-existing chronic hepatitis B virus infection, hepatitis D virus infection becomes persistent in almost 90% of the patients. Persistent infection with both hepatitis D virus and hepatitis

B virus may have clinical implications. For example, some studies of chronic hepatitis B virus carriers with hepatitis D virus superinfection suggest a higher rate of liver disease progression (70% to 80%) compared to those with hepatitis B virus mono-infection (15% to 30%), although this is not borne out in all population-based studies. An interesting virus–virus interaction may also occur in the course of hepatitis D virus superinfection with marked inhibition of hepatitis B virus replication during the early phase of hepatitis D virus superinfection. In fact, hepatitis D virus superinfection in a minority of patients may lead to clearance of HBsAg and resolution of the hepatitis B virus infection. This phenomenon may be permanent or it may be transient as the hepatitis D virus infection wanes.

Diagnosis

Typically, tests for hepatitis D virus will be performed in individuals presenting with acute hepatitis or in those known to have chronic hepatitis presenting with an apparent flare. In addition to the laboratory tests for hepatitis D virus infection, it is important to establish the phase of hepatitis B virus infection since this will determine the risk for fulminant hepatic failure and for developing chronic infection. The gold standard in diagnosis of hepatitis D virus infection is the detection of hepatitis D virus RNA in the serum or hepatitis D antigen (HDAg) in liver tissue. It is also possible to perform serologic tests for anti-HDV IgM and IgG. The presence of HBsAg is necessary to establish hepatitis D virus infection. Presence of anti-HBc IgM suggests acute hepatitis B virus/hepatitis D virus co-infection, rather than superinfection.

Clinical picture

The clinical picture of hepatitis D virus infection depends on the state of the hepatitis B virus infection, the interaction between hepatitis D virus and hepatitis B virus, and the host's immune response as discussed above. When symptomatic, hepatitis B virus/hepatitis D virus infection will present as icteric acute hepatitis. In this situation, it is easy to miss the diagnosis of hepatitis D virus if it is not tested for.

Complications

The risk of hepatocellular carcinoma in patients chronically infected with hepatitis B virus/hepatitis D virus is similar to that for hepatitis B virus alone. In one series from Greece, hepatocellular carcinoma was detected in 40% of patients with hepatitis D virus/hepatitis B virus cirrhosis.

Treatment

The treatment of hepatitis D virus consists of interferon alpha. Generally, the response rate to interferon therapy is less than 50%. In cases of decompensated liver disease, liver transplantation may be life saving. Transplantation for hepatitis D virus/hepatitis B virus infection actually carries a better prognosis than transplantation for other forms of viral hepatitis.

Prevention

Effective vaccination against hepatitis B virus will prevent infection with hepatitis D virus.

Further reading – hepatitis delta virus

Bonino F, Heermann KH, Rizzetto M, Gerlich WH. Hepatitis delta virus: protein composition of delta antigen and its hepatitis B virus-derived envelope. *J Virol* 1986; 58(3): 945–950.

Negro F, Lok AS. Diagnosis of hepatitis D infection. *UpToDate* 2002.

Negro F, Lok AS. Pathogenesis and clinical manifestations of hepatitis D virus infection. *UpToDate* 2002.

Rizzetto M, Canese MG, Arico S, *et al*. Immunofluorescence detection of new antigen–antibody system (delta/anti-delta) associated to hepatitis B virus in liver and in serum of HBsAg carriers. *Gut* 1977; 18(12): 997–1003.

Taylor JM. Hepatitis Delta virus. *Intervirology* 1999; 42: 173–178.

HEPATITIS C

Non-A non-B hepatitis was first recognized in 1975. However, it was not until 1989 that its causative agent was cloned, sequenced, and named the hepatitis C virus.

The virus

Hepatitis C virus is a hepatotropic RNA virus belonging to the Flaviviridae family with a single positive strand RNA genome that is approximately 9.5 kilobases in length (Figure 3.6). The viral genome consists of a single open reading frame coding for the viral polyprotein flanked by the 5′ and 3′ non-coding regions that are vital to the hepatitis C virus life cycle. The hepatitis C virus polyprotein consists of both structural and non-structural proteins. Sequentially from N- to C-terminus, these proteins include the hepatitis C virus core (viral nucleocapsid), E1 and E2 (variable envelope glycoproteins), p7, NS2, NS3 (serine protease and helicase), NS4A (protease cofactor), NS4B, NS5A, NS5B (viral RNA polymerase).

A notable feature of the hepatitis C virus is its sequence heterogeneity due to the high error rate of the viral RNA polymerase, resulting in at least six different genotypes with intergenotypic sequence variation up to 33% and well over 100 different hepatitis C virus subtypes. The major genotypes differ in their geographical distribution. Genotypes 1, 2, and 3 have a worldwide distribution, while genotype 4 is more prevalent in India and Egypt, genotype 5 in South Africa, and genotype 6 in southeast Asia. In the US, 65% to 70% of all hepatitis C virus infections are genotype 1, 14% genotype 2, 5% genotype 3, and 1% genotype 4. Within each patient, hepatitis C virus also exists as a swarm of quasispecies or a population of closely related but genetically distinct viral species. The extensive genetic diversity is believed to contribute to the pathogenesis of hepatitis C virus infection by selection of variants that evade the host immune surveillance or antiviral therapy.

Epidemiology

The world prevalence of hepatitis C virus infection is estimated at 3% according to the World Health Organization, although there are regional variations. Hepatitis C virus accounts for 30 000 new infections each year, 70% of all cases of chronic hepatitis, and 90% of all non-A non-B hepatitis cases. In the US, hepatitis C virus antibody is detectable in 1.8% of the general population. Hepatitis C virus seroprevalence varies in different ethnic and sociodemographic groups. For example, hepatitis C virus infection is observed in 3.2% of

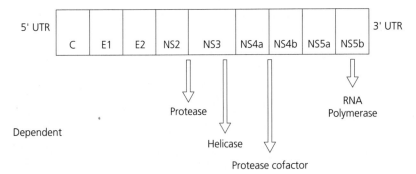

Figure 3.6 Hepatitis C virus genome. E = envelope protein; NS = non-structural protein; C = core protein; UTR = untranslated regions.

African-Americans, 2.1% in Mexican-Americans, and 1.5% in non-Hispanic whites. Hepatitis C virus infection may also be more prevalent among the US veterans receiving care at various Veterans Affairs Medical Centers with some sites showing seroprevalence over 10%. Because of the shared parenteral risk factor, hepatitis C virus infection can be found in a third of all HIV-infected patients (particularly those with history of transfusion or drug use) and as many as 20% of patients on hemodialysis.

In the US, chronic hepatitis C virus infection accounts for 10 000 deaths annually and is the leading indication for orthotopic liver transplantation. While the actual incidence of new hepatitis C virus infection is now declining, the long-term hepatitis C virus-related morbidity and mortality is expected to double or triple in the next two decades with a greatly increased economic burden. For example, the proportion of hepatitis C virus-infected patients with cirrhosis is estimated to increase from 15.6% in 1988 to more than 28.9% by 2018. Moreover, hepatic decompensation may increase by 85% and hepatocellular carcinoma by 60%, with a subsequent tripling of the death rate.

tion has also been associated with intranasal cocaine use. Before the mid-1980s, 40% of all new cases of hepatitis C virus resulted from blood transfusion. However, with the routine testing of blood donors, the risk of hepatitis C virus infection due to transfusion is now less than 1 in 103 000 transfused units. With the decrease in transfusion-associated hepatitis C virus infection, injection drug use accounts for the majority of the new infections reported annually, followed by sexual exposure and work-related accidents (e.g. needle-stick accidents) in health care professions according to the Centers for Disease Control. Although hepatitis C virus may be transmitted sexually, its efficiency is low compared to hepatitis B. Thus, the risk of transmission of hepatitis C virus via sexual activity for patients in a stable monogamous relationship is apparently low, although a greater number of sexual partners and a history of sexually transmitted diseases are associated with hepatitis C virus infection. The estimated rate of mother-to-infant transmission is 1% to 5% and maternal risk factors for increased transmission include history of intravenous drug abuse, co-infection with HIV, and high maternal viral load. Mode of delivery and breast feeding do not significantly influence transmission rates.

Transmission

Hepatitis C virus transmission is primarily parenteral through contaminated blood. Although hepatitis C virus RNA has been found in saliva, urine, semen, and ascitic fluid, transmission through these bodily secretions is less efficient. The risk factors for hepatitis C virus infection include intravenous drug use, history of blood transfusion (before 1991), hemodialysis, tattooing, high-risk sexual behavior, health care work, and organ transplants from hepatitis C virus-positive donors. Hepatitis C virus infec-

Natural history

Hepatitis C virus causes both acute and chronic hepatitis, similar to hepatitis B virus. The acute phase of hepatitis C virus infection is mostly subclinical and does not result in fulminant hepatic failure. Unlike hepatitis B virus, however, hepatitis C virus infection becomes chronic in 50% to 70% of infected individuals. The basis of this high rate of chronicity in otherwise immune competent individuals is not fully elucidated, although the rapid viral mutation that escapes the host immune response may play a role. Persistent hepatitis C virus infection is then associated with chronic hepatitis that can progress to cirrhosis (20% to 25%) and hepatocellular carcinoma (5%) over many years. The clinical features of acute and chronic hepatitis C are described later.

Diagnosis

Diagnostic tests for hepatitis C virus infection include serologic tests measuring the antibody response to hepatitis C virus antigen and molecular tests that detect the circulating viral nucleic acid (Table 3.3). Unlike hepatitis B virus infection in which detection of anti-HBs implies resolution of acute disease and/or protective immunity, antibody response to hepatitis C virus generally indicates exposure with ongoing infection. However, confirmation of ongoing hepatitis C virus infection requires sensitive molecular tests that demonstrate hepatitis C virus viremia, i.e. detection of hepatitis C virus RNA in a patient's serum. Additional molecular assays can also provide hepatitis C virus RNA quantitation and genotyping. The various serologic and molecular assays used in hepatitis C virus diagnostics are described below.

Serologic tests

Screening assays

The main screening assay for detecting anti-hepatitis C virus antibodies is the multi-antigen EIA. The second generation EIA-2 (based on the hepatitis C virus core, NS3, and NS4 antigens) has a sensitivity of 92% to 95% with a positive predictive value of 90% to 95% among high-prevalence populations and 50% to 60% in low-prevalence populations. The third generation hepatitis C virus EIA-3 tests for antibody response to an additional antigen (HCV NS5) as well as to the core, NS3, and NS4 antigens. The EIA-3 is higher in sensitivity and specificity, with an earlier detection of hepatitis C virus seroconversion during acute infection (2 to 3 weeks) and a lower false positive rate in low-prevalence populations than the EIA-2. Both EIA-2 and EIA-3 are currently available in the US. False positive results may occur in patients without any hepatitis C virus risk factors and those with high globulins perhaps due to non-specific immunoglobulin binding. False negatives can occur in immunocompromised patients (e.g. HIV, renal failure, hypogammaglobulinemia) and in acutely infected patients before seroconversion. A positive antibody response does not distinguish between prior or ongoing infection, is of no benefit in assessing recovery after antiviral treatment, and may even be lost in patients who spontaneously clear hepatitis C virus after 1 to 2 decades. Detection of a positive antibody response warrants further testing with molecular assays for the presence of serum hepatitis C virus RNA, distinguishing between infection, previous infection followed by clearance, or false positive response.

Supplemental tests for detecting anti-hepatitis C virus

The recombinant immunoblot assay (RIBA, Chiron, Emeryville, CA) was developed as a supplemental test to resolve false positive EIAs in low-risk groups. It determines the specificity of hepatitis C virus antibody response to each individual hepatitis C virus antigen (e.g. core, NS3, and NS4). The RIBA is considered positive if antibodies are detected against two or more antigens, indeterminate if antibodies are detected against only one antigen, and negative if no antibodies are detected.

Table 3.3 Interpretation of various hepatitis C virus (HCV) tests

Anti-HCV enzyme immunoblot assay	HCV RNA	Recombinant immunoblot assay	Interpretation
−	+	−	False negative anti-HCV result in early acute hepatitis C
+	−	−	False positive
+	+	+	HCV infection (acute or chronic)
+	−	+/indeterminate	Recovery from HCV infection*

*following spontaneous HCV clearance, the HCV antibody response may wane after many years (1-2 decades) thus yielding an indeterminate or negative HCV antibody response despite true exposure. This profile can appear as negative or indeterminate anti-HCV antibody result in high risk persons without HCV RNA viremia.

The RIBA may be used to distinguish false positive versus cleared infection. In patients with a positive EIA, but negative hepatitis C virus RNA, a positive RIBA suggests prior exposure to hepatitis C virus with subsequent viral clearance. However, with the enhanced sensitivity and specificity of EIA and the hepatitis C virus RNA tests, the utility of RIBA is currently limited.

Molecular tests

Molecular tests are an integral part in the work-up and management of hepatitis C virus infection, and they are used in

1. qualitative assays to establish the presence of hepatitis C virus RNA
2. quantitative assays to measure the level of hepatitis C virus RNA
3. hepatitis C virus genotyping assays to classify the dominant hepatitis C virus isolate in the patient.

Three different methods to detect and quantify hepatitis C virus RNA in the blood are commercially available. These include RT-PCR (Roche COBAS Amplicor HCV Monitor 2.0, Roche Diagnostics, Branchburg, NJ; HCV Superquant®, National Genetics Institute, Culver City, CA), transcription-mediated amplification assay (TMA, Versant® HCV RNA Qualitative assay, Bayer Diagnostics, Emeryville CA), and branched DNA assay (Quantiplex® HCV RNA 2.0 assay and Versant HCV RNA 3.0 assay, Bayer Diagnostics). Both the RT-PCR and TMA require amplification of viral nucleic acid to enhance their sensitivity. In contrast, the branched DNA assay involves direct hybridization of the viral nucleic acid to specific probes which are then further amplified for detection. Although all assays were initially expressed in different units (e.g. copies or genome equivalents specific to each assay), the current recommendation is to standardize all assays in international units.

Currently, the presence or absence of hepatitis C virus viremia is established best with the sensitive PCR- or TMA-based methods rather than the less sensitive branched DNA assay. Most hepatitis C virus-infected patients will have measurable hepatitis C virus RNA by the less sensitive quantitative RT-PCR assays (sensitivity 500 IU/mL) and can be monitored with these assays after initial establishment of hepatitis C virus viremia.

However, the best assurance for a lack of hepatitis C virus RNA (e.g. spontaneous clearance, treatment response, or false positive HCV Ab test) requires the most sensitive qualitative RT-PCR (sensitivity 50 IU/mL) or TMA (sensitivity 5 to 10 IU/mL).

The infecting viral genotype can be established in various ways, including laborious sequence analysis, genotype-specific RT-PCR using specific PCR primers, restriction fragment length polymorphism of PCR products and hybridization of PCR products with genotype-specific probes. While the first three methods are used in research settings, the last method (InnoLipa®, Innogenetics) is readily available commercially and is utilized most frequently in the clinical setting to determine the treatment regimen and likelihood of treatment response.

Liver biopsy

Liver biopsy is not required for the diagnosis of hepatitis C virus infection. Rather, it is used to stage the extent of liver inflammation and fibrosis as well as to exclude other causes of chronic liver disease in patients with chronic hepatitis C virus infection. Frequent findings include prominent portal lymphoid aggregates, steatosis, and sinusoidal lymphocytic infiltration. There are no predictive markers of fibrosis; moreover, there is an inconsistent relationship between the degree of serum transaminase elevation and the severity of disease as defined histologically. Studies have demonstrated that patients with mild hepatitis and without fibrosis on initial biopsy have a 10% risk of cirrhosis over the next 10 years compared to 70% of those with initial severe hepatitis or septal fibrosis.

Diagnosis of acute hepatitis C infection

The diagnosis of acute hepatitis C remains a clinical challenge, partly because of its rare clinical presentation and its variable course. Notably, hepatitis C virus RNA may be detected in the blood within 1 week of exposure while hepatitis C virus antibody seroconversion occurs much later (typically 8 to 10 weeks, but ranging between 3 to 21 weeks). Thus, in a patient presenting with acute hepatitis, the lack of hepatitis C virus antibody does not rule out acute hepatitis C virus infection. Moreover, hepatitis C virus RNA titers may fluctuate during acute infection becoming undetectable, only to become detectable once again on future testing. Thus, a single negative hepatitis C virus RNA test obtained during the acute infection should not be interpreted as evidence for sustained viral clearance.

The diagnosis should be entertained in any person with acute hepatitis while excluding other causes (e.g. other viral, toxic, and immunologic causes) and while conducting a detailed history for potential hepatitis C virus exposure (e.g. needle-stick injury, medical or surgical procedures, high-risk sexual exposure, or any contact with potentially contaminated body fluids). Initial screening for acute hepatitis C should include both hepatitis C virus RNA and hepatitis C virus antibody tests. Typically, this will identify patients with hepatitis C virus viremia in the absence of anti-hepatitis C virus antibody early on, and the subsequent hepatitis C virus seroconversion (i.e. rise in anti-hepatitis C virus antibody) will be diagnostic for acute hepatitis C. Patients with acute hepatitis C should be monitored closely for clinical and virological outcome (e.g. hepatitis C virus persistence versus clearance), and may be considered for antiviral therapy. Liver biopsy is not generally indicated to diagnosis acute hepatitis C virus infection, but rather to examine other causes that need to be assessed.

Diagnosis of chronic hepatitis C infection

The diagnosis of chronic hepatitis C virus infection is made on the basis of anti-hepatitis C virus antibodies and persistent serum hepatitis C virus RNA. In most cases, the diagnostic work-up begins with hepatitis C virus antibody testing of patients with abnormal liver function tests or known risk factors for hepatitis C virus infection and during screening for blood donation. If positive for hepatitis C virus antibody, hepatitis C virus viremia (i.e. infection) is established by sensitive molecular assays testing for serum hepatitis C virus RNA. With the exception of patients presenting with acute hepatitis C or undergoing antiviral therapy, multiple positive hepatitis C virus RNA tests are not required to establish the chronicity of hepatitis C virus infection since most hepatitis C virus

viremic patients remain viremic. The liver enzymes and relevant liver function tests may vary depending on the patient and extent of liver disease progression.

Clinical picture

Acute hepatitis C

Although asymptomatic (or at best with vague or non-specific symptoms) in most cases, acute hepatitis C can present with symptoms characteristic of the other viral hepatidities including nausea, vomiting, right upper quadrant pain, and malaise. Less than 25% of cases of acute hepatitis C are associated with jaundice. Fulminant liver failure due to acute hepatitis C is extremely rare, although cases have been reported. Observational data suggest that those persons presenting with clinically evident acute hepatitis C are much more likely to clear the virus spontaneously, perhaps because of a more vigorous immune response against the virus that may also be responsible for their symptoms. After exposure to hepatitis C virus, it may be 2 to 12 (mean of 7) weeks before symptoms become apparent, if they are recognized at all.

Typically, patients show serum transaminase elevations in the range of several hundreds to a thousand and variable degrees of hyperbilirubinemia. The overall laboratory parameters of liver dysfunction are not as severe as acute hepatitis B in which ALT elevations can reach 2 to 3000 IU/dL with marked jaundice and coagulopathy. The presenting symptoms and laboratory abnormalities may last for 2 to 12 weeks. During the initial flare of acute hepatitis, hepatitis C virus antibody may be of little use since hepatitis C virus antibody seroconversion may not yet have occurred. However, a negative test at this time followed by a positive antibody test is invaluable in documenting hepatitis C virus seroconversion during acute hepatitis C. As mentioned earlier, some patients have a fluctuating course with initial loss of viremia accompanied by ALT normalization, only to have a recurrent viremia and ALT flare thereafter. Such fluctuations in clinical disease and viremia have been associated inversely with antiviral T-cell responses, suggesting a helpful role for virus-specific T cells in viral clearance and resolution of clinical liver disease.

The acute infection is spontaneously cleared in a certain proportion of patients. The specific percentage is unclear because of the difficulty in identifying and prospectively monitoring patients with acute hepatitis C, since most are asymptomatic and do not present to medical attention. Although previous studies suggested a spontaneous hepatitis C virus clearance rate of approximately 15%, more recent longitudinal cohort studies have suggested a higher rate, at least in certain groups. For example, in a cohort of Irish women who received hepatitis C virus-contaminated immunoglobulins almost two decades, spontaneous hepatitis C virus clearance was noted in 45% of individuals.

Chronic hepatitis C

Hepatitis C virus infection becomes chronic in 50% to 70% of patients after a mostly subclinical acute phase, and chronic hepatitis may develop in 55% to 85% of those chronically infected (Figure 3.7). Most patients in the chronic phase of hepatitis C virus infection are asymptomatic and may be diagnosed by the incidental finding of elevated aminotransferases or through screening at the time of blood donation. Non-specific symptoms such as fatigue, myalgias, arthralgias, weight loss, malaise, anorexia, and right upper quadrant pain may develop in approximately 20%, although these symptoms generally do not correlate with disease activity. Some patients display extrahepatic manifestations of hepatitis C virus infection (e.g. vasculitic rash associated with cryoglobulinemia, thyroid disease, Sjögren's syndrome, and glomerulonephritis). Others may show signs and

symptoms of liver failure due to hepatitis C virus-associated liver cirrhosis. As for the clinical laboratory parameters, chronic hepatitis C virus infection may be associated with only mildly abnormal serum transaminase activity. In fact, up to a third of patients will have a normal ALT activity and only about 25% will have serum ALT activity more than twice the normal level. Although the serum ALT activity may not accurately predict the severity of histological liver disease, normal ALT activity was associated with a 50% reduction in the rate of liver fibrosis progression compared to patients with elevated ALT activity.

The rate of progression of hepatitis C virus remains controversial and problematic to study because of the difficulties in determining its onset, its long indolent course and the variable results obtained in different studies. In one study of 131 patients with chronic hepatitis C virus infection following transfusion 22 years ago, the disease was shown to take an aggressive course with 23% of patients developing chronic active hepatitis, 51% cirrhosis, and 5% liver cancer. In contrast, among the 917 Irish women who received contaminated anti-D immunoglobulin, only half remained viremic and only 0.4% developed cirrhosis after 20 years. In a study of US military recruits, the rates of liver disease and liver-related mortality of seventeen hepatitis C virus seropositive recruits were 11.8% and 5.9%. Overall, less than 15% progressed to overt chronic liver disease over this time period. The reasons for these apparently contradictory results in the natural history of hepatitis C virus infection are not well understood. However, factors predictive of progression include age at infection greater than 40 years, duration of infection, post-transfusion acquisition, daily alcohol consumption of 50 grams or more, severity of injury, degree of damage on initial liver biopsy, and male gender. Other factors that may influence disease progression include co-infection with hepatitis B virus or HIV, and the presence of an elevated ALT.

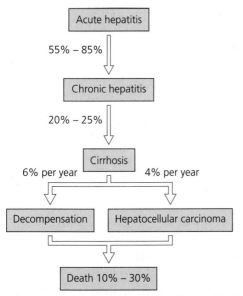

Figure 3.7 Natural history of hepatitis C virus.

Complications

Cirrhosis and liver failure

Cirrhosis may develop in at least 25% of patients with long-term chronic hepatitis C virus infection and approximately 10 000 deaths per year are related to hepatitis C virus liver disease. Hepatitis C virus, alone or in combination with alcohol, is currently the leading indication for adult liver transplantation in the US. In patients with compensated cirrhosis, about 20% will develop decompensation over a 5-year period. Importantly, the 5-year survival is about 90% among patients with compensated cirrhosis whereas it falls to 50% after decompensation develops. As in decompensated liver cirrhosis from any other causes, hepatitis C virusassociated chronic liver failure is associated with liver synthetic and metabolic dysfunction (prolonged prothrombin time, hyperbilirubinemia, hypoalbuminemia) and portal hypertension (varices, ascites, encephalopathy).

Hepatocellular carcinoma

The overall prevalence of hepatocellular carcinoma is 5% in patients with hepatitis C virus. The risk of hepatocellular carcinogenesis is significantly increased with the presence of cirrhosis: 7% to 20% in patients with hepatitis C virus-related cirrhosis with an annual incidence of 3% in compensated cirrhosis compared to 1% to 4% per 20 years in patients without cirrhosis. Conversely, the prevalence of hepatitis C virus infection among patients with hepatocellular carcinoma is 10% to 75%. Thus, all patients with cirrhosis should be screened with bi-annual alpha-fetoprotein and abdominal imaging study (e.g. ultrasound, MRI, or CT scan). The mechanism of hepatocarcinogenesis in patients with hepatitis C virus remains unknown, although some of the viral proteins (e.g. hepatitis C virus core antigen) have been implicated.

Extrahepatic manifestations

Hepatitis C is associated with a myriad of extrahepatic manifestations and illnesses. The association is strongest with essential mixed cryoglobulinemia, membranoproliferative glomerulonephritis, and porphria cutanea tarda. Other manifestations include arthritis, keratoconjunctivitis sicca, lichen planus, thyroiditis, Raynaud's syndrome, Mooren corneal ulcers, Sjögren's syndrome, pulmonary fibrosis, diabetes mellitus, psoriasis, lymphoma, and polyarteritis nodosa.

Mixed cryoglobulinemia

Cryoglobulinemia is the predominant extrahepatic manifestation of hepatitis C virus, with a prevalence of 1% to 2%. Up to 55% of patients with hepatitis C virus will have cryoglobulins but are asymptomatic. The presence of cryoglobulins does not appear to be related to hepatitis C virus genotype or disease duration. Mixed cryoglobulins are antigen–antibody complexes in the serum that precipitate at cold temperatures and redissolve with warming. The complexes are composed of viral particles and anti-hepatitis C virus antibodies linked by pentameters of IgM and rheumatoid factor. They have been characterized according to the clonal composition of immunoglubulins into type I (monoclonal), type II (mixed monoclonal and polyclonal), and type III (polyclonal only). Both hepatitis C virus antibody and RNA are concentrated to 10- and 100-fold in type II cryoprecipitates. The cryoglobulins themselves are not pathogenic but may deposit in small- and medium-sized blood vessels thus leading to neutrophil infiltration and increased vascular permeability.

The syndrome of mixed essential cryoglobulinemia is characterized by recurrent episodes of vasculitic rash (palpable purpura) on the extremities (Figure 3.8), arthralgias, weakness, and features of glomerulonephritis (see below). Other symptoms include headaches, fatigue, leg ulcers, and Raynaud's syndrome. Cryoglobulinemia may be the initial presentation of hepatitis C. Interferon has been effective in treating this syndrome.

Renal disease

Glomerulonephritis is a well-known, but still poorly understood, complication of hepatitis C virus infection. Chronic hepatitis C virus infection may account for up to 20% of all cases of membranoproliferative glomerulonephritis and less frequently, membranous nephropathy. The mechanism of hepatitis C virus induced damage is not well understood although essential mixed cryoglobulinemia is present in most cases of membranoproliferative glomerulonephritis. Interferon treatment is beneficial in some patients with membranoproliferative glomerulonephritis. However, sustained response after treatment cessation is unusual, and maintenance therapy may be required. Other treatment modalities include strreoids, cytotoxic agents, and plasmaphoresis.

Porphyria cutanea tarda

Hepatitis C virus infection is present in 75% of patients with a sporadic form of porphyria

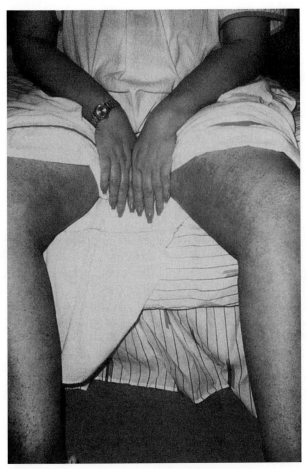

Figure 3.8 A maculopapular rash indicating cutaneous vasculitis over the lower extremities in a patient with hepatitis C virus infection.

Lichen planus

Hepatitis C virus infection has been associated with lichen planus, a benign disease that is associated with pruritic, violaceous, and flat-topped papules distributed in a generalized fashion and which may include the mucus membranes, hair, and nails. The histology reveals degeneration of basal cell layer keratinocytes and dense infiltration of lymphocytes in the upper dermis. Although 10% to 40% of patients are positive for hepatitis C virus antibody, causality has not been established. Treatment with interferon has been associated with an exacerbation of lichen planus.

Diabetes

An association between hepatitis C virus and diabetes mellitus has been observed (regardless of the degree of liver damage), with a prevalence of 25% to 60%. Using data from the NHANES III, a cross-sectional study, persons over the age of 40 years with hepatitis C virus infection were more than three times more likely than those without hepatitis C virus infection to have type 2 diabetes mellitus. Conversely, there was an increased prevalence (3% to 4%) of hepatitis C virus infection in patients with type 2 diabetes mellitus. A clear biological link between hepatitis C virus and type 2 diabetes mellitus has not yet been established.

Autoantibodies

Hepatitis C virus infection is associated with a high prevalence (20%) of autoantibodies such as rheumatoid factor, antismooth muscle cell, antithyroglobulin, anti-GOR, and anticardiolipin antibodies. Antinuclear antibodies (in low titer) are present in up to 40% of patients, suggesting an autoimmune pathogenesis for the liver disease. In patients with autoimmune hepatitis, anti-hepatitis C virus EIA may yield false positive results in up to 40% of cases. Chronic viral hepatitis may also induce secondary autoimmune liver damage. Because of the overlap with hepatitis C and autoimmunity, a liver biopsy is necessary to clarify the dominant process and the treatment option. Classic autoimmune hepatitis is more common in females, is associated with elevated globulins, responds to steroids, and may worsen with interferon. Hepatitis C, on the other hand, does not respond to steroids.

cutanea tarda, with histology ranging from mild hepatitis to frank cirrhosis. Porphyria cutanea tarda, the most common form of porphyria, is caused by reduced activity of uroporphyrinogen decarboxylase. It is characterized by the development of cutaneous lesions, increased skin fragility, bruising, and the appearance of vesicles and bullae. The enzymatic defect is essential but not sufficient for the clinical expression of porphyria cutanea tarda. The basis for this association between hepatitis C virus and porphyria cutanea tarda is not known, although hepatitis C virus may act as a trigger for porphyria cutanea tarda in genetically predisposed hosts. Viral load, but not hepatitis C virus genotype, may be related to the development of porphyria cutanea tarda. However, there are no reported data regarding the efficacy of interferon.

Antibodies to hepatitis C virus have also been reported in patients with type II autoimmune hepatitis characterized by antibodies to liver-kidney-microsome type 1 (anti-LKM1), particularly in Europe. In contrast to the typical LKM-positive autoimmune hepatitis patient, these anti-hepatitis C virus-positive patients tended to be older males with less inflammatory activity and lower LKM antibody titers. Interestingly, the LKM antibodies in patients with hepatitis C virus infection do not often recognize the same epitope (amino acid sequence 254–71) on cytochrome P450 2D6 as LKM1 antibodies in patients with autoimmune hepatitis (recognized in 70% to 95% of patients with type 2 autoimmune hepatitis, but only in 20% of patients with LKM1-positive hepatitis C virus). Although patients with hepatitis C virus infection and anti-LKM1 antibody may benefit from interferon-based treatment, a close follow-up during interferon therapy is warranted to monitor for flare of autoimmune hepatitis.

Treatment

Treatment of hepatitis C virus infection has evolved considerably over the last decade and will continue to evolve in the future. While the ultimate goals of treatment remain prevention of long-term complications of chronic hepatitis C virus infection (e.g. cirrhosis, liver cancer, extrahepatic manifestation) and overall improvement in quality of life, much of the treatment studies focus on more immediate biochemical and virological results. Initial studies (before the development of reliable and sensitive RT-PCR methods) relied on biochemical response based on normalization of ALT activity. Currently, the treatment response is defined in virological terms, as sustained virological response which is generally defined as sustained hepatitis C virus clearance identified by sensitive RT-PCR 6 months after treatment cessation. This has generally been associated with concurrent normalization of biochemical liver disease (i.e. ALT activity) and histological improvement. The hope is that the elimination of the agent that perpetuates liver inflammation will ultimately prevent or reduce cirrhosis and hepatocellular carcinoma while improving the quality of life. The following is a brief overview of the existing treatment options that will undoubtedly change as research progresses.

Treatment of acute hepatitis C virus

For those individuals with recent onset of acute hepatitis C without spontaneous hepatitis C virus clearance, interferon treatment may be appropriate. Recent studies suggest that interferon may be much more effective during the acute phase than during the established chronic phase. In one large German study, interferon monotherapy within several months of acute hepatitis was associated with viral clearance in up to 98% of individuals. Although there was no untreated control group to assess spontaneous recovery in this study, this clearly represented a dramatic improvement from 40% to 50% virological response observed after 12 months of interferon and ribavirin combination therapy for chronic infection. Since some patients do clear spontaneously, one approach is to carefully monitor patients for 6 months from the start of the acute infection and treat only those who remain viremic after that time. Also, the comparison of using interferon monotherapy versus interferon and ribavirin combination therapy in the acute phase of infection has not yet been investigated.

Treatment of chronic hepatitis C virus

Minimal criteria for the treatment of hepatitis C virus include the presence of serum hepatitis C virus RNA, abnormal ALT activity, compensated liver disease, an ability to comply with the treatment regimen, at least 6 months of abstinence from ongoing illicit drug and alcohol use, and liver biopsy indicating moderate inflammation and/or portal fibrosis. In addition, when considering for interferon-based treatment, patients must be in a stable psychiatric condition without active ongoing depression and/or suicidal thoughts. The role of antiviral therapy is less clear for patients with normal ALT, chronic renal failure on hemodialysis, decompensated cirrhosis, hemoglobinopathies, and liver and renal transplantation.

Currently, the mainstay of therapy is a two-drug regimen of interferon alpha injection and oral ribavirin. However, treatment is lengthy (24 to 48 weeks), costly, not always effective, and fraught with side effects. Therefore treatment should be individualized and the risks and benefits carefully assessed. All forms of interferon, i.e. interferon alpha-2b, interferon alpha-2a, and consensus interferon, appear to have a similar efficacy in hepatitis C virus. Early side effects of interferon include fatigue, myalgias, headache, anorexia, low-grade fevers, rigors, impaired concentration, difficulty sleeping, retinopathy, and injection-site reactions. Late side effects include weight loss, hair loss, bone-marrow suppression, autoantibody formation, hypothyroidism, anxiety, depression, psychosis, and clinical decompensation. Ribavirin causes a dose-related hemolytic anemia, cough, dyspnea, rash, pruritus, elevated uric acid, insomnia, and anorexia. In addition, ribavirin is a teratogen and patients must be counseled to use two forms of contraception, including a barrier method, and continue this for up to 6 months after treatment has been discontinued. Up to 10% of patients will discontinue treatment because of the side effects.

Contraindications to antiviral therapy include severe neuropsychiatric illness, pregnancy, unstable coronary artery disease, decompensated liver disease, hemolysis, anemia, autoimmune disease, active alcohol or illicit drug use, and an inability to practice contraception.

Interferon monotherapy

Historically, a 6- to 12-month course of interferon alpha monotherapy at 3 MU subcutaneously three times weekly has led to a virological end-of-treatment response rate of 30% to 40% and a sustained virological response rate of only 10% to 15%. Induction therapy does not lead to a better response rate.

Interferon plus ribavirin

Because of the limited efficacy of monotherapy, interferon was combined with other antiviral, immunomodulatory, and anti-inflammatory agents. Although the exact mechanism of action has not been established, the addition of ribavirin, a nucleoside analog, has significantly enhanced the rate of hepatitis C virus clearance. Overall sustained response rates with 48 weeks of therapy for treatment of naïve patients, relapsers, and non-responders to monotherapy are 38% to 43%, 49%, and 10% to 30% respectively. Extending the duration of interferon and ribavirin from 24 to 48 weeks does not enhance the end-of-treatment response but it did improve the sustained virological response, indicating that extending the duration of treatment decreases the relapse rate.

Favorable predictors of antiviral treatment response include hepatitis C virus RNA less than 2 million, age less than 40 years, female gender, white race, genotype 2 or 3, lower fibrosis stage (0–1), treatment duration, and compliance. Genotype is the best predictor of response and patients infected with genotypes 2 or 3 display a sustained viral clearance of 80% after only 24 weeks of therapy. Patients with hepatitis C virus genotype 1 infection derive additional benefit from an additional 24 weeks of treatment. Thus, total treatment duration is 24 weeks for patients with genotype 2 or 3 infection. In contrast, patients with hepatitis C virus genotype 1 infection should continue treatment for an additional 24 weeks if a significant response is observed by 24 weeks (i.e. hepatitis C virus RNA clearance or reduction by 2–3 log fold). Therapy may be stopped for patients without sustained virological response at 24 weeks as the likelihood of sustained viral clearance is very low. However, our current therapeutic approach may be modified by the results of studies that are currently ongoing, including the National Institutes of Health sponsored multi-center study examining the effect of long-term interferon therapy in reducing hepatic fibrosis and liver cancer development. Ninety-five percent of patients who achieve sustained virological response remain free of detectable RNA with normal liver function tests and improvement in histology when followed for up to 5 to 10 years. Late relapse will occur in 5% of cases.

Pegylated interferon

Because standard interferon is administered three times a week, drug clearance between doses may lead to troughs in drug concentration and activity that may lead to breakthrough viral replication and selection of drug-resistant variants. The development of pegylated interferons with covalently attached polyethylene glycol (an inert non-toxic and water-soluble molecule) resulted in delayed absorption, reduced clearance, enhanced solubility, and weekly dosing with a more sustained level of interferon activity. Pegylated interferon monotherapy was shown to be more effective than shorter acting interferon monotherapy. However, a combination of pegylated interferon and ribavirin is more efficacious than pegylated interferon monotherapy or interferon and ribavirin combination therapy, particularly for the genotype 1 patients. For example, pegylated interferon alpha-2b given at a dose of 1.5 µg/kg weekly and ribavirin 800 mg/day for 48 weeks resulted in an overall sustained virological response rate of 54% compared to 47% with standard interferon and ribavirin therapy. For the different genotypes, the sustained virological response was 42% for genotype 1 (better than 34% for interferon and ribavirin) and 82% for genotype 2 and 3 (no different from standard interferon and ribavirin). Patients receiving more than 10.6 mg/kg ribavarin daily demonstrated an increased sustained virological response of 88% for genotype 2 or 3, and 48% for genotype 1. Another combination therapy that has been evaluated is pegylated interferon alpha-2a as a fixed dose of 180 mcg weekly subcutaneously and ribavirin orally at either 1000 mg or 1200 mg daily based on body weight, for 48 weeks. The overall sustained virological response rate with this combination therapy was 56%. Genotype 1 patients achieved a sustained virological response of 46% and those with genotype 1 and high viral load had a sustained virological response of 41%. Pegylated interferon and ribavirin had many of the same side effects, except perhaps a greater rate of neutropenia, as standard interferon and ribavirin therapy. Currently, it is likely that pegylated interferon and ribavirin may provide better efficacy for genotype 1 infection but not for genotypes 2 or 3, compared to standard interferon and ribavirin therapy. Therefore, treatment should be individually based for each patient after careful discussion about the pros and cons of the available treatment options.

Role of interferon on hepatocellular carcinoma and fibrosis progression

Maintenance therapy with interferon may reduce the degree of fibrosis and decrease the risk of hepatocellular carcinoma, even in the presence of persistent viremia. This suggests that treatment should be continued even if there is no virological response. There have been a number of studies in the literature examining the effect of interferon therapy on the prevention of hepatocellular carcinoma. Interferon therapy is associated with a reduced risk for hepatocellular carcinoma (adjusted risk ratio 0.5), especially in patients with sustained virological response (risk ratio 0.2), persistently normal serum ALT levels (risk ratio 0.2), and ALT levels less than twice the upper limit of normal (risk ratio 0.4). However, current evidence that interferon prevents hepatocellular carcinoma is far from being conclusive. Indeed, almost all studies have used a *post hoc* analysis of previously collected data from treatment trials, development of hepatocellular carcinoma has not generally been the studies' primary or secondary end point, surveillance methods for hepatocellular carcinoma have been variable, and randomization methods (if any) are unclear. Prospective studies are currently ongoing to examine the role of interferon as maintenance therapy.

Future therapy

Unfortunately, more than 50% of hepatitis C virus-infected patients fail to respond to current antiviral therapies. However, several classes of drug are on the horizon, including direct antiviral agents (e.g. inhibitors of hepatitis C virus helicase, protease, polymerase) as well as immune modulators (e.g. thymosin α-1, interleukin-2, interleukin-10), IMPDH inhibitors (similar to ribavirin), and amantadine. The utility of these agents, either alone or in combination, remains to be determined.

Treatment recommendations

Laboratory tests that should be obtained prior to initiation of therapy include baseline liver function tests, biochemistry panel, complete blood count, thyroid stimulating hormone, hepatitis C virus RNA titer, and hepatitis C virus genotype. A liver biopsy prior to the initiation of therapy is recommended, but its utility, especially in genotypes 2 or 3, is debatable. In patients over the age of 50 years, one should consider a cardiac work-up. Patients with diabetes should be optimized in their management of blood-glucose levels and referred for a routine eye examination. A complete cell count with differential should be obtained every 1 to 2 weeks during the first month of therapy and every 4 to 6 weeks thereafter. A reduction in hemoglobin or white blood cell count will require an adjustment in the dose of ribavirin or interferon. Alternatively, epogen or neupogen treatment can be considered. Thyroid function should be monitored every 3 months. At 6 months of therapy, hepatitis C virus RNA titer should be measured (quantitative PCR) and consideration given to stop therapy if the viral titer is not reduced significantly from pretreatment levels. Patients should be monitored for signs of depression. The benefit of treatment adherence should be stressed. The viral load should be rechecked at completion of therapy and then again 6 months after discontinuation of treatment. The final confirmation of viral clearance should be done using the most sensitive test available (e.g. qualitative RT-PCR).

Health maintenance

Patients with chronic hepatitis C virus should be tested for immunity for hepatitis B virus and hepatitis A virus, and receive prophylactic vaccination if not immune. Vaccine response in patients with cirrhosis may be low (about 50%) and accelerated high-dosing schedules may be necessary. Patients should also given Pneumovac and annual influenza vaccine. Patients should also be advised to abstain from alcohol, refrain from donating blood, organs, tissues, or semen, and avoid sharing razor blades or toothbrushes with members of their household. Patients in a long-term monogamous relationship do not need to change their sexual practices, although partners of infected patients may be tested for anti-hepatitis C virus. Patients should be educated on the natural history of hepatitis C virus including the likelihood of a normal life span in the absence of cirrhosis. Currently, there is no effective vaccine for preventing hepatitis C virus infection and passive immunization with immunoglobulin has not shown any benefit.

Screening recommendations

The Centers for Disease Control lists the following people as being at high risk for hepatitis C and testing is necessary

- injection drug users (past and current)
- recipients of blood products prior to1992
- hemodialysis patients
- patients with persistently abnormal liver function tests
- recipients of organ transplants prior to 1992
- infants more than1 year of age born to hepatitis C virus-positive mothers
- health care workers who suffer needle-stick accidents.

Based on available data, hepatitis C virus testing is of uncertain need for the following people

- people who have body piercing or tattoos
- people with multiple sexual partners or sexually transmitted diseases

- long-term partners of individuals infected with hepatitis C virus
- intranasal cocaine and non-injection illegal drug users
- recipients of transplanted tissue.

Routine testing is not necessary unless the following people have a risk factor for infection

- health care workers
- emergency medical personnel
- public safety workers
- pregnant women
- non-sexual household contacts of individuals infected with hepatitis C virus
- the general population.

Further reading – hepatitis C virus

Alter HJ, Houghton M. Clinical Medical Research Award. Hepatitis C virus and eliminating post-transfusion hepatitis. *Nat Med* 2000; 6(10): 1082–1086.

Alter MJ, Kruszon-Moran D, Nainan OV, *et al*. The prevalence of hepatitis C virus infection in the United States, 1988 through 1994. *N Engl J Med* 1999; 341: 556–562.

Centers for Disease Control and Prevention. Recommendations for prevention and control of hepatitis C (HCV) infection and HCV-related chronic disease, *MMWR* 1998; 47: 1–38.

Fried MW, Shiffman ML, Reddy KR, *et al*. Peginterferon alfa-2a plus ribavirin for chronic hepatitis C virus infection. *N Engl J Med* 2002; 347(13): 975–982.

Heathcote EJ, Shiffman ML, Cooklsey GE, *et al*. Peginterferon alfa-2a in patients with chronic hepatitis C and cirrhosis *N Engl J Med* 2000; 343: 1673–1680.

Kenny-Walsh E. Clinical outcomes after hepatitis C infection from contaminated anti-D immune globulin. *N Eng J Med* 1999; 340: 1228–1233.

Manns MP, McHutchison JG, Gordon SC, *et al*. Peginterferon alfa-2b plus ribavirin compared with interferon alfa-2b plus ribavirin for initial treatment of chronic hepatitis C: a randomised trial. *Lancet* 2001; 358: 958–965.

National Institutes of Health Consensus Development Conference Panel. Statement: management of hepatitis C., *Hepatology* 1997; 26(S1): 2S–10S.

Poynard T, Bedossa P, Opolon P. Natural history of liver fibrosis progression in patients with chronic hepatitis C. The OBSVIRC, METAVIR, CLINIVIR, and DOSVIRC groups. *Lancet* 1997; 349: 825–832.

Poynard T, Marcellin P, Lee SS, *et al*. Randomised trail of interferon α2b plus ribavirin for 48 weeks or for 24 weeks versus interferon α2b plus placebo for 48 weeks for treatment of chronic infection with hepatitis C virus. *Lancet* 1998; 352: 1426–1432.

Reddy KR, Wright TL, Pockros PJ, *et al*. Efficacy and safety of pegylated (40-kd) interferon (α-2a in noncirrhotic patients with chronic hepatitis C. *Hepatology* 2001; 33: 433–438.

Seeff LB. Natural history of hepatitis C. *Hepatology* 1997; 26(S1): 21S–28S.

Seeff LB, Miller RN, Rabkin CS, *et al*. 45-year follow-up of hepatitis C virus infection in healthy young adults. *Ann Intern Med* 2000; 132: 105–111.

Serfaft L, Aumaitre H, Chazouilleres O, *et al*. Determinants of outcome of compensated hepatitis C virus-related cirrhosis. *Hepatology* 1998; 27: 2435–2440.

Zeuzem S, Feinman SV, Rasenack J, *et al*. Peginterferon alfa-2a in patients with chronic hepatitis C. *N Eng J Med* 2000; 343: 1666–1672.

HEPATITIS E

Hepatitis E was formerly referred to as enterically transmitted non-A non-B hepatitis, it was first recognized as a distinct clinical entity in the 1980s, and the viral genome was elucidated in 1990. The hepatitis E virus is responsible for causing an acute, self-limited hepatitis that historically has caused severe disease in pregnant hosts.

The virus

The hepatitis E virus has an icosahedral shape and measures 32 to 34 nanometers in diameter. It is a single stranded RNA virus with a genome length of approximately 7.5 kilobases and some morphological features similar to the Caliciviridae. There are three genotypes of the hepatitis E virus which are geographically distinct, they include the Burma strain (southeast Asia), the China strain (north and central Asia), and the Mexico strain (North America). The three genotypes share approximately 75% of sequence homology and may induce partial cross-protection.

Epidemiology

The epidemiology of hepatitis E virus infection is similar to that of hepatitis A virus, although hepatitis E virus appears to cause fewer infections with a smaller worldwide distribution. The hepatitis E virus is endemic in Asia, Africa, the Middle East and central America (Figure 3.9). The largest recorded outbreak occurred in the Xinjiang region of China between 1986 and 1988. Since it is not

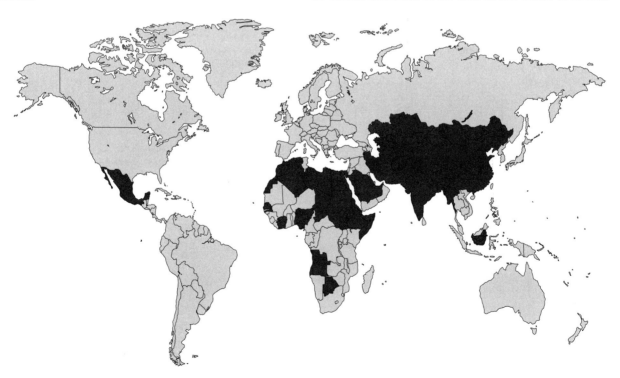

■■■ Outbreaks or confirmed infection more than 25% of sporadic non-ABC hepatitis

Figure 3.9 Geographic distribution of hepatitis E virus infection. From Centers for Disease Control and Prevention (www.cdc.gov)

endemic in the US, most cases identified in the US are associated with a history of travel to areas where hepatitis E virus is endemic.

Transmission

Hepatitis E virus is transmitted by the fecal–oral route. Most often hepatitis E virus outbreaks are related to exposure to contaminated water. Unlike hepatitis A virus, person-to-person contact is not an efficient route for hepatitis E virus transmission. In endemic regions, hepatitis E virus tends to occur as large outbreaks that affect several hundred to several thousand people. In India, hepatitis E virus is estimated to cause 50% to 70% of all cases of sporadic viral hepatitis. Often outbreaks will follow heavy rains and floods that facilitate the contamination of water with fecal matter. Notably, epidemics may occur in the summer months in regions where common water sources are used for drinking, cooking, and personal hygiene, perhaps with an increased risk of fecal contamination as the water level decreases. In certain parts of the world, a recurrent pattern of hepatitis E virus epidemics has been observed. This recurrent pattern may be related to seasonal changes and unchanging conditions that facilitate the fecal contamination of water. There has not been extensive research investigating the risk of vertical transmission of hepatitis E virus. In one study evaluating eight pregnant women with hepatitis E virus, it appeared that vertical transmission was possible with significant perinatal morbidity and mortality.

Natural history

The clinical picture of hepatitis E virus is that of acute hepatitis only. Hepatitis E virus is self-limited and does not evolve into a chronic hepatitis, cirrhosis, or hepatocellular carcinoma.

Diagnosis

The diagnosis of hepatitis E virus relies on either serologic tests to detect antibodies against the virus or molecular tests to detect viral RNA directly using reverse transcriptase techniques.

Serologic tests

The most commonly employed assay for the detection of anti-hepatitis E virus antibodies is the EIA. During acute infection, IgM anti-hepatitis E virus appears first and may last for 4 to 5 months. The IgG anti-hepatitis E virus [anti-HEV IgG] usually arises a few days after IgM and its titer increases into the convalescent phase. This IgG anti-hepatitis E virus titer may remain high from 1 to 4.5 years following acute infection. The precise duration of IgG antihepatitis E virus is not known (Figure 3.10).

Molecular tests

The advent of molecular techniques such as RT-PCR has made it possible to detect hepatitis E virus RNA in body fluids including stool or serum. Hepatitis E virus RNA may be detected in the stools of infected individuals starting approximately 2 weeks after the onset of illness. In a subset of cases, hepatitis E virus RNA may be detected for considerably longer than this. Similarly, hepatitis E virus RNA can be found in the serum of infected individuals for approximately 2 weeks after the onset of illness. Prolonged viremia lasting 4 to 16 weeks has also been described.

Liver biopsy

In acute hepatitis E virus, the liver histology may show the classic pattern of acute inflammation similar to other causes of acute viral hepatitis, or it may appear quite different. Nearly half of patients with hepatitis E virus may demonstrate a cholestatic picture on liver biopsy characterized by canalic-

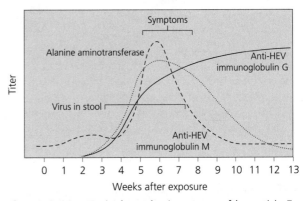

Figure 3.10 Typical serologic course of hepatitis E virus (HEV) infection. Centers for Disease Control and Prevention (www.cdc.gov)

ular bile stasis and glandular transformation of parenchymal cells. Consistent with the classic histological features of acute viral hepatitis, the biopsy may be characterized by focal or confluent hepatocyte necrosis as well as hepatocyte ballooning and acidophilic degeneration.

Clinical picture

The incubation period for hepatitis E virus ranges from 4 to 5 weeks following oral exposure to hepatitis E virus in human volunteers. During acute hepatitis E virus outbreaks, it has also been reported to range between 15 to 60 days. The attack rate is highest in individuals aged 15 to 40 years old. If an individual acquires hepatitis E virus, it is unlikely that they will transmit it to household contacts since the incidence of person-to-person transmission is rare. The clinical signs and symptoms of acute hepatitis E virus infection are very similar to those of other acute viral hepatidities, and may include jaundice, malaise, anorexia, nausea, vomiting, abdominal pain, fever and hepatomegaly. Less commonly, acute hepatitis E virus may be characterized by arthralgias and pruritus. The illness is usually self-limited, lasting 1 to 4 weeks. The clinical picture of hepatitis E virus includes the spectrum from completely asymptomatic disease to acute fulminant and fatal liver failure. In a subset of individuals, the hepatitis E virus infection can take a prolonged cholestatic course lasting 2 to 6 months, presenting a diagnostic challenge. Other infected individuals will present with more severe disease with fulminant or subacute liver failure. It appears that illness severity increases with age and the overall case fatality rate in disease-endemic countries ranges from 0.5% to 4%.

There is a high attack rate among pregnant women who are exposed to the virus, particularly in the second and third trimesters. In pregnant women, hepatitis E virus infection also follows a more severe course with mortality rates as high as 15% to 25%. The reason for this propensity for more severe disease in pregnant hosts is not well understood. In addition to causing severe liver disease and mortality in the mother, hepatitis E virus infection is associated with a higher incidence of abortions, stillbirths, and perinatal deaths.

Complications

Complications of acute hepatitis E virus infection include acute or subacute hepatic failure.

Treatment

Treatment is supportive in cases of acute hepatitis E treatment as no specific therapy exists.

Prevention

The cornerstone of prevention of hepatitis E virus transmission is preventing exposure to fecally contaminated water supplies. On a community level, this requires strict attention to sewage disposal. For individuals in endemic areas this entails boiling water before drinking. For travelers to endemic areas, the Centers for Disease Control recommends avoiding water (and beverages with ice) of unknown purity, uncooked shellfish, uncooked vegetables or fruits not peeled or prepared by the traveler. There is little information regarding the risks or benefits of pre- and post-exposure prophylaxis using pooled anti-hepatitis E virus immune globulin nor the nature of protective immunity to hepatitis E virus. To date, pooled immune globulin is not recommended. Currently there is no vaccine against hepatitis E virus.

Further reading – hepatitis E virus

Krawczynski K, Aggarwal R, Kamili S. Hepatitis E. *Infect Dis Clin North Am* 2000; 14(3): 669–687.

Krawczyncski K, Bradley DW. Enterically transmitted non-A, non-B hepatitis: identification of virus-associated antigen in experimentally infected cynomologus macaques. *J Infect Dis* 1989; 159: 1042.

Reyes GR, Purdy MA, Kim JP, *et al*. Isolation of a cDNA from the virus responsible for enterically transmitted non-A, non-B hepatitis. *Science* 1990; 247(4948): 1335–1339.

Umashanker R, Chorpra S. Hepatitis E virus infection. *UpToDate* 2002.

HEPATITIS G

The hepatitis G virus is an RNA virus of the Flaviviridae family. Another isolate of the same viral species is called the GB virus C, based on the initials of the person whose blood was used to study the virus. Although hepatitis G virus has been labeled as a hepatitis virus, it is controversial whether the virus is truly hepatotrophic and whether it even replicates in the liver. The clinical implications of the virus are equally unclear.

Hepatitis G virus has been recognized in patients with chronic liver disease but the role that this virus plays in the pathogenesis of liver disease has not been fully demonstrated.

Epidemiology

Hepatitis G virus appears to have a worldwide distribution. Its highest prevalence is among individuals with frequent opportunities for parenteral exposure, particularly to blood products.

Transmission

The primary mode of transmission for hepatitis G virus is parenteral. It may also be transmitted sexually and perinatally.

Natural history

Most patients with evidence of exposure to hepatitis G virus do not develop clinically apparent liver disease. Thus, hepatitis G virus infection is not definitively associated with either acute or chronic hepatitis.

Diagnosis

Hepatitis G virus can be detected by sensitive RT-PCR which detects hepatitis G virus RNA in the serum.

Clinical picture

Since hepatitis G virus has not been clearly linked to hepatitis, it is difficult to characterize a clinical picture if one exists. Interestingly, some recent studies have found that hepatitis G virus infection is common in individuals with HIV infection and it may be associated with decreased mortality related to HIV. Further investigations are underway to determine the significance of this association.

Treatment

Primary treatment for hepatitis G virus mono-infection is not usually undertaken. In individuals who are co-infected with hepatitis C virus and hepatitis G virus, treatment with interferon may be appropriate. Based on small studies, interferon may result in decreased levels of hepatitis G virus RNA although this effect may not be lasting. The presence of hepatitis G virus along with hepatitis C virus does not affect the response to therapy for hepatitis C virus.

OTHER VIRUSES THAT MAY INVOLVE THE LIVER

In addition to the well-known hepatotrophic viruses such as hepatitis A through E, it is important to consider other viruses that may involve the liver and cause liver injury. Some viruses that may cause hepatitis include the Epstein–Barr virus, yellow fever, Ebola virus, Marburg virus, Lassa fever, Rift Valley fever, adenoviruses, influenza, and enteroviruses. There may be considerable variation in the degree to which these viruses cause liver disease. The age and immune status of the host will also influence the course.

Further reading – hepatitis G virus and others

Alter HJ. The cloning and clinical implications of HGV and HGBV-C. *N Eng J Med* 1996; 334: 1536.

Chopra S. Current status of hepatitis G infection. *UpToDate* 2002.

Linnen J, Wages J Jr, Zhang-Keck ZY, *et al*. Molecular cloning and disease association of hepatitis G virus: a transfusion-transmissible agent. *Science* 1996; 271(5248): 505–508.

Schiff ER, Sorrell MF, Maddrey WC. *Schiff's Diseases of the Liver* 8th edn. Philadelphia PA, 1999.

Simons JN, Leary TP, Dawson GJ, *et al*. Isolation of novel virus-like sequences associated with human hepatitis. *Nat Med* 1995; 1(6): 564–569.

Tillman HL, Heiken H, Knapik-Botor A, *et al*. Infection with BG virus C and reduced mortality among HIV-infected patients. *New Eng J Med* 2001; 345(10): 715–724.

Xiang J, Wunschmann S, Diekema *et al*. Effect of coinfection with GB virus C on survival among patients with HIV infection. *New Eng J Med* 2001; 345(10): 707–714.

Chapter 4

Alcoholic Liver Disease and Non-Alcoholic Fatty Liver Disease

Anne Burke

Introduction

Fatty liver is defined as a liver where more than 5% of the liver mass is made of fat, usually triacylglycerol (triglyceride). Excessive fat can accumulate for a variety of reasons. It is traditionally classified as either alcoholic or non-alcoholic fatty liver. These conditions share a common pathological appearance and it is likely that they share, at least in part, a common pathophysiological pathway. However the disease mechanisms are incompletely understood and for the purpose of this chapter, other than the following sections on histopathology, the two conditions will be considered separately.

Common pathology

Alcoholic and non-alcoholic fatty liver disease encompass a spectrum of severity from bland steatosis (fatty liver) to inflammation (steatohepatitis), to fibrosis and cirrhosis. They share common features on histology and this will be reviewed briefly here. Further details can be found in Chapter 2.

Steatosis

Steatosis (fatty liver) can be described as macrovesicular or microvesicular. In macrovesicular steatosis, the fat is commonly in one large droplet which displaces the nucleus and is easily seen on hematoxylin and eosin stain. Microvesicular steatosis is manifest as numerous small cytoplasmic droplets which are poorly seen on hematoxylin and eosin stain, and which do not displace the nucleus. It thus requires special lipid stains or electron microscopy for diagnosis.

The steatosis of alcoholic and obesity-related non-alcoholic fatty liver disease is a macrovesicular steatosis. A large fat droplet in the hepatocyte displaces the nucleus eccentrically. It is a non-specific finding and whereas it is most commonly seen in alcohol and non-alcohol-related fatty liver, it may also occur with hepatitis C, ingestion of corticosteroids or other drugs, and with Wilson's disease. In alcohol and obesity-related liver disease, the fat tends to be concentrated in the perivenular region of the hepatic lobule. Mallory bodies may also be present. They are eosinophilic aggregations of tubular or fibrillar structures and are believed to represent modified tubulin fibrils. They are more conspicuous with alcohol-related liver disease but may also be seen in fatty liver of other etiologies. Megamitochondria may also be seen, again these are more typical of alcohol rather than non-alcohol-related liver disease.

Steatohepatitis

This is not merely a combination of macrovesicular steatosis and inflammatory features as the name would suggest. Rather there are other signs of injury including ballooning degeneration of hepatocytes, apoptotic cells, and a lobular inflammatory infiltrate. This is a more severe lesion than bland steatosis and commonly "chicken-wire" fibrosis will be seen with deposition of collagen in the sinusoids.

Fibrosis

As the liver disease progresses, fibrosis becomes more extensive and rather than the fine chicken-wire appearance, broader bands develop eventually leading to bridging fibrosis. Again, the fibrosis tends to be more extensive in the perivenular region with alcohol-related liver disease but this distribution is neither sensitive nor specific to this condition. It is not unusual for extensive fibrosis to occur with remarkably little inflammation.

Cirrhosis

Eventually, broad bands of fibrosis and associated nodule formation demonstrate the features of cirrhosis. Commonly, at this stage the features of cirrhosis predominate over those of steatosis. There is little steatosis or Mallory's hyaline and the etiology of the liver disease must be established by other means.

Alcoholic liver disease

The distinction between alcoholism and alcoholic liver disease

Alcohol use is widespread in the US with approximately 75% of the population consuming alcohol at least occasionally. Approximately 10% of this group abuse alcohol or are alcohol dependent. Alcoholism is a psychiatric diagnosis which should be made by a professional person who is experienced in addiction. A diagnosis of alcohol abuse and dependence requires evidence of deleterious effects on social and role functioning, not merely the presence of medical illness. Similarly, only 71% of patients transplanted for alcohol-related liver disease met the Diagnostic and Statistical Manual of Mental Disorders IV (DSM IV) criteria for alcohol dependence, and more than 50% of patients with alcohol-related liver disease undergoing evaluation for liver transplantation stop drinking without any formal treatment or support group. Indeed many of these patients have difficulty accepting the diagnosis of "alcoholic liver disease".

Although it is widely assumed that patients with alcohol-related liver disease are alcoholics this assumption should be made cautiously and for the remainder of this chapter, in order to emphasize this distinction, the term "alcohol-related liver disease" will be used.

Etiology

Alcohol intake

The etiology of alcohol-related liver disease is poorly understood. Although it is clear that alcohol consumption is a prerequisite, it is not the only factor involved. Approximately 17% of excessive drinkers develop alcohol-related liver disease, therefore 83% do not. Furthermore, whereas the risk of alcohol-related liver disease increases with alcohol consumption, injurious effects can be seen at remarkably low levels of exposure. A Danish population study with a 12-year follow-up showed that the relative risk of alcohol-related liver disease in women drinking 7 to 13 drinks per week was 2.6 that of those drinking 1 to 6 drinks per week. Although the rate of alcohol-related liver disease among this group was still low (2%), it should be borne in mind that two drinks or fewer per day is considered safe and perhaps is even cardioprotec-tive. Similar rates of alcohol-related liver disease (2.3%) were seen in men who consumed 14 to 27 drinks per week and this was 1.5 times the risk of those drinking 1 to 6 drinks per week.

Metabolism of ethanol

Ethanol is metabolized by alcohol dehydrogenase to acetaldehyde which is rapidly metabolized by acetaldehyde dehydrogenase to acetone and water. There are five isoforms of alcohol dehydrogenase and two of acetaldehyde dehydrogenase. Many studies have looked for a correlation between iso-forms of these enzymes and the risk for liver dis-ease but there have been no significant findings.

With chronic "heavy" ethanol consumption and persistent saturation of alcohol dehydrogenase, there is increasing induction of cytochrome $P450_{2E1}$. This pathway also metabolizes ethanol to acetaldehyde and acetone. However, there is greater generation of free radicals by the cytochrome $P450_{2E1}$ system compared to the alcohol and acetaldehyde dehydrogenase pathway. It is notewor-thy that cytochrome $P450_{2E1}$ is confined to the few layers of hepatocytes nearest the central vein and this is the area most vulnerable to alcohol-induced liver injury.

Ethanol consumption both acutely and chroni-cally increases the hepatocyte fat content causing macrovesicular steatosis. This is believed to be due to ethanol-induced increased lipolysis in adipose tissue leading to increased delivery of free fatty acids to the liver, increased hepatic levels of glyc-erol-3-phosphate, a substrate for triacylglycerol syn-thesis, and with chronic ethanol consumption, impaired oxidation of fatty acids within the liver. However, macrovesicular steatosis in isolation is a relatively benign lesion. It is the presence of microvesicular steatosis and steatohepatitis that herald more severe liver disease. The accumulation of microvesicular steatosis is attributed to severe impairment of mitochondrial β-oxidation of fatty acids. This leads to the accumulation of free fatty acids, decreased energy sources in the liver, and uncoupling of oxidative phosphorylation to produce heat rather than adenosine triphosphate (ATP) from oxidation of fat and carbohydrate.

Co-factors

Given that 83% of excessive drinkers do not develop liver disease, other factors must be involved. Despite much research the nature of these factors remains elusive. Some risk factors are outlined in Table 4.1. The presence of another liver disease clearly increases the risk of injury from alcohol. The mech-anism whereby women are more at risk of alcohol-related liver disease at a given level of ethanol consumption is not clear. Differences in body weight or body fat composition do not explain it and although women have slower rates of hepatic ethanol metabolism, this seems to be offset by more rapid rates of gastric ethanol metabolism. Likewise the studies of various polymorphisms of alcohol dehydrogenase, acetaldehyde dehydrogenase and cytochrome $P450_{2E1}$ do not predict the risk of devel-oping alcohol-related liver disease.

There is increasing evidence that oxidative stress is central to the injury of alcohol-related liver dis-ease, and that polymorphisms in antioxidant enzymes may play a role in an individual's propen-sity to develop alcohol-related liver disease. This is discussed further in the next section.

Oxidative stress and alcohol-related liver disease

Oxidative stress denotes an upset in the redox state of the intracellular milieu in favor of oxidation.

Table 4.1   Risk factors for alcohol-related liver disease (ALD)

Risk factors for alcohol-related liver disease	Factors NOT shown to increase the risk of alcohol-related liver disease

Heavy alcohol consumption
Sex Men (more likely to drink heavily)
      Women (more likely to develop
      ALD for a given dose of ethanol)
Chronic viral hepatitis
Other chronic liver diseases
Hereditary hemachromatosis
Malnutrition
Obesity
	Polymorphisms of alcohol dehydrogenase
	Polymorphisms of acetaldehyde dehydrogenase
	Polymorphisms of cytochrome $P450_{2E1}$

From Ewing, JA. Detecting alcoholism: the cage questionnaire. JAMA 1984; 14: 1905–1907.

Typically, free radicals, which are highly reactive chemical species interact non-enzymatically with cellular components, thereby altering their structure and function. The cellular machinery includes antioxidant pathways and repair mechanisms to minimize the consequences of free radical attack. If these are overwhelmed then injury ensues. Cytochrome $P450_{2E1}$ is seen as a "leaky" enzyme in that it generates more free radicals per unit substrate metabolized than other enzymes performing similar reactions, for example alcohol dehydrogenase.

Studies have shown that levels of isoprostanes, markers of lipid peroxidation or free radical attack on lipids, are increased by ethanol consumption. This can be seen with even a single dose of ethanol in social drinkers. The levels are increased further in those with alcoholic cirrhosis and particularly in those with alcoholic hepatitis. In an experimental model, the level of isoprostane production correlated with the severity of the liver injury. Human and animal studies have also shown depletion of endogenous antioxidants, vitamins C and E, and glutathione in regular consumers of ethanol.

The injury of alcohol-related liver disease includes an autoimmune component. Ethyl-protein adducts and acetaldehyde-protein adducts are immunogenic and are found in the serum of alcohol-related liver disease patients. Mallory bodies, typical of alcohol-related liver disease, are collections of acetaldehyde-tubulin adducts (NB they are seen in other liver diseases also and are *not* pathognomonic of alcohol-related liver disease). There is evidence from animal studies using electron microscopy that mitochondrial injury is an early lesion in alcohol-related liver disease. Mitochondria are the main sources of free radicals in eukaryotic cells. Finally, reactive oxygen and nitrogen species are chemoattractant for neutrophils and are involved in the signaling pathways for fibrosis.

Two recent publications add to the evidence of the role of oxidative stress in alcohol-related liver disease and also may provide an insight into why some individuals are at greater risk than others of developing alcohol-related liver disease. Manganese superoxide dismutase (Mn-SOD), is important for detoxifying reactive oxygen species which are generated in the mitochondria. Ethanol increases mitochondrial reactive oxygen species generation. A dimorphism for Mn-SOD has been described with alanine replacing valine at position minus 9. The frequency of Ala/Ala, Ala/Val and Val/Val genotypes in the white population has been estimated to be 21%, 50%, and 29% respectively. However Ala/Ala homozygosity has been demon-strated to be over-represented in those with alcohol-related liver disease, occurring in 17% of those with macrovesicular steatosis but 69% of those with alcohol-induced cirrhosis. This study has since been refuted. A larger study of 281 patients with advanced alcohol-related liver disease and 218 drinkers without liver disease showed no differences in either the heterozygote (55% vs 50%), or the homozygote (19% vs 23%) frequency for the alanine allele (see Stewart et al 2002)[1] Surprisingly, it is the Ala/Ala variant that is associated with improved translocation into the mitochondrial matrix, whereas the Val/Val subtype is partly blocked at the inner membrane import pore. In a related study, over-expression of Mn-SOD in rats protected against alcohol-induced liver disease. At the time of writing, studies evaluating the relative activity of the different isoforms of Mn-SOD in humans have not been done.

The role of tumor necrosis factor

There is evidence to suggest that tumor necrosis factor (TNFα) may play a role in the pathogenesis of alcoholic hepatitis. It could regulate many of the metabolic derangements seen in this condition, including fever, neutrophilia, and anorexia as well as causing liver injury. Serum levels of TNFα correlate with severity in patients admitted with alcoholic hepatitis, and a TNFα promoter polymorphism has been linked to alcoholic hepatitis. Rats chronically fed ethanol have higher TNFα production in response to endotoxin and TNFα receptor-1 knock-out mice are resistant to alcohol-induced liver injury.

Progression of alcohol-related liver disease

It is clear that the presence of macrovesicular steatosis in isolation need not herald progressive liver disease, even in the presence of persistent ethanol consumption. However, the presence and severity of steatosis is a more accurate predictor of progression of alcohol-related liver disease than the presence or absence of ethanol consumption. The onset of microvesicular steatosis suggests the presence of oxidative stress. The metabolic perturbations associated with this indicate increasing difficulty at a cellular level to maintain homeostasis and increased risk of cell death. Reactive oxygen species are involved in the cellular signaling of

[1]Stewart SF *et al* Hepatology 2002; 36: 1355–1360

inflammation, apoptosis, and fibrosis, and this signaling can be triggered by or can occur independently of cell death. Increasing inflammation is followed by increasing fibrosis and eventually nodule formation and cirrhosis. Acute alcoholic hepatitis almost invariably progresses to fibrosis in those individuals who survive the acute injury.

Alcohol-related liver disease and hepatitis C

It is estimated that approximately 4 million people in the US (1.6% of the population) are infected with the hepatitis C virus (HCV). Since 1991, routine screening of the blood pool means that intravenous drug use is the most common route of acquisition of HCV infection. Approximately 70% of injection drug users are HCV positive, and approximately 10% of these HCV-positive individuals will develop cirrhosis. Of patients with alcohol-related liver disease requiring transplantation, 30% to 60% also have HCV, the majority of these acquired through injection drug use. In 1995, alcohol-related liver disease accounted for 27% of liver transplants (the most common indication), and one third of these cases also had HCV. There have been some reports of an increased risk of hepatocellular carcinoma in HCV-positive patients who consume excessive amounts of ethanol. However, these epidemiological based studies were unable to control for the severity of liver disease. Thus, it remains unclear if excessive ethanol consumption is an additional risk factor for hepatocellular carcinoma, once the severity of liver disease has been controlled for in patients with viral hepatitis.

Clinical features

Typical of many liver diseases, alcohol-related liver disease can be remarkably silent and it is not unusual for a patient's first presentation to be an acute variceal hemorrhage or other manifestation of end-stage liver disease. Earlier signs of alcohol-related liver disease include a palpable liver from steatosis induced hepatomegaly. Usually this is painless, but it may be tender if there is stretching of the liver capsule or if steatohepatitis is present. More commonly, vague abdominal discomfort, if present, may be attributable to alcohol-induced gastritis. It is also quite common for a patient to be referred for evaluation of elevated transaminases,

which were drawn as part of an evaluation for life-insurance rather than for any symptoms. Although it is generally stated that in alcohol-related liver disease, the asparagine transferase level is greater than the alanine transferase level, this occurs less commonly in the outpatient setting and alanine transferase greater than asparagine transferase is more common. This feature may represent hepatic steatosis. The transaminases are relatively more increased than the alkaline phosphatase.

With progression to cirrhosis, the liver may become smaller and no longer be palpable and manifestations of cirrhosis and its complications predominate, for example splenomegaly and spider nevi. If decompensation occurs, ascites and hepatic encephalopathy may ensue.

Alcoholic hepatitis

Although considerably less common, acute alcoholic hepatitis is a serious illness. The classic presentation is the combination of anorexia, malaise, fever, jaundice, tender hepatomegaly, splenomegaly, ascites, and encephalopathy. As with all classic syndromes, the full array of symptoms and signs is seldom seen. Patients have often been abstinent for several days prior to presentation. Leukocytosis is common. Patients are prone to infection, but frequently the fever and increased white blood count represent a response to the hepatitis. Transaminases are elevated often 100 to 200 IU/L but rarely exceed 300 IU/L. The ratio of asparagine transferase to alanine transferase is approximately 2:1 or greater. Low levels of potassium and magnesium may be seen and should be repleted. Albumin may be decreased and prothrombin time is prolonged. Bilirubin may also be increased. The presence of increased bilirubin and increased prothrombin time are worrisome for severe disease, which has a high mortality. Maddrey's Discriminant Function (DF) is defined as

$$DF = 4.6 \times (\text{prothrombin time} - \text{control}) + \text{bilirubin (mg/dL)}$$

is commonly used to stratify patients, those with a DF greater than 32 having a high mortality, 50% in Maddrey's original study. The clinical course can be relentlessly progressive and treatment options are limited.

Concomitant illnesses

The patient with alcohol-induced liver disease is susceptible to extrahepatic manifestations of alcohol injury, particularly chronic calcific pancreatitis, peripheral neuropathy, cardiomyopathy, organic brain injury, hypertension, Dupuytren's contracture, parotid enlargement, and pseudo-Cushing's syndrome. There is also an increased rate of smoking among those who drink heavily, and increased rates of smoking-related illnesses including ischemic heart disease, chronic obstructive lung disease, and cancer of the lung and head and neck. It should be remembered that patients who habitually consume alcohol are more susceptible to the toxic effects of acetaminophen and fulminant hepatic failure has been reported at high therapeutic doses.

Diagnosis

As with the diagnosis of any disorder, evaluation should include the components of history and physical examination and directed laboratory and radiological investigations (Table 4.2). Although not indicated in all patients, liver biopsy is very useful to establish the diagnosis of alcohol-related liver disease (although there are no pathognomonic features on biopsy), rule out other liver diseases and establish the severity of liver disease, particularly the presence or absence of cirrhosis.

Because of the subtle nature of early liver disease, the patient presenting with a history suggestive of excessive alcohol consumption should be assessed for alcohol-related liver disease. The CAGE questionnaire (Box 4.1) provides a useful screening tool for alcohol with a sensitivity of 21% to 71% for one positive answer.

Harmful drinking and alcohol abuse is often diagnosed in the primary care setting with patients presenting with vague physical or psychological complaints or simply for the annual check-up. Patients who present with the consequences of harmful drinking, including accidents, marital or family problems, or depression should be screened for the medical consequences of excessive drinking including liver disease. Likewise those with a diagnosis of alcohol abuse are seven times more likely to abuse other substances and 37% of patients with an alcohol disorder also have a concomitant psychiatric disorder. Because of the interaction of alcohol-related liver disease with other liver diseases, patients with a liver disease of another etiology should be advised against alcohol consumption.

Treatment

The treatment of alcohol-related liver disease centers on abstinence from alcohol, correction of mal-

nutrition, and, in certain cases, the use of corticosteroids.

Management of alcohol abuse

Central to the therapy for alcohol-related liver disease is abstinence from ethanol. Patients with advanced liver disease have a considerably decreased capacity for ethanol metabolism and even small amounts of ethanol can have relatively persistent effects. It is likely that much of the improvement seen in patients with decompensated liver disease who stop drinking is because of a reversal of hepatic steatosis and consequent portal hypertension rather than to any decrease in fibrosis or cirrhosis. Options to help patients maintain abstinence are only recently receiving critical investigation. There is some evidence that programs with combined medical and alcohol-dependence treatments achieve better abstinence rates than separate programs for those with alcohol dependence and significant medical morbidity. In particular, these combined programs are successful in engaging patients who are interested in following up for medical illnesses but would be disinclined to receive treatment for alcoholism. For the patient with hazardous drinking but without a diagnosis of alcohol abuse or dependence, brief intervention strategies in the primary care setting are useful. These include education regarding the level of alcohol consumption and its medical consequences, feedback on clinical assessment and recommendations for drinking limits, and regular follow-up. Patients with alcohol dependence or abuse require detoxification. This can frequently be done in an outpatient setting ideally under the supervision of an addiction professional. It should include correction of nutritional and electrolyte disturbances, and monitoring for withdrawal symptoms. Detoxification should be followed by ongoing addiction counseling and therapy. The main types of therapy are cognitive behavioral therapy, motivational enhancement therapy, and twelve-step facilitation. Whereas one study has shown cognitive behavioral therapy and twelve-step facilitation to be superior to motivational enhancement therapy among an unselected population of excessive drinkers motivational enhancement therapy may be more useful in the patient with significant alcohol-related liver disease who frequently does not recognize the severity of his alcohol problem.

Supportive care

Nutritional support remains the mainstay of therapy of alcohol and non-alcohol-related liver disease.

Table 4.2   Investigation of a patient with suspected alcohol-related liver disease

Test	Indication	
History	Establish effects of alcohol consumption on the liver and other systems.	
	Establish levels of alcohol consumption currently and in the past.	
	Screen for other psychiatric disorders and abuse of other substances, particularly intravenous drug use.	
Physical examination	Seek manifestations of liver disease.	
	Seek evidence of decompensated liver disease.	
	Seek evidence of extrahepatic consequences of alcohol-induced injury.	
Laboratory tests	CBC	Macrocytosis, thrombocytopenia.
	Transaminases	AST > ALA.
	Bilirubin, albumin, INR, α feto-protein	Impaired synthetic function.
	Anti-HCV antibody	Development of hepatoma in cirrhotic patient.
	Hepatitis B surface antigen	Concomitant hepatitis C infection.
	Serum iron, TIBC, and ferritin	Concomitant hepatitis B infection.
		Hereditary hemochromatosis.
	AMA, ANA	
	α_1 anti-trypsin level and phenotype	Primary biliary cirrhosis, auto-immune hepatitis α_1 anti-trypsin deficiency.
Radiology	Ultrasound	Fatty liver
	Magnetic resonance imaging and gadolinium	Features of cirrhosis
		Presence of iron overload
		Presence of hepatoma
Liver Biopsy		Establish etiology/etiologies.
		Establish severity of liver disease including presence of cirrhosis.

CBC = complete blood count.
AST = asparagine transferase.
ALA = alanine transferase.
INR = international normalized ratio.
TIBC = total iron binding capacity.
AMA = anti-mitochrondrial antibody.
ANA = anti-nuclear antibody.

Box 4.1   The "CAGE" questionnaire

Have you ever felt you should **C**ut down on your drinking?
Have people **A**nnoyed you by criticising your drinking?
Have you ever felt **G**uilty about your drinking?
Have you ever taken an "**E**yeopener"?

The vast majority (100% in some studies) of patients with advanced alcohol-related liver disease have protein-calorie malnutrition. This is compounded by their having increased protein and calorie requirements. Furthermore, ethanol increases the daily requirements of folate, thiamine, pyridoxal-5-phosphate, and choline. Although poor nutritional status is associated with increased mortality, and several studies show improved liver function with parenteral nutrition, nutritional intervention has not been associated definitively with improved survival. Studies have also attempted to address the efficacy of branch chain amino acid supplementation. The rationale for this being that patients with advanced liver disease and hepatic encephalopathy have a decreased ratio of branch chain amino acid to aromatic amino acids. The sum of available data suggests that it is maintenance of a positive protein balance rather than the provision of particular amino acids used which is of most importance, and nutritional support should be used to achieve this. The recommendations of the American College of Gastroenterology are to provide nutritional support to correct or prevent protein-calorie malnutrition, but specific branch chain amino acid formulations are not recommended. Direct dietary intervention is preferable to enteral feeding, which in turn is preferable to parenteral nutrition. It must be emphasized that patients with advanced liver disease have increased protein and energy requirements, up to 1.5 to 2 g protein and 40 to 45 cal/kg of body weight during acute illness. Sodium should be restricted and in those developing hypernatremia, free water restriction may also be required. Vitamins, particularly thiamine, folate, and pyridoxine, should also be supplemented. The role of antioxidants in the treatment of alcohol-related liver disease, although theoretically attractive, has not been adequately tested

Attention should be paid to the management of end-stage liver disease as appropriate, for example the use of β-blockers as primary prevention of esophageal variceal hemorrhage and the management of hepatic encephalopathy and ascites.

Specific therapy

The history of specific therapies for alcohol-related liver disease, particularly alcoholic hepatitis, is notable for its lack of success. Some of the agents investigated over the years are discussed below.

Corticosteroids The use of corticosteroids to treat alcoholic hepatitis dates back to 1960 and remains controversial today. Corticosteroids have been shown in some studies to decrease mortality in patients with alcoholic hepatitis, but reports have been mixed and the use of meta-analyses has failed to resolve the issue completely. Studies have largely been confined to those with more severe illness and without evidence of infection, gastrointestinal bleeding, or concomitant medical conditions. Even in the studies showing improved survival with corticosteroids, mortality frequently is above 30% in the treated group. Given that prednisone requires hepatic metabolism to the active prednisolone, there is some theoretical appeal to the use of prednisolone in preference to prednisone. In general, it is recommended that corticosteroids (prednisolone 40 mg/day for 4 weeks followed by a 2 to 4 week taper), be given to those with severe alcoholic hepatitis (DF > 32) or hepatic encephalopathy, who have no significant contraindications to steroid therapy. Unfortunately, patients with acute alcoholic hepatitis often have concomitant infection or gastrointestinal bleeding which are contraindications to steroid therapy.

Colchicine The role of colchicine in alcoholic and viral hepatitis was recently the focus of a Cochrane systematic review. The basis for the use of colchicine in alcoholic hepatitis is that it has anti-inflammatory and antifibrotic properties. Unfortunately, several studies involving more than 1000 subjects failed to show any improvement in mortality, liver-related mortality (OR 0.9, 95% CI 0.63–1.69) or several markers of liver injury and liver function. Indeed the only finding of note was

an increase in minor adverse events (OR 4.9, 95% CI 2.7–9.1). Therefore, colchicine is not indicated in the treatment of patients with alcoholic liver disease.

Propylthiouracil Alcohol has been shown to increase hepatic oxygen consumption, and propylthiouracil to decrease cellular oxygen consumption. Short-term propylthiouracil (46 days) has not been shown to decrease mortality in patients hospitalized with acute alcoholic hepatitis and is not recommended in this setting. A single study investigating long-term (2 years) propylthiouracil in an outpatient population of 310 patients with alcohol-related liver disease, showed improved mortality in those who were compliant with therapy and abstinence from alcohol. This study requires confirmation before long-term propylthiouracil can be recommended as standard therapy.

Oxandralone The beneficial effects of this anabolic steroid seem to be related to the concomitant use of nutritional supplementation. It is not recommended for routine use in patients with alcoholic hepatitis.

Pentoxyphiline This is the newest agent to undergo significant investigation as a therapy for alcoholic hepatitis. This agent is currently used to treat intermittent claudication as it increases erythrocyte deformability. Relevant to alcoholic hepatitis is that pentoxyphiline has been shown to decrease TNFα gene transcription. It inhibits several effects of the cytokine and inflammatory response pathways. It has been shown to decrease liver injury in animal studies and has been used as an anti-inflammatory agent in Beçhet's disease in humans. In a randomized double-blinded study of 101 patients with severe alcoholic hepatitis (DF > 32), mortality was 12.4% in the 49 patients randomized to pentoxyphiline and 46% in the 51 patients randomized to placebo. Placebo was chosen as the control arm as the study predated the American College of Gastroenterology recommendations for the use of steroids in alcoholic hepatitis. The majority of deaths in the placebo group (22 of 24) were due to hepatorenal syndrome, versus 6 of the 12 deaths in the pentoxyphiline group. Pentoxyphiline use was associated with a marked decreased risk in the development of hepatorenal syndrome. Whether this was a direct protective effect of pentoxyphiline on the kidneys or secondary to preserved hepatic function is unknown. This study has been greeted with enthusiasm but caution. Should the above findings be confirmed, pentoxyphiline could be more effective than corticosteroids in alcoholic hepatitis and may provide a therapy for hepatorenal syndrome in non-alcohol-related liver disease. Further studies are recommended on this agent.

Liver transplantation

The role of liver transplantation for alcohol-related liver disease remains controversial. This stems largely from social and cultural argument rather than scientific data. There is no doubt that there are insufficient cadaveric liver donors to meet the needs of the current liver transplant waiting list. In 1999, approximately 13 000 patients were awaiting liver transplantation, 4 500 cadaveric transplants were performed and 1 700 patients died whilst awaiting liver transplant. Despite increasing numbers of transplants, the list grows by over 1 000 new patients each year. Thus, the question of organ allocation arises. It has been argued that since alcohol-related liver disease is the result of chronic self-inflicted substance abuse, that patients with alcohol-related liver disease should not be transplanted as this automatically denies the liver to another patient with end-stage liver disease through no fault of their own. This thesis fails when one remembers that alcohol-related liver disease and alcoholism are distinct conditions and that there must be other genetic or environmental factors at play leading to progression of liver disease in the 20% of excessive drinkers who develop end-stage liver disease. Concern has also been raised that patients with alcohol-related liver disease are likely to return to drinking, leading to poor compliance with immunosuppression and graft loss from chronic rejection or recurrent alcohol-related liver disease. To date several small to moderate size studies have attempted to look at this problem. Most are limited by small numbers of subjects, short duration of follow-up, or incomplete follow-up of all relevant subjects – particularly important when failure to follow-up of an eligible patient with alcohol-related liver disease may be linked to non-compliance with abstinence or immunosuppression therapy. Despite these limitations, the studies consistently report 1, 3, and 5-year post-liver transplant patient and graft survival comparable to those of non-alcohol etiologies and better than that for viral hepatitis. Rates of return to drinking vary widely but seem to increase with duration since transplant. Post-transplant rates of consumption of "any alcohol" are estimated to be 30% to 40% at 5 years with 10% to 15% returning to "problem drinking". Nevertheless, these data

compare favorably with those in the non-transplant alcoholic population. Few alcohol treatment programs in the non-transplant population achieve 50% sobriety at 5 years, even though sobriety under these programs is more liberally defined than the return to "any drinking" used in the liver transplant studies. Rates of return to work, a surrogate marker of "success", vary from 16% to 59%. Return to work rates tend to be lower for patients with alcohol-related liver disease compared with non-alcohol-related liver disease controls but there is insufficient data at present to adequately assess this area.

Many programs have a "six-month rule" i.e. only patients who have been abstinent for 6 months or longer, will be transplanted, and in the US, most third party payers will not pay for a liver transplant for chronic alcohol-related liver disease unless the recipient has been abstinent for a minimum of 6 months. This is on the grounds that

- patients with end-stage alcohol-related liver disease, who abstain from alcohol may regain sufficient function to avoid transplant
- patients with longer pre-transplant sobriety are more likely to remain abstinent post-transplant.

However the duration of pre-transplant sobriety has not been shown to adequately predict post-transplant sobriety and the 6-month rule should not be a deciding factor in transplanting a patient for end-stage alcohol-related liver disease.

On a practical note, the waiting times for most patients is now greater than 6 months and any patient with advanced liver disease who is not actively drinking at present should be considered for liver transplantation.

The role of liver transplantation for acute alcoholic hepatitis is even more controversial. Patients with severe alcoholic hepatitis (DF > 32) have a high short-term mortality and may not survive 6 months.

On the other hand, there is great reluctance to transplant patients with acute alcoholic hepatitis. This stems from the belief that those patients with severe alcoholic hepatitis who are developing progressive liver disease have high rates of infection and renal impairment and are high-risk candidates. Furthermore, as a group they will tend to have less insight into the role of alcohol in their disease than patients with more chronic alcohol-related liver disease, higher rates of post-transplant harmful ethanol consumption, and poor compliance with post-transplant medical regimens. Consequently, alcoholic hepatitis is considered by most transplant programs to be a contraindication to transplantation, and our program does not transplant for acute alcoholic hepatitis at this time. However, given that acute alcoholic hepatitis is an exclusion criterion for most programs, there is a paucity of data to support these arguments. Most studies evaluating this question are small retrospective case series, but they have suggested survival benefit to the recipient. In more recent years the 6-month rule and the long waiting times made the question of liver transplantation for acute alcoholic hepatitis moot, but this will soon need to be addressed in a systematic fashion. The increasing practice of live-donor liver transplantation allows for patients to be transplanted independent of the cadaveric list waiting times. The new MELD (Mayo Clinic End-Stage Liver Disease) scoring system for organ allocation also has had a significant impact on prioritizing patients awaiting liver transplantation. Indeed those with alcoholic hepatitis (high bilirubin and elevated prothrombin time) especially with the onset of renal impairment – a particularly poor prognostic sign – would score very highly in the MELD system, and were they accepted for listing would likely be transplanted after a short waiting period.

Two questions need to be answered

1. do patients with severe alcoholic hepatitis do significantly better if transplanted compared to those receiving best available medical management?
2. do patients who are transplanted for severe alcoholic hepatitis have significantly different outcomes to those transplanted for other reasons?

The only way to adequately address this issue is through a randomized controlled trial of liver transplant versus medical management. Such a trial will require a multi-center approach and the backing of the transplant community as a whole.

Prognosis

The outcome of patients with alcohol-related liver disease depends on the severity of the liver disease and degree of abstinence. Assuming that the patient has macrovesicular steatosis only, no other underlying liver disease, and maintains abstinence, full recovery is likely. However, ongoing alcohol consumption in the face of moderate to severe steatosis is associated with a greater than 20% risk of cirrhosis at 10 years. Even for the patient with

established cirrhosis, the benefits of abstinence are considerable. The 5-year prognosis for a compensated cirrhotic patient who is abstinent is more than 90%. Even those who had decompensated liver disease have over 60% 5-year survival if abstinent. This is in contrast to the prognosis of patients with decompensated liver disease from other causes or in those who continue to drink. Their 1-year survival is less than 70%, and in patients with compensated cirrhosis who continue to drink, the 7-year prognosis is less than 70%. Furthermore, in those who present with decompensated acute alcoholic steatohepatitis, 1-month mortality rates of 50% have been reported.

Non-alcoholic fatty liver disease

Non-alcoholic fatty liver disease is estimated to be present in 20% of the general population and is currently the most prevalent liver disease in the US. Non-alcoholic fatty liver disease covers a spectrum of disease from bland steatosis, through steatohepatitis, fibrosis, and cirrhosis. There are a variety of well recognized risk factors, but the pathophysiology and the reasons why it progresses in some cases but not in others are poorly understood. It is likely that it represents a variety of liver diseases sharing, at least in part, aberrant metabolic pathways. What is lacking is an understanding of a unifying mechanism linking these disparate conditions. The nomenclature is currently under review and will probably change from a "single" condition of "non-alcoholic fatty liver disease" to a term describing the etiology and severity of the disease, for example obesity-induced steatohepatitis. The terms non-alcoholic fatty liver disease (NAFLD) and non-alcoholic steatohepatitis (NASH) will be used here.

Pathophysiology

Etiology of non-alcoholic fatty liver disease

The pathogenesis of NAFLD is not understood but it likely represents a series of partially related conditions. Table 4.3 outlines some risk factors for NAFLD.

In an attempt to link the various etiologies of NASH and to explain why not all who have steatosis develop steatohepatitis, Day and James proposed the idea of "two hits", represented schematically in Figure 4.1. The first hit is the presence of excessive amounts of fat in the liver. This

Table 4.3   Risk factors for non-alcoholic fatty liver disease (NAFLD)

Association	Putative mechanism
Insulin resistance/metabolic syndrome	
Acute starvation	probably excessive peripheral lipolysis
Poorly controlled type I diabetes mellitus	probably excessive peripheral lipolysis
Drugs	probably interfere with mitochondrial β-oxidation
amiodarone	
valproate	
corticosteroids	
high-dose estrogen/ tamoxifen	
calcium channel blockers	
salicylates	may lead to Reye's syndrome
HAART	deranged oxidative phosphorylation
Endotoxin	
short bowel syndrome	
blind loop syndrome	
post-bariatric surgery	
Multifactorial	
prolonged total parenteral nutrition	
Inborn errors of metabolism	
lipoatrophic diabetes	
abetalipoproteinemia	
Mauriac syndrome	
Niemann–Pick disease	
Cryptogenic cirrhosis	possibly undiagnosed NAFLD

HAART = highly active anti-retroviral therapy.

can be caused by the deranged metabolism seen in insulin-resistance syndromes, or with certain drugs. The second hit is a source of free radicals. This too can be from certain drugs which impair electron transfer along the respiratory chain, alcohol, iron, mitochondrial enzyme defects, or increased activity of cytochrome $P450_{2E1}$. Indeed, among the very obese, steatohepatitis is more likely to occur during periods of rapid weight loss induced by overly stringent dieting.

Influx of lipid

Dietary lipid   Dietary lipids are absorbed by the small intestine and enter the chyle as reassembled triacylglycerol (triglyceride), carried in chylomicrons. Although some of this is taken directly into the liver, triacylglycerol is removed from the circulation largely by muscle cells where it is used as an energy source and by adipocytes where stored for later use. In order to be utilized by peripheral tissues, fatty acids must be released from triacylglycerol by the action of endovascular lipases at the peripheral sites. Endovascular lipoprotein lipase is made by monocytes and adipocytes, it then attaches to vascular endothelial cells. The lipoprotein lipase associated with muscle tissue is largely constitutive and increases modestly with fasting, whereas the lipoprotein lipase associated with adipose tissue is hormone sensitive and is increased in the fed state by the action of insulin. Under the action of these enzymes, triacylglycerol from chylomicrons is largely depleted within 10 minutes of entering the circulation and triacylglycerol from hepatic very low-density lipoproteins is largely cleared within 1 hour.

Lipid from adipocytes   Lipoprotein lipase is also responsible for the release of triacylglcyerol from adipocytes into the circulation in response to intracellular levels of cyclic adenosine monophosphate (cAMP). Intracellular levels of cAMP are increased by the presence of epinephrine, corticosteroids, glucagon, and caffeine, all of which serve to stimulate lipolysis. The released fatty acids are bound to albumin. In the fed state, insulin increases phosphodiesterase activity, depletes intracellular cAMP, and inhibits peripheral lipolysis whilst promoting uptake of fatty acids from circulating lipoproteins.

Disposal of hepatic lipid

Beta-oxidation of fatty acids   On entering the hepatocyte, fatty acids are bound to coenzyme-A to make acyl-CoA. In order to enter the

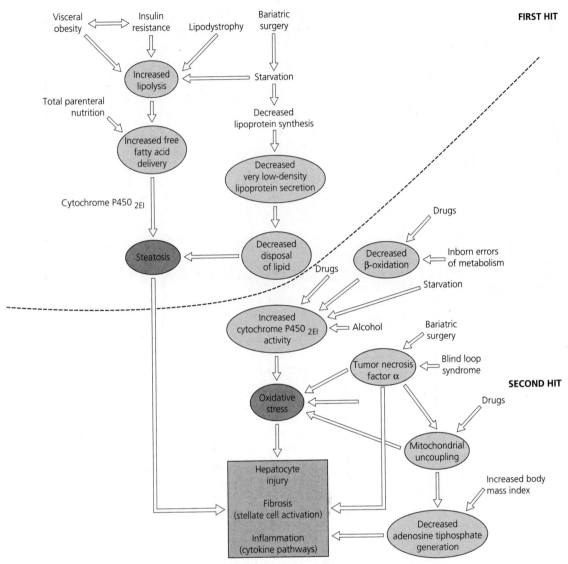

Figure 4.1 Schema of the two-hit theory of non-alcoholic fatty liver disease.

mitochondria, the free fatty acid must pass via a carnitine shuttle as the mitochondria are impermeable to acyl-CoA. Acyl-CoA is reassembled in the mitochondria and is then hydrolysed, two carbons at a time, to generate acetyl-CoA which can enter Kreb's cycle to produce ATP. This source of energy is important in the fasted state.

Secretion of very low-density lipoproteins

In the fed state there are ample stores of hepatic glycogen and the entering free fatty acids along with excessive glucose and amino acids are converted back into triacylglycerol. Triacylglycerol is combined with cholesterol, apolipoprotein B-100 and a variety of other molecules to form very low-density lipoproteins which are secreted from the liver to be taken up by adipocytes or other tissues. The complex assembly of very low-density lipoproteins is the rate limiting step in the transport of lipid from the liver. Fatty acids are also consumed in the synthesis of phospholipids, cholesterol and its by-products.

Hepatic steatosis occurs when delivery of lipid to the liver exceeds the liver's capacity to metabolize and secrete it. The uptake or release of free fatty acids by adipocytes is tightly regulated by various hormones. In contrast, the uptake of free fatty acids by the liver is largely unregulated and is dependent on the ambient levels of albumin-bound free fatty acid in the circulation.

Obesity, insulin resistance, and non-alcoholic fatty liver disease

Obesity is the single most important risk factor for hepatic steatosis. It is defined as a body mass index (BMI) greater than 30 kg/m^2, it is present in 23% of the population and this is expected to reach 40% by the year 2025. It is estimated that 40% to 70% of the variance of BMI among the general populace is attributable to polygenic factors, the remainder being due to societal and environmental factors including changes in dietary composition, portion sizes, and physical activity patterns. Not only is the degree of obesity important but studies dating back to the 1940s demonstrate the significance of the distribution of the fat. The insulinresistance syndrome, which is continuously being redefined (Box 4.2), is associated with visceral adiposity. Given that visceral (intra-abdominal) fat accounts for only 6% to 20% of total adipose volume in obese subjects, its significance is noteworthy. Those with increased gynoid (gluteal–femoral) distribution of fat do not appear to suffer at increased rates from insulin resistance, atherosclerosis, or diabetes mellitus. Visceral fat exposes the liver to high levels of free fatty acids. It is relatively resistant to the lipotrophic effects of insulin but is sensitive to the lipolytic effects of catecholamines, thus maintaining a supply of free fatty acids not only to the liver but also to the systemic circulation, even in the post-prandial state.

A common feature of NAFLD is resistance to insulin. This leads to increased lipolysis in the adipocytes and delivery of lipid to the liver. Furthermore, there is impaired oxidation of fatty acids by mitochondria and accumulation of fatty acids in the hepatocyte. Non-alcoholic fatty liver disease, although not yet considered part of the insulin-resistance syndrome, is continually gaining credence as such. Two recent publications linked

insulin resistance with biopsy proven NASH, independent of weight or the presence of diabetes mellitus, and demonstrated that the increased insulin levels were from increased pancreatic secretion rather than decreased hepatic extraction.

It is likely that visceral adiposity is a permissive factor exacerbating an underlying propensity to the insulin-resistance syndrome. However, the nature of the primary defect leading to increased visceral adipose tissue, increased insulin resistance, and its consequence is unknown. Laboratory studies have shown that adipocytes secrete "resistin", a peptide which impairs insulin action *in vivo* in mice and *in vitro* in an adipocyte cell line. Its role in human type II diabetes remains to be confirmed.

Non-alcoholic fatty liver disease independent of insulin resistance

Non-alcoholic fatty liver disease is associated with prolonged total parenteral nutrition. This may represent a combination of excessive circulating lipid compounded by increased endotoxin levels from the disorder leading to gastrointestinal insufficiency requiring the total parenteral nutrition. Protein-calorie malnutrition and acute starvation are believed to impair the synthesis of lipoproteins and export of triacylglycerol from the liver as well as increase peripheral lipolysis and delivery of free fatty acids to the liver as a fuel source.

Inborn and acquired errors of metabolism associated with hepatic steatosis Unlike the obesity-related macrosteatosis, much of the steatosis seen with inborn errors of metabolism is microvesicular. The mechanism(s) behind this distinction is unclear. Defects in the carnitine shuttle are associated with early childhood hepatic steatosis and an intolerance to fasting. Acute fatty liver of pregnancy, (see below), is believed to involve a partial defect in long-chain hydroxyacyl-CoA dehydrogenase, an enzyme required for the β-oxidation of long-chain (> 16 carbon) fatty acids. Acquired defects in β-oxidation from toxic valproate intermediates or hypoglycine ingested in unripe ackee fruit, leading to microvesicular steatosis and hypoglycemia, which are characteristic of valproate liver injury and Jamaican vomiting sickness.

Phospholipidoses also lead to microvesicular steatosis, for example Niemann–Pick disease and amiodarone toxicity. These conditions are characterized by lamellar bodies which are accumulations of phospholipid in lysosomal membranes. The exact mechanism whereby these conditions lead to

---

Box 4.2   Features of the insulin-resistance syndrome

Diabetes mellitus type II or impaired glucose tolerance
Hypertension
Elevated triglycerides
Decreased high-density lipoprotein cholesterol
Polycystic ovarian syndrome
Hyperuricemia
Hyperinsulinemia
Obesity

---

microvesicular steatosis is unclear but it probably involves impaired intracellular processing and trafficking of very low-density lipoproteins.

The lipodystrophies are rare conditions characterized by marked mobilization of lipid from adipocytes and a habitus defined by diminished peripheral adipose. The excessive amounts of circulating free fatty acids lead to hepatic steatosis.

The use of highly active antiretroviral therapy in the treatment of acquired immunodeficiency syndrome (AIDS) requires special mention. Several of these medications are associated with lipodystrophy, hyperlipidemia, and insulin resistance. Their use is associated with a high risk of liver toxicity requiring discontinuation of therapy. Whether this is due to NAFLD or a variety of liver disorders is not yet clear. However the hepatic toxicity of one of the nucleoside analogs, stavudine, has received some recent attention. Stavudine is a potent inhibitor of mitochondrial DNA and it is hypothesized that depletion of mitochondrial DNA leads to depletion of the components of the electron transport chain, uncoupling of oxidative phosphorylation, lactic acidosis, oxidative stress, and deranged lipid metabolism in the liver. A selection for viral nucleosides relative to mitochondrial DNA is associated with a more favorable toxicity profile.

Acute fatty liver of pregnancy Acute fatty liver of pregnancy is a rare disorder and much of the published material involves case reports and reviews of the literature. It is believed to occur in between 1 per 6 600 and 1 per 13 000 births. It is a life-threatening condition and although the prognosis has improved markedly with improved management of the critically ill, maternal and fetal deaths still occur.

The etiology of acute fatty liver of pregnancy is unknown. Much attention has been paid to errors in mitochondrial β-oxidation of lipids. Fetal long-chain 3-hydroxyacyl-coenzyme A dehydrogenase (LCHAD) deficiency is the most commonly diagnosed metabolic disorder in acute fatty liver of pregnancy but is neither sufficient nor required, in that mothers of children subsequently found to be LCHAD deficient have had uneventful pregnancies and infants of mothers with acute fatty liver of pregnancy have been shown to have normal LCHAD function. In some of these infants, other lipid-metabolizing enzymes have been shown to be abnormal but a percentage of cases remains without adequate explanation.

Electron microscopy of acute fatty liver of pregnancy livers reveals microvesicular lipid deposition and giant mitochondria. Studies of pregnant mice or of non-pregnant female mice given high doses of estrogen or progesterone lead to distortions in the appearance of mitochondria, decreased β-oxidation of fatty acids and decreased mitochondrial energy production. However, hepatic steatosis was not seen in these experiments. It is theorized that acute fatty liver of pregnancy is the result of a combination of insults

- toxic intermediates from impaired fetal lipid metabolism
- less efficient maternal lipid peroxidation
- putative environmental toxins
- putative viral infections (TNFα also impairs mitochondrial function) in the permissive milieu of the pregnant liver.

Acute fatty liver of pregnancy is seen toward the end of the third trimester, typically presenting between 30 weeks gestation and term. Symptoms are non-specific and diagnosis usually relies on a combination of clinical and laboratory data. Although the full-blown syndrome is easily recognized, the vague prodromal symptoms often prevent early diagnosis.

The most common symptoms are nausea and vomiting (70%), malaise (65%), fever (25%), and cholestasis (20%). Hypertension (>140/90 mmHg) is common (70%) as is renal impairment manifesting as elevated creatinine (90–100%). Pre-existing pre-eclampsia has been reported in 46% of subjects with acute fatty liver of pregnancy.

Laboratory abnormalities are very common. Transaminases are typically 200 to 600 IU/L. Levels greater than 1000 IU/L are rare but have been reported. Bilirubin is elevated 11 ± 9 mg/dL. Prothrombin time is nearly always prolonged and disseminated intravascular coagulation occurs in approximately 70% of patients. However, clinically significant bleeding is rare in the absence of surgery or trauma during delivery. The measurement of individual clotting factors, for example antithrombin III levels, has received much attention. These levels are nearly always low in cases of acute fatty liver of pregnancy, and retrospective analysis of stored plasma has shown the levels to be decreased up to 2 weeks prior to clinical presentation of acute fatty liver of pregnancy. However, it remains to be decided how this information can be used in a clinical setting. Finally, hypoglycemia is common and remains an important clinical problem in patients with acute fatty liver of pregnancy. Aggressive glucose repletion is usually required during the period of liver failure. Radiological studies are usually unhelpful with a very high falsenegative rate for fatty liver. Although liver biopsy with special stains for microvesicular fat is definitive, most diagnoses are based on the compilation of clinical and laboratory findings.

The only specific management of acute fatty liver of pregnancy is prompt delivery of the infant. It is not uncommon for women to present with spontaneous labor and then to be diagnosed with acute fatty liver of pregnancy. In those in whom labor is proceeding well, it can be allowed to continue. In those who are not yet in labor or labor is not progressing well, it may be necessary to deliver the infant by cesarean section. There is a high rate of fetal compromise (25%) manifesting as abnormal fetal heart tracings during labor, meconium, *in utero* death, or stillbirth. Thus, fetal monitoring is strongly advised. Because of the presence of disseminated intravascular coagulation, trauma to the birth canal during delivery can result in prolonged bleeding and there is an increased risk of wound infection following cesarean section.

Following delivery, it is common for further deterioration to occur in the mother's condition. Indeed, many cases of acute fatty liver of pregnancy do not manifest until the early post-partum days. Management is supportive. Glucose levels should be closely monitored with 1 to 2 hourly glucometer readings, and attention given to maintaining glucose levels. Many patients require prolonged 10% dextrose infusions combined with intermittent boluses of 50% dextrose. Volume resuscitation is also important to preserve renal function. Approximately 50% of patients will require blood products, 25% requiring multiple transfusions of multiple blood products. Hepatic encephalopathy is common and the patient should be monitored by serial neurological examinations. Given the fulminant nature of acute fatty liver of pregnancy, patients with hepatic encephalopathy are at risk of cerebral edema and may require mannitol, phenobarbital, or hyperventilation to protect central nervous system perfusion and function. Another common complication is infection. Patients with acute fatty liver of pregnancy commonly have preceding fever or elevated leukocyte count related to the acute fatty liver of pregnancy rather than infection, thus infection may be masked and vigilance must be maintained. Most recently reported deaths from acute fatty liver of pregnancy are secondary to sepsis in this compromized population rather than a direct consequence of hepatic failure.

Prompt delivery of the fetus and improved intensive care support have improved fetal and maternal mortality from more than 80% to less than 20%. Acute fatty liver of pregnancy on subsequent pregnancy is rare but has been reported. Children born of acute fatty liver of pregnancy mothers should be tested for errors in lipid metabolism in particular, not only LCHAD deficiency. Those positive for such errors are at risk of cerebral, cardiovascular, and musculoskeletal dysfunction, which may present very acutely during the first year, and up to the fifth year, of life.

Putative role of tumor necrosis factor

Many types of acute liver injury are associated with an increase in the production of TNFα. Exposure to TNFα is increased by bacterial overgrowth seen in patients with abnormal gastrointestinal tracts requiring chronic total parenteral nutrition, or following bariatric surgery or even non-operative rapid weight loss.

Studies suggest that this exposure is important in triggering the c-JUN pathway which leads to hepatocyte proliferation and liver repair. However an aberrance in the response to TNFα can lead either to activation of the caspase pathway and apoptosis or to the induction of sphingomyelinase pathway and cell necrosis. Interestingly, both of these cell-death pathways target the mitochondria. The factors which lead to the one TNFα response over another are unclear but it is likely that the levels of other cytokines, antioxidants, and ATP play an important role. It is important to note, however, that much of the above work was done in the mouse model. Mice demonstrate much higher levels of TNFα production in adipose tissue than humans.

Cryptogenic cirrhosis and non-alcoholic fatty liver disease
Cryptogenic cirrhosis, a condition where no etiology can be found despite intensive investigation, accounts for approximately 10% of patients undergoing liver transplantation. It has been proposed that NAFLD may be one of the underlying etiologies. However, as the fat content decreases with advancing fibrosis, this diagnosis is difficult to make in those with advanced liver disease. Nevertheless, obesity and diabetes are independent risk factors for progression of hepatitis C liver disease, alcohol-related liver disease and NAFLD. In a case control study of 49 patients with cryptogenic cirrhosis, and 98 controls (all patients with known NAFLD having been excluded), the prevalence in the cryptogenic cirrhosis group of obesity (47%) and diabetes mellitus (47%) was twice that seen in the control group, 24% and 22% respectively.

Hepatitis C and non-alcoholic fatty liver disease
Liver disease is associated with impaired glucose tolerance, and obesity is an independent

risk factor for liver disease as well as for diabetes mellitus. Having controlled for obesity, age, and socioeconomic status, the NHANES (National Health and Nutritional Examination Survey) demonstrated a threefold increase in the risk of diabetes mellitus in patients with hepatitis C who were over 40 years old. In addition, steatosis is commonly seen in the liver biopsies of patients with hepatitis C and is associated with an increased risk of fibrosis in these patients. Although the topic continues to be evaluated, the sum of the evidence, at present, suggests that significant steatosis occurring in patients with hepatitis C is more reflective of obesity (or ethanol consumption) and is not an independent manifestation of HCV infection (infection with genotype 3 may be an exception to this). Therefore, we should consider steatosis to be an independent risk factor for progressive liver disease in those with hepatitis C, and controlling weight and diabetes should be part of the therapeutic approach to these patients.

The role of oxidative stress

Regardless of the etiology, the accumulation of hepatic lipid is considered to represent the "first hit" in the development of NAFLD. However, hepatic steatosis is relatively bland and additional factors are required to lead to progressive liver disease. Patients with NAFLD are shown to have increased markers of oxidative stress, particularly those with NASH. Oxidative stress and subsequent lipid peroxidation is currently considered the most likely "second hit" and it may arise through several different mechanisms.

Cytochrome $P450_{2E1}$, which is believed to play a significant role in the oxidative stress associated with alcohol-related liver disease, is upregulated in people with NASH. More compelling is the evidence that the distribution of immuno-staining for cytochrome $P450_{2E1}$ correlated with the distribution of steatosis, and the fibrosis of NASH commences in the perivenular region where the concentration of cytochrome $P450_{2E1}$ is highest. *In vitro* studies have demonstrated that cytochrome $P450_{2E1}$ is upregulated by fatty acids. Starvation also upregulates cytochrome $P450_{2E1}$. Several drugs which cause NAFLD impair mitochondrial β-oxidation leading to decreased ATP formation and increased reactive oxygen species generation. Not only are the reactive oxygen species directly toxic, but the decreased ATP generation leaves hepatocytes more vulnerable to other injurious stimuli (e.g. exposure to endotoxin or surgery). Interestingly, patients with NAFLD compared with healthy control subjects demonstrate impaired recovery of hepatic ATP following its depletion in an experimental setting. Furthermore, hepatic ATP repletion is correlated with BMI in both patients and control subjects. Whereas the role of TNFα as a "first hit" in NAFLD is controversial, its role as an instigator of oxidative stress is more plausible. Many of the cytokine pathways promoted by TNFα lead to increases in reactive oxygen species particularly by interfering with normal mitochondrial function.

Oxidative stress is known to play a significant role in recruiting inflammatory cells and cytochrome $P450_{2E1}$ derived reactive oxygen species have been shown to activate hepatic stellate cells *in vitro* leading to increased collagen production. The role of oxidative stress as a mediator of hepatic fibrosis has been reviewed elsewhere.

The role of hepatic iron in NASH is no longer considered to be of major etiological importance. Clearly iron is capable of promoting oxidative stress and several studies have demonstrated increased stainable iron in the livers of patients with NASH and in patients with iron overload, increased hepatic iron is an independent risk factor for progressive liver disease. More recent studies, however, have failed to demonstrate convincingly increased hepatic iron content in NASH patients, increased prevalence of hemachromatosis genes, and they have failed to rule out liver inflammation as the cause rather than the consequence of the increased iron seen. It is prudent to rule out iron overload in patients with NASH as phlebotomy is appropriate in those with iron overload. Iron chelation to improve insulin sensitivity has been reported to be beneficial in subjects with NAFLD, even in those without genetic hemachromatosis or documented iron overload. However, this has not yet been substantiated in multiple centers and is not yet common practice.

Co-factors

As with alcohol-related liver disease, the coexistence of NAFLD and liver disease of other etiologies increases the likelihood of significant injury. This has been demonstrated clearly in patients with hepatitis C viral hepatitis. Furthermore, obesity is recognized to be an independent risk factor for progression of liver disease.

Clinical features

Non-alcoholic fatty liver disease, once considered an uncommon disease, is now being increasingly recognized. This is probably because of a combination of earlier and more intensive investigation as a result of the increased use of liver enzymes as screening tests in asymptomatic individuals as well as an increase in the prevalence of risk factors (obesity, bariatric surgery, total parenteral nutrition, and predisposing medications). The true prevalence of NAFLD is unknown. It has been estimated to occur in 3% to 20% of normal individuals and in 20% to 80% of obese persons, with NASH occurring up to 3% and 15% of these individuals respectively, i.e. 15% to 20% of those with NAFLD develop NASH. It is clear, however, that the prevalence of NAFLD increases with the degree of obesity. It can occur at any age and more recent studies indicate that it is equally prevalent in men and women. In keeping with the theory that it commonly reflects a state of insulin resistance, the risk in those with central obesity is greater than those with peripheral obesity for a given percentage of body fat.

Non-alcoholic fatty liver disease is usually silent and is most often discovered incidentally. The most common presentation is aberrant hepatic biochemical tests, which have been drawn for investigation for life insurance, or to monitor an individual taking lipid-lowering or other medications. Alternatively, increased echogenicity of the liver is noticed on an ultrasound done to investigate the presence of gallstones, which are more prevalent in obese individuals, and many patients with NAFLD have normal liver enzymes. In general, alanine transferase is greater than asparagine transferase and alkaline phosphatase is within twice the upper limit of normal levels. For those who do develop symptoms, non-specific right upper quadrant discomfort or fatigue are the most common. Unlike ALD where portal hypertension can occur in the presence of alcoholic hepatitis, the presence of portal hypertension in NAFLD usually indicates a progression to cirrhosis. Manifestations of advanced or end-stage liver disease are rare but can occur. For those who progress from bland steatosis to NASH, the risk of progression to advanced liver disease is markedly increased. Likewise, physical examination, other than the manifestations of obesity, is usually unremarkable unless there are manifestations of end-stage liver disease.

Diseases concomitant to obesity in the NAFLD patient include cardiovascular disease, hypertension, hyperlipidemia, and diabetes mellitus. There are also increased rates of osteoarthritis among the obese, and those who have end-stage liver disease should be reminded to avoid non-steroidal analgesics because of their adverse effects on renal and platelet function.

Investigations

Ultrasound, computed tomography (CT), particularly non-contrast, and magnetic resonance imaging (MRI) all display features strongly suggestive of steatosis. However, none of these modalities can distinguish bland steatosis from more ominous steatohepatitis – this distinction usually requiring a liver biopsy.

Treatment

There is no proven therapy for the treatment of NAFLD. Obese patients are advised to lose weight and diabetic patients are advised to maintain tight glycemic control. Patients taking medications associated with fatty liver are advised to discontinue them. Although there is much common sense behind these recommendations, they have not been tested in randomized controlled trials.

Diet

One controlled non-randomized study of 25 NASH patients followed for 1 month on a weight-reducing diet combined with exercise showed a mean weight loss of 8 kg (9.6%), a borderline decrease in steatosis, and significant decreases in transaminase levels. A non-controlled study of 10 diabetic men receiving dexfenfluramine for 12 weeks showed decreased liver fat by MRI evaluation in association with increased insulin sensitivity. This group demonstrated a mean weight reduction of 3 kg but this was not associated with a change in hepatic steatosis.

Most of the research on diet relates to cardiovascular disease risk. In those with increased visceral adiposity, an energy-deficient diet is associated with preferential mobilization of central adipose tissue before that of peripheral abdominal tissue. Thus, modest (5%–10%) weight reduction may be associated with a significant improvement in metabolic profile, 30% to 60% increased sensitivity to insulin which is greater than that seen with insulin sensitizing medication. The ideal content of this energy deficient diet remains controversial – at least in part because of a lack of controlled studies. Studies suggest that monounsaturated fats in preference to saturated fatty acids may be beneficial in reducing insulin resistance. The effects of high fiber and low-glycemic index foods on insulin sensitivity remain unclear even though these foods are beneficial to blood glucose levels. Despite the hypothesized role of oxidative stress in the pathogenesis of NAFLD, and in particular in NASH, the use of antioxidant vitamins in this condition has not been studied. The goals of dietary therapy for NAFLD are outlined in Table 4.4.

The goals outlined in Table 4.4 are largely met by conforming to the diet in the "US Dietary Food Guide Pyramid". This emphasizes a diet based on whole grains, fruits, and vegetables, with meat, dairy products, and sweets comprising the apex of the pyramid. For the general practising physician, this provides a starting point. Ongoing and more specific dietary advice and monitoring should be done by a licensed dietician. Although small quantities of alcohol have been shown to be beneficial in lowering triacylglycerol and increasing high-density lipoprotein cholesterol, it cannot be recommended in the NAFLD patient because of the existent liver disease.

In a nation obsessed by appearance and weight control, advertised weight reduction diets and programs rapidly gain popularity. Despite their ability to promote weight loss by switching to energy inefficient ketogenesis, ketogenic, low-carbohydrate high-fat diets such as the popular "Atkins" diet do not meet these goals and ostensibly could promote fatty liver by increasing the rate of delivery of free fatty acids to the liver faster than the liver could oxidize them.

The details of weight management are beyond the scope of this article and have been reviewed elsewhere *http://www.nhlbi.nih.gov/guidelines/ obesity/practgde.htm*

Exercise

Exercise training has also been shown to be beneficial for NAFLD patients. A program of regular exercise is recommended to prevent decreased metabolic rate which occurs with calorie restriction in the absence of exercise, and to maintain muscle mass. The recommendations for cardiovascular fitness of at least 30 minutes of moderately vigorous exercise three times weekly may be beyond the capacity of an obese population with liver disease. From a metabolic point of view, it would seem that overall energy expenditure is more important than changes in maximal oxygen consumption $(V_{O2\,max})$, and improvement in lipoprotein profiles, insulin resistance, and blood pressure have been seen in those engaging in regular exercise despite no reduction in body weight or fat. Thus, longer periods of lower intensity exercise may be more appropriate for patients with NAFLD.

Pharmacological agents and surgery

Some animal studies and small human pilot studies suggest a role for antidiabetic medications, in particular metformin and the thiazolidinediones. However, it should also be noted that a case of fulminant hepatic failure attributed to a thiazolidinedione has been reported. Paradoxically, it is patients with the most recalcitrant obesity who are at biggest risk of NAFLD who are also at greatest risk of post-bariatric-surgery complications, in particular the change from bland steatosis to NASH. Therefore, bariatric surgery should be undertaken, in those with NAFLD, with great caution and as part of an overall obesity management plan. Nevertheless, 69 patients in a cohort of 505 patients undergoing gastroplasty for severe obesity, had pre- and post-surgery liver biopsies (the second biopsy was taken 27 ± 15 months after surgery). This group had a mean weight loss of 32 kg between the two biopsies. There was a marked increase in the number of patients with normal liver biopsies (45% after surgery versus 13% before), a marked decrease in the grade of steatosis, but also a small but significant increase in the number of patients with steatohepatitis (26% after surgery versus 14%

Table 4.4 Goals of various dietary modifications in non-alcoholic fatty liver disease patients

Goal	Dietary modification
Increased insulin sensitivity	mono-unsaturated fat in preference to saturated fat
Decreased blood glucose levels	low glycemic-index foods high-fiber diet
Decreased blood pressure	lower sodium higher potassium
Decreased triglyceride levels	higher ω–3 fatty acids lower saturated fats
Energy deficient diet	less energy-dense foods including beverages and sweets (NB overly zealous calorie restriction promotes loss of muscle tissue and increases insulin resistance)

before). Other tried but untested remedies include the use of ursodeoxycholic acid, and vitamins C and E. A multi-center National Institutes for Health funded study is due to commence shortly to rigorously investigate these agents.

Finally, in those with progressive NAFLD, liver failure may require liver replacement by orthotopic liver transplantation. Little data is available on those undergoing this procedure for NAFLD, but of all orthotopic liver transplantation recipients, morbid obesity (BMI > 40 kg/m^2) is associated with increased early and late mortality. Non-alcoholic steatohepatitis has also been shown to recur after orthotopic liver transplantation.

Liver transplantation

For the minority of patients who progress to decompensated end-stage liver disease, orthotopic liver transplantation remains an option. It is likely that approximately 50% of patients transplanted for cryptogenic cirrhosis have indeed burnt-out NAFLD. As with patients with liver disease of any other etiology, they must be assessed for the presence of extrahepatic disease which would preclude transplantation. They have a higher prevalence of hypertension, diabetes, and hyperlipidemia compared with lean controls with decompensated liver disease. As with morbidly obese patients undergoing non-transplant-related abdominal surgery, the risks of local wound infection and difficulty weaning from the ventilator are also increased. Finally, although the number of patients transplanted for NAFLD remains small, follow-up reports in these patients have documented recurrence of NAFLD and in some subjects this was associated with progressive liver disease requiring retransplantation. Whether this is merely a recurrence of the underlying metabolic state or compounded by the presence of corticosteroids and tacrolimus which increases the risk of diabetes mellitus and hyperlipidemia is not yet clear.

Prognosis

There are no large, long-term follow-up studies of patients with NAFLD and prognosis must be inferred from indirect observations. In a study of 132 patients with NAFLD diagnosed by liver biopsy and over 8 years mean follow-up, 49 patients had fatty liver alone and 83 had fatty liver and evidence of inflammation or fibrosis. Four per cent of the 49 patients with fatty liver alone developed cirrhosis and there was one liver-related death. In contrast the liver-related mortality for the 83 patients with fatty liver associated with inflammation or fibrosis was 10% – considerably higher than the age-adjusted rate of 1% for the US population.

Summary

Alcoholic liver disease and NAFLD represent a broad spectrum of disease from bland steatosis through progressive necroinflammatory liver disease and cirrhosis. Progressive liver disease probably occurs in 15% to 20% of both groups but there is no effective means of predicting which individuals with steatosis will develop end-stage liver disease.

Oxidative stress likely plays a role in the pathogenesis of both conditions. Insulin resistance is of major importance in NAFLD. There is little specific therapy for either condition and therapy is based largely on removing the offending agent, i.e. abstinence from alcohol or weight reduction to reduce insulin resistance.

Further reading

Alcohol-related liver disease

Akriviadis E, Botla R, Briggs W, *et al*. Pentoxyphiline improves short-term survival in severe acute alcoholic hepatitis: a double-blind, placebo-controlled trial. *Gastroenterology* 2000; 119(6): 1637–1648.

Burke A, Lucey MR. Liver transplantation for alcoholic liver disease. *Clin Liver Dis* 1998; 2(4): 839–850.

Eaton S, Record CO, Bartlett K. Multiple biochemical effects in the pathogenesis of alcoholic fatty liver. *J Clin Invest* 1997; 27: 719–722.

Karnam US. A toast to pentoxifylline. *Am J Gastroenterol* 2001; 96(5): 1635–1637.

Koretz RL. *ACP Journal Club* 2001; Jul–Aug; 135(1): 4.

Lucey MR. Is liver transplantation an appropriate treatment for acute alcoholic hepatitis? *J Hepatol* 2002; 36(6): 829–831.

McCullough AJ, O'Connor JFB. Alcoholic liver disease: proposed recommendation for the American College of Gastroenterology. *Am J Gastroenterol* 1998; 93(11): 2022–2036.

Morgan TR, McClain CJ, Pentoxifylline and alcoholic hepatitis. *Gastroenterology* 2000; 119(6): 1787–1791.

Non-alcohol-related liver disease

Chitturi S, Abeygunasekea S, Farrell GC, *et al*. NASH an insulin resistance: insulin hypersecretion and specific association with the insulin resistance syndrome. *Hepatology* 2002; 35(2): 373–379.

Day CP, James OFW. Steatohepatitis: a tale of two hits? *Gastroenterology* 1998; 114(4): 842–845.

Fromenty B, Berson A, Pessayre D. Microvesicular steatosis and steatohepatitis: role of mitochondrial dysfunction and lipid peroxidation. *J Hepatol* 1997; 26 (suppl. 1): 13–22.

Luyckx FH, Desaive C, Thiry A, *et al*. Liver abnormalities in severely obese subjects: effect of drastic weight loss after gastroplasty. *Int J Obes Relat Metab Disord* 1998; 22(3): 222–226.

Marchesini G, Forlani G. NASH: from liver diseases to metabolism and back to clinical hepatology. *Hepatology* 2002; 35(2): 497–499.

Neuschwander-Tetri BA. Fatty liver, non-alcoholic steatohepatitis. In: Bacon BR, Di Bisceglie AM, (eds) *Liver Disease: Diagnosis and Management*. Churchill Livingston, Philadelphia PA, 2000: pp. 127–139.

Pagano G, Pacini G, Musso G, Gambino *et al*. Non-alcoholic steatohepatitis, insulin resistance, and metabolic syndrome: Further evidence for an etiologic association. *Hepatology* 2002; 35(2): 367–372.

Chapter 5

Metabolic Liver Diseases

Kirti Shetty

CHAPTER OUTLINE

Introduction

The metabolic liver diseases encompass a wide spectrum of disorders with varying presentations and modes of onset. Many of these diseases manifest in childhood, often with non-specific findings of growth retardation and failure to thrive. Others present in adolescence or adulthood, usually with evidence of chronic liver disease. Box 5.1 provides an outline of some of the more common inherited diseases of the liver, although it is by no means a comprehensive list. This discussion will focus on the more important of these disorders encountered in adult clinical practice.

Disorders of metal metabolism

These disorders include the iron overload syndromes, such as hereditary hemochromatosis, as well as those involving copper dysmetabolism, such as Wilson's disease.

Iron-overload syndromes

Iron-overload disorders may be either primary due to a genetic defect, for example hereditary hemochromatosis, or may occur secondarily as a result of increased turnover of red blood cells (because of frequent transfusions or hemolysis) (Box 5.1). The following discussion will deal primarily with hereditary hemochromatosis.

Disorders of metal metabolism

Iron-overload states
Hereditary hemochromatosis (HFE-related)
Juvenile hemochromatosis
Autosomal dominant hemochromatosis
Secondary iron overload
chronic liver diseases – hepatitis C virus, hepatitis B virus, alcohol, porphyria cutanea tarda
hemolytic anemias, ineffective hematopoiesis, transfusion overload
Dietary iron excess
Miscellaneous causes
African iron overload
aceruloplasminemia
congenital atransferrinemia

Disorders of copper metabolism
Wilson's disease
Menke's disease

Alpha-1-antitrypsin deficiency

Disorders of heme biosynthesis
The hereditary porphyrias

Glycogen storage disorders affecting the liver
Types I, III, IV, VI, VIII, IX

Sphingolipidoses
Gaucher's disease
Niemann–Pick disease
Tay–Sach's disease

The prevalence of hereditary hemochromatosis in a given population reflects the frequency of the specific genetic mutation. The gene frequency in populations of European descent is as high as 1 in 10, but is much rarer in Asian and African populations. The phenotypic expression of the genetic abnormality is a subject of debate. In studies examining the incidence of the C282Y mutation in populations with iron overload, a wide variability has been noted depending on the area of the world. In the US this mutation accounts for approximately 85% of iron overload, in Italy only 65%, while in Australia it is present in nearly 100% of the population.

Pathophysiology of iron overload The physiologic regulatory mechanism for iron homeostasis operates by modulation of iron absorption from the gastrointestinal tract. Normally, 1 to 2 mg/day of iron is absorbed in the duodenum. In states of iron deficiency, increased intestinal iron uptake (up to 10 mg/day) is seen.

Iron absorption is regulated by three important mediators

- transferrin, the major transporter of iron
- the transferrin receptor
- ferritin, the intracellular storage form of iron.

The transferrin receptor is a key protein in iron transport, and modulation of its expression controls iron uptake. The production of transferrin receptor is regulated by iron regulatory proteins which directly sense the intracellular iron level. When iron levels are low, iron regulatory proteins bind to RNA stem-loops known as iron-responsive elements. This results in a more stable messenger RNA and thus an increase in the amount of transferrin receptor on the cell membrane, increasing iron uptake. The amount of intracellular ferritin decreases simultaneously, decreasing iron storage. The converse happens in conditions of iron excess.

Cellular uptake and transport of iron also occurs by mechanisms independent of transferrin and the transferrin receptor. These mechanisms have recently been elucidated and involve the divalent metal transporter (DMT1). Mutations in the DMT1 gene are detrimental to transport of free iron from the intestinal lumen and of transferrin receptor-cycled iron from the endosome. While the precise defects in iron-overload states remain to be elucidated, it is believed that the DMT1 plays a critical role in the process of iron uptake at the cellular level.

Our present level of understanding suggests that the normal role of the HFE gene product present in

Hereditary hemochromatosis

Prevalence and mode of inheritance Hereditary hemochromatosis is the most common identifiable genetic disease in Caucasians. The defect within the newly discovered HFE gene (localized to the short arm of chromosome 6) has been well-characterized. This is a missense mutation leading to the substitution of tyrosine for cysteine at the 282 amino acid position (C282Y). Another mutation (H63D), in which aspartate is substituted for histidine has also been identified, but has not been associated with the same degree of iron loading as the C282Y mutation. The C282Y homozygous state is almost invariably associated with iron overload. Compound heterozygotes for C282Y or H63D sometimes manifest the hemochromatosis phenotype.

the duodenal crypt cells is to modulate the uptake of iron by these cells. In hereditary hemochromatosis, an impairment in transferrin receptor-mediated iron uptake sends the false signal that iron stores are low. As a result, the differentiating enterocytes migrating up to the villus tip increase the production of DMT1 and hence enhance iron uptake.

The intestinal absorption of iron therefore proceeds at rates comparable to those in iron-deficient patients, that is at 10 to 20 times the basal levels, despite the continual accumulation of iron within the reticuloendothelial system, and later in other body sites. This accumulation is toxic to the liver because of the generation of hydroxyl radicals with resultant membrane lipid peroxidation and disruption of cellular function. Other effects include the induction of collagen synthesis, contributing to hepatic fibrosis and cirrhosis. Direct DNA damage may also occur, leading to an increased risk for the development of hepatocellular carcinoma.

Pathology The major pathologic findings in the advanced stages of hemochromatosis relate to the massive amounts of iron deposited in the parenchymal cells of various organs, in particular the liver, pancreas, heart, and endocrine glands. Macroscopically, the liver is enlarged and nodular. Histologic examination shows large amounts of iron in the parenchymal cells, and, in the late stage, in Kupffer cells, macrophages, and biliary epithelial cells. At a critical level of hepatic iron, fibrosis develops, starting in a periportal distribution, and ultimately bridging from portal tract to portal tract. A mixed macronodular–micronodular cirrhosis eventually develops.

Cardiac deposition of hemosiderin occurs both in the heart muscle fibers, and in the conducting fibers of the atrioventricular node. Other organs with hemosiderin deposition are the pancreas, endocrine glands such as the pituitary and the adrenals, and the skin. The characteristic "bronzed" hue of the skin is imparted by the increased melanin (with or without iron) in the dermis, in association with an atrophic epidermis.

Clinical manifestations The classical presentation of hereditary hemochromatosis patients with the triad of diabetes mellitus, skin pigmentation ("bronze diabetes"), and hepatomegaly, is becoming increasingly uncommon in this era of increased awareness of the disease. Individuals are usually detected at an asymptomatic stage on the basis of either abnormal iron studies or screening of family members.

If untreated, this condition is thought to evolve in a series of stages, the first of which consists of clinically insignificant iron accumulation (at 0 to 20 years of age, 0 to 5 grams parenchymal iron), advancing to a stage of iron overload without disease (at 20 to 40 years of age, 10 to 20 grams parenchymal iron), and culminating in iron overload with organ damage (over 40 years of age, over 20 grams of parenchymal iron).

Patients usually present with one or more of the following symptoms: fatigue, skin pigmentation, loss of libido, joint pain, or features of diabetes. The most prominent physical signs include skin pigmentation, hepatomegaly, testicular atrophy, and arthropathy. Symptoms occur approximately ten times more frequently in men than in women because of physiological blood loss in the latter group.

Hepatomegaly is the most frequently encountered abnormality, and is present in over 95% of symptomatic patients. Diabetes mellitus develops in 30% to 60% of those with advanced disease. Loss of libido is common, and is believed to be related to hypothalamic or pituitary failure, with selective impairment of gonadotropin or gonadotropin-releasing hormone.

Arthropathy is noted in 30% to 70% of symptomatic patients, and is characterized by the deposition of calcium pyrophosphate (chondrocalcinosis). Its course occurs independent of the degree of iron overload, and is not often impacted by therapeutic phlebotomy.

Cardiac symptoms may be the initial manifestation in 5% to 15% of patients, although electrocardiogram abnormalities are present in about 30% of patients. The most common cardiac complications are those of biventricular failure and cardiac arrhythmias.

Hepatocellular carcinoma is the most common cause of death in patients with hereditary hemochromatosis. Those individuals with hereditary hemochromatosis-related cirrhosis are at a 200-fold higher risk of developing hepatocellular carcinoma than the general population. This risk is related to the degree of iron overload, and is especially marked in males over 40 years old, with concomitant alcohol and tobacco abuse. The lifetime risk of developing hepatocellular carcinoma in a male with hereditary hemochromatosis is approximately 30%. Rare cases of hepatocellular carcinoma have been described in non-cirrhotic patients. However, for practical and screening purposes, we may assume that underlying cirrhosis is essential for hepatocellular carcinoma development in cases of hereditary hemochromatosis.

Diagnosis of hereditary hemochromatosis

The aim of diagnosing hereditary hemochromatosis is to detect the disease and initiate treatment before irreversible organ damage occurs. Studies have demonstrated that the prognosis of hereditary hemochromatosis and the development of complications such as decompensated cirrhosis, hepatocellular carcinoma, and cardiac disease, depend on the amount and duration of iron excess. Intervention at the pre-cirrhotic stage will therefore impact favorably on overall survival.

Diagnostic approach The diagnosis of hereditary hemochromatosis is based on demonstrating increased iron stores, namely increased hepatic iron concentration, associated with elevated serum ferritin levels.

Diagnostic strategies are twofold.

1. Identification of high-risk groups such as those with evidence of target organ damage (liver, heart, endocrine glands), a family history of hereditary hemochromatosis, or abnormal biochemical and radiological tests suggesting iron overload.
2. Screening the general population. Increasing evidence supports the cost-effectiveness of performing phenotypic screening (utilizing standard markers) on the general population. A recent study comparing the screening of blood donors using both phenotypic and genotypic methods concluded that phenotypic screening, followed by genotypic confirmation of abnormal tests, was a viable strategy in a population with a high genetic frequency of hereditary hemochromatosis, such as in the US. Further studies are required to confirm the widespread application of such a strategy.

Diagnostic studies Iron studies An elevated transferrin saturation is the earliest abnormality in hereditary hemochromatosis. It is usually measured as a ratio of the fasting serum iron, and the total iron-binding capacity. The latter is not an automated test, however, and makes this method relatively expensive. Transferrin saturation may also be expressed as the ratio of serum iron to the calculated total iron-binding capacity, derived from summing the serum iron and the unsaturated iron-binding capacity. This method reduces costs and is more suitable for large-scale screening.

Transferrin saturation is most accurate when measured in the fasting state. If a cut off of 45% is used, 98% to 100% of C282Y homozygotes are cor-

rectly identified. However, the false positive rate has been reported to range between 22% and 44%. Hence, other groups with secondary iron overload may be identified and will need further careful clinical evaluation. Serum iron and serum ferritin when used alone lack specificity in the diagnosis of hereditary hemochromatosis, as ferritin acts as an acute-phase reactant, and is often elevated in other disease states. However, the addition of the serum ferritin to the transferrin saturation confers a negative predictive value of 97%, and exceeds the accuracy of any single test. In confirmed hereditary hemochromatosis, a level of serum ferritin above 1000 ng/mL accurately predicts the presence of hepatic fibrosis or cirrhosis.

Genotypic testing: Testing for the HFE mutations C282Y and H63D can now be done by PCR using whole-blood samples. Fasting transferrin saturation less than 45% and a normal serum ferritin require no further evaluation. Genotype testing is indicated in those individuals with abnormal studies, and in those who are first-degree relatives of identified homozygotes.

Liver biopsy: Histologic analysis of the liver is useful in documenting the presence of cirrhosis, to exclude iron overload in the presence of equivocal serum markers, and to detect other possible etiologies of liver disease.

The importance of age in determining the progression of hereditary hemochromatosis to fibrosis and cirrhosis has been confirmed in several studies. Cirrhosis is rarely, if ever, seen in any patient less than 40 years of age. Hence, liver biopsy is indicated in those C282Y homozygotes over the age of 40 years, those with serum ferritin levels greater than 1000 ng/mL, and in those with clinical evidence of liver disease (abnormal hepatic biochemical tests or hepatomegaly) or with other risk factors for hepatic involvement such as alcohol abuse.

Iron stores may be assessed by liver biopsy. Qualitative iron determination may be done using a Perls' Prussian blue stain. If increased iron stores are suggested, quantitative determinations are indicated. The hepatic iron index (hepatic iron concentration in micromoles per gram dry weight divided by age in years) may be calculated from such a determination. A level in excess of 1.9 μmol g^{-1} year^{-1} is strong evidence of homozygous hemochromatosis. However, up to 15% of C282Y homozygotes lack this characteristic feature, and it is no longer considered essential for diagnosis. Liver biopsy is also useful in compound or C282Y heterozygotes with elevated transferrin saturation, in order to determine the etiology of the abnormal iron studies.

Figure 5.1 summarizes a suggested approach to the diagnosis and management of hereditary hemochromatosis.

Treatment Indisputable evidence supports the fact that prevention of iron deposition in target organs significantly reduces the morbidity and mortality attributable to hereditary hemochromatosis. Once the diagnosis is made, a course of iron depletion and monitoring should be initiated. Initially, patients should undergo once or twice weekly therapeutic phlebotomy with regular monitoring of hemoglobin and hematocrit values. Each unit of blood is equal to 250 milligrams of iron, and in some patients with total iron stores greater than 30 grams, adequate reduction of iron stores may take up to 3 years to achieve. The target ferritin level should be below 50 ng/mL, and transferrin saturation under 30%. At the point when these criteria are reached, a maintenance schedule may be initiated.

One caution to be kept in mind is the recognition that the risk of cardiac dysrhythmias is particularly high during periods of rapid iron mobilization. Pharmacologic doses of vitamin C accelerate mobilization of iron, and should be avoided during this period.

While phlebotomy improves or reverses some of the manifestations of hereditary hemochromatosis such as fatigue, skin pigmentation, and insulin requirements, other manifestations such as cirrhosis, arthopathy, and hypogonadism are rarely improved. Most studies report that the risk of developing hepatocellular carcinoma does not decrease after adequate iron removal. Thus, cirrhotic patients should continue careful surveillance for hepatocellular carcinoma, although the optimal method or frequency for surveillance remain

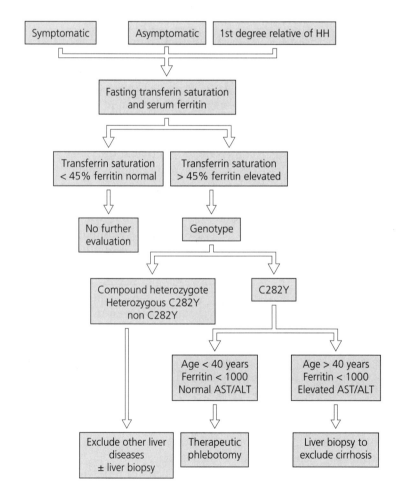

AST = Aspartate aminotransferase
ALT = Alanine aminotransferase

Figure 5.1 Proposed algorithm for the diagnosis and management of hereditary hemochromatosis (HH) (modified from AASLD Practice Guidelines. *Hepatology* 2001;33;1321-1328).

unclear. At the present time, annual or 6-monthly alpha-fetoprotein with abdominal ultrasound is an accepted screening modality.

Liver transplantation is indicated for those with advanced disease. Some evidence suggests that these individuals have significantly diminished post-transplant survival rates, although more recent studies dispute this finding.

Other iron overload states

Hematological disorders Chronic hemolytic anemias such as thalassemia major, and conditions characterized by ineffective erythropoiesis such as sideroblastic anemia, are both characterized by excessive iron stores. This occurs because of increased gut absorption, as well as the parenteral iron load delivered by multiple blood transfusions. Iron loading can be controlled by the use of chelating drugs. Desferrioxamine is the most effective practical chelating agent. However, it is poorly absorbed orally, and for best results, must be administered as a subcutaneous pump. Prospective studies have demonstrated the utility of desferrioxamine in reducing iron stores, and hence the risk of diabetes, cardiac disease, and early death in those with hemolytic anemia. Its utility is greatly limited by its mode of administration and difficulties encountered in achieving adequate compliance amongst its users. Research efforts are underway in the development of oral iron chelators.

Iron overload in chronic liver disease It is thought that cirrhosis alone may cause iron accumulation in the liver, although the pathophysiology behind this is unclear. Explant studies have demonstrated increased hepatic iron concentrations in approximately 20% of those with cirrhosis. Serum and hepatic iron stores have also been found to be increased in those with chronic hepatitis C. It is believed that iron overload may interfere with response to antiviral therapy in hepatitis C, and that repeated phlebotomy may be of therapeutic benefit, although this remains unproven.

Iron overload associated with metabolic disorders It is believed that conditions such as obesity, hyperlipidemia, abnormal glucose metabolism, and hypertension, may be associated with a non-human leukocyte antigen-linked iron-overload syndrome. Studies have demonstrated that these individuals have evidence of hepatic iron overload with elevated serum ferritin levels, and normal transferrin saturation. The overall significance and

long-term prognosis of this condition remains to be elucidated.

Disorders of copper metabolism

Wilson's disease

This is a genetic disorder characterized by the accumulation of copper in the liver and brain, secondary to an inherited defect in the biliary excretion of copper.

Genetics and pathophysiology Wilson's disease is inherited in an autosomal recessive fashion. The isolation and identification of the gene for Wilson's disease, designated ATP7B, has led to a greater understanding of the aberrations in copper metabolism caused by mutations in this gene. Copper is an essential co-factor for many enzymes. Approximately 50% of ingested copper (1.5 to 3 mg/day) is absorbed in the upper small intestine. This absorbed copper is extracted from the portal circulation by hepatocytes. Intracellular copper is subsequently utilized for metabolic needs, incorporated into the secretory glycoprotein ceruloplasmin, or excreted into bile. This last route is the most crucial in the excretion of copper as it undergoes minimal enterohepatic recirculation.

The transport of hepatocellular copper to bile is thought to involve a pathway that is dependent on ATP7B function. The absence or reduced function of ATP7B results in a decrease in biliary copper excretion, and hence the hepatic accumulation of this metal. The latter feature is pathognomic of Wilson's disease.

The synthesis of ceruloplasmin is also believed to be dependent on ATP7B, which mediates copper incorporation into the ceruloplasmin molecule. Defective ATP7B function results in the production of a non-copper-containing apoprotein which is less stable, and therefore manifests as reduced circulating levels of ceruloplasmin.

Copper is known to be hepatotoxic at excess levels. The toxic effects of copper include the generation of free radicals, lipid peroxidation of membranes and DNA, inhibition of protein synthesis, and altered levels of cellular antioxidants.

When the storage capacity of the liver for copper is exceeded, or when hepatocellular damage results in the release of cellular copper into the circulation, levels of non-ceruloplasmin-bound copper in the circulation become elevated. It is from this pool of copper that the extrahepatic deposition of copper is thought to occur. The brain is the most important site for the extrahepatic accumulation of copper. Copper-induced neuronal injury is responsible for many of the neurologic and psychiatric manifestations of Wilson's disease.

Pathology The main organ systems involved in disorders of copper metabolism are the liver, brain, kidneys, eyes, and joints.

Hepatic pathology In the early stages, the liver may be only mildly enlarged. Light microscopic changes at this stage are non-specific and consist of macro- and microsteatosis with glycogenated nuclei. On electron microscopy, distinctive mitochondrial changes may be identified. These consist of enlargement and widening of intercristal spaces, and increased matrix granularity. With progression of the disease, copper-protein is sequestered in lysosomes, and may be detected as granules on copper immunohistochemistry.

The intermediate stage of Wilson's disease is characterized by the features of chronic active hepatitis consisting of periportal inflammation, interface hepatitis, and bridging fibrosis. Cirrhosis in either a micronodular or a mixed macronodular–micronodular histologic pattern is seen next. Mallory bodies may be present in up to half of all biopsies. In patients with fulminant hepatic failure, parenchymal necrosis may overshadow other histologic features. Histochemical confirmation of copper deposition may be helpful when positive, but its absence does not exclude copper overload.

Neuropathology Macroscopically, most of the overt changes occur in the lenticular nuclei which show atrophy and discoloration, with cystic degeneration. Microscopic changes occur most commonly in the thalamus, followed by the putamen and cerebral cortex. Characteristic neuroglial changes occur with an increase in astrocytes which are distinctive for Wilson's disease, known as Opalski cells. The swollen glia are subject to liquefaction creating small cavities.

Miscellaneous pathologic changes Functional changes in the kidneys are disproportionate to any microscopic changes. Proximal or distal tubular dysfunction is common, and leads to tubular proteinuria, metabolic acidosis, aminoaciduria, glycosuria, hyperphosphaturia, uricosuria, and hypercalciuria.

Bone pathology is observed, with the spine and knee joints being most commonly involved. Osteo-porosis, osteomalacia, adult rickets, chondrocalcinosis, and subchondral cyst formation can be noted.

Ophthalmologic changes include the Kayser–Fleischer rings which are due to granular deposition of elemental copper on the inner surface of the cornea in Descemet's membrane. The sunflower cataract, another manifestation of Wilson's disease, is due to copper deposition in the anterior and posterior lens capsule. Both these manifestations are reversible with effective therapy.

Clinical manifestations Many of the early symptoms of Wilson's disease are subtle and nonspecific, accounting for the frequency of delayed diagnoses. Symptoms are rare in the first 5 years of life, but about half of all affected individuals become symptomatic by their teens. Early symptoms are usually hepatic, with the full-blown syndrome becoming apparent after deposition of copper in other organs, primarily the central nervous system and the cornea. Most individuals who are affected manifest the disease by the age of 40 years, and delayed diagnosis beyond this age is rare.

The major clinical syndromes associated with Wilson's disease may be summarized as follows.

Asymptomatic stage This is of variable duration. It is usually identified in individuals with a family history of Wilson's, or in the course of the work-up of abnormal hepatic biochemistries. Physical examination usually discloses hepatomegaly, splenomegaly, or corneal Kayser–Fleischer rings.

Acute Wilsonian hepatitis This is characterized by the sudden onset of hemolytic anemia and gastrointestinal symptoms, subsiding within 1 to 2 weeks. Even though a moderate indirect hyperbilirubinemia is often noted at this stage, liver biopsy is rarely performed, and the diagnosis is often overlooked.

Fulminant hepatic failure A dramatic manifestation of Wilson's disease is that of acute liver failure. If timely liver transplantation is not performed this condition is uniformly fatal. There are several unique features of this form of fulminant hepatitis. These include an associated non-immune hemolytic anemia, markedly elevated serum copper levels, modest transaminitis given the severity of the decompensation, hypoalbuminemia, and low alkaline phosphatase.

Chronic active Wilsonian hepatitis/cirrhosis Some young individuals present with chronic liver disease indistinguishable from other types of chronic hepatitis, often associated with fever, polyarthralgias, amenorrhea, and delayed puberty. If unrecognized, this progresses to cirrhosis, characterized by the many manifestations of decompensated liver disease. The development of hepatocellular carcinoma, once considered a rarity, has now been recognized to occur in at least 15 patients.

Neurologic Wilson's This is almost invariably associated with cirrhosis. Patients with neurologic involvement are often older than those who present with hepatic symptoms. Neurologic manifestations are varied, and include Parkinsonian characteristics of dystonia, hypertonia, and rigidity, along with chorea, tremors, and dysarthria. A variety of psychologic disturbances may be noted, ranging from mild memory impairment to overt psychosis.

Diagnostic modalities

The criteria for the confirmation of Wilson's disease vary according to the patient's age and mode of presentation.

The following tests have been found to be the most useful in either confirming or excluding Wilson's disease as the etiology for liver disease.

Ophthalmic evaluation A slit-lamp examination of the cornea may detect a golden-greenish granular deposition within Descemet's membrane, designated as the Kayser–Fleischer ring (Figure 5.2). In association with characteristic neurologic symptoms, the Kayser–Fleischer ring is diagnostic of Wilson's disease. Conversely, its absence in a patient with neurologic manifestations, virtually excludes the disease. However, the Kayser–Fleischer ring is not specific for Wilson's disease, and may also be present in individuals with cholestatic syndromes leading to copper retention. Therefore, in the asymptomatic patient, additional tests would be necessary to confirm Wilson's disease.

Serum ceruloplasmin Two types of assays are available for the measurement of serum ceruloplasmin.

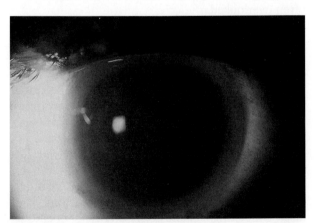

Figure 5.2 Kayser–Fleischer ring. Copper deposition in Descemet's membrane in the cornea is responsible for this classic finding in Wilson's Disease *(see plate section for color).*

The immunologic assay tends to give higher readings, caused by the antibody reaction with not only circulating apoceruloplasmin, but also holoceruloplasmin. The enzymatic assay which measures ceruloplasmin by its oxidase activity toward various substrates is more accurate, and is preferred in clinical practice. A concentration lower than 20 mg/dL is found in 96% of those with Wilson's disease. However, such a result alone is not diagnostic, as 10% of heterozygous carriers who never manifest the disease, also have values under 20 mg/dL. Levels of ceruloplasmin are also decreased in states of severe copper deficiency, in patients with severe fulminant hepatitis, significant protein-losing nephropathy or enteropathy, and in the rare disorders of hereditary hypoceruloplasminemia or aceruloplasminemia. Ceruloplasmin is an acute-phase reactant, and may be elevated in inflammatory states, pregnancy, or in response to the exogenous administration of estrogens.

Serum free copper concentration Total serum copper is the sum of ceruloplasmin copper (90%) and non-ceruloplasmin copper (10%). The former fraction is decreased in the presence of hypoceruloplasminemia, leading to low measured levels of total copper, despite an elevation in free copper levels. The latter may be calculated by subtracting ceruloplasmin copper (typically three times the serum ceruloplasmin) from the total copper. Normally, the free copper level is under 10 mcg/dL. In Wilson's disease, levels of free copper are typically greater than 25 mcg/dL.

Urinary copper This is increased to more than 100 mcg per 24 h in most symptomatic patients. The addition of penicillamine administration prior to the urine collection dramatically increases the urinary copper content to above 1500 mcg per 24 h, and may be utilized as an adjunctive test to help establish the diagnosis of Wilson's disease.

Hepatic copper Determination of hepatic copper content remains the standard test for the diagnosis of Wilson's disease, and a liver biopsy is considered essential before subjecting an individual to lifetime therapy. A hepatic copper concentration greater than 250 mcg/g dry tissue (normal is less than 50 mcg/g) is diagnostic of Wilson's disease, especially in association with characteristic histologic findings.

Genetic studies The large number of disease-specific mutant alleles of ATP7B limits the practical application of genetic screening for the disease. Within a family in which a specific defective gene has been identified, such testing may replace liver biopsy in the diagnostic work-up.

Diagnostic approach

Symptomatic patients

Neurologic presentation: The disease may be relatively easy to confirm in those who have a neurologic mode of presentation. Almost all such patients exhibit Kayser–Fleischer rings, and 95% of them have serum ceruloplasmin concentrations below 20 mg/dL.

Hepatic presentation: These patients are younger than those with neurologic symptoms, and corneal copper deposits are not necessarily present. The ceruloplasmin concentrations are not as reliable, as about 10% to 15% of these individuals have levels in the low-normal range (up to 30 mg/dL). Rings similar to the Kayser–Fleischer ring may be seen in the corneas of those patients with cholestatic syndromes. A liver biopsy is often crucial in resolving the diagnostic dilemma.

Asymptomatic patients Screening family members of affected individuals is mandatory. Unexplained transaminemia or an incidentally discovered Kayser–Fleischer ring may also provide a basis for screening. Screening tests involve corneal slit-lamp examination and determination of the serum ceruloplasmin concentration. A value under 20 mg/dL is highly suspicious for Wilson's, and one over 30 mg/dL virually excludes the diagnosis, except for pregnant women and those taking estrogens. These conditions may cause the ceruloplasmin to rise to within the normal range.

Treatment Therapy should be started as soon as the diagnosis is confirmed and should be continued for life.

Pharmacologic therapy British Anti-Lewisite (BAL) Also known as 2,3-dimercapto-1-propanol, is now mainly of historic interest. It is a chelating agent which works by promoting cupriuresis. Its use is limited by its intramuscular mode of administration and unfavorable side-effect profile. Its only utility now is in the rare patient with severe neurologic disease who is refractory to therapy with other agents. However, some experts question even that role.

D-penicillamine (3-mercapto-D-valine) This is an orally administered chelating agent capable of markedly reducing the effects of copper toxicity. The daily dose ranges from 750 milligrams to 2 grams in divided doses. Importantly, this is the first medication that was shown to effectively prevent disease progression, and to reverse some of the neurologic and hepatic manifestations of the disease. Side effects of penicillamine may be grouped either as early or late-occurring. Sensitivity reactions occur in about 10% of patients and consist of fever, cutaneous eruptions, lymphadenopathy, neutropenia, or thrombocytopenia. These reactions should prompt discontinuation of the medication. Late reactions include nephrotoxicity, a lupus-like syndrome, Goodpasture's syndrome, and dermatologic toxicities including progeric skin changes, pemphigoid lesions, and lichen planus. Very late side effects include polymyositis, myasthenia gravis, and serous retinitis.

The clinical response may often be delayed for months, and there may be an initial worsening of neurologic symptoms in 10% to 50% of patients. Worsening hepatic enzymes have also been reported with the medication. However, most individuals tolerate the medication well and can be maintained on it for several decades.

In the past, patients who experienced allergic reactions underwent hyposensitization, then gradual re-introduction of the medication along with steroid administration. The emergence of safer and better tolerated alternative therapies has made this approach unnecessary.

Trientine dihydrochloride This is an alternative chelating agent, which has a more favorable side-effect profile than D-penicillamine, and has been demonstrated to be as clinically effective. The daily dose is 1 to 2 grams in divided doses. Sideroblastic anemia is a rare side effect in patients receiving more than 2 grams of trientine daily, and is thought to be secondary to copper deficiency. It is easily reversible with a reduction of the dose.

Trientine is useful both as initial therapy in patients with severe neurologic and hepatic disease, as well as in maintenance regimes.

Zinc salts Zinc salts – acetate, gluconate, and sulphate – can block the intestinal absorption of copper by inducing metallothionein in enterocytes. Copper is therefore chelated in enterocytes, which are later shed naturally along with the ingested copper in the feces. The rate at which copper is depleted is slow. Hence, zinc is not recommended as the sole agent for the initial therapy of symptomatic patients. However, it is an effective maintenance therapy and recent studies substantiate earlier claims of its long-term effectiveness. The average dose is 50 milligrams of elemental zinc three times daily. Common side effects include headaches and gastrointestinal upsets. Zinc acetate may be better tolerated than other formulations.

Thiomolybdate This is an investigational drug used primarily for initial treatment before switching to trientine or zinc; it is used to avoid the neurologic deterioration that accompanies chelation treatment in some patients. It is presently undergoing a comparison study with the combination of trientine and zinc for effectiveness in patients with neurologic Wilson's disease.

Combination therapy There are few published data available on combining agents in the treatment of Wilson's disease. One approach is to combine two medications with different and complementary modes of action, for example zinc with another oral chelating agent such as trientine. This concept is now undergoing formal testing as part of a trial of initial therapy for neurologic Wilson's disease. The potential role of tetrathiomolybdate as an alternative combination therapy awaits formal approval and commercial production in this country.

Dietary measures These are of limited utility in Wilson's disease. It involves the avoidance of certain copper-containing foods such as shellfish, liver, nuts, mushrooms, and chocolate.

Liver transplantation This is indicated in patients with Wilsonian fulminant hepatitis, whether it is occurring as the first manifestation of the disease, or as a result of therapeutic non-compliance. It may also be indicated for severe hepatic insufficiency that is not responsive to several months of intensive chelation treatment. Transplant recipients have an excellent long-term prognosis, with 1-year survival rates reported in the 80% range.

Treatment during pregnancy Therapy should be maintained during pregnancy, although the doses of D-penicillamine or trientine should be reduced to 0.5 to 0.75 grams daily during the last trimester, as the fetus sequesters some of the excess copper. There have been reports of more than 100 successful pregnancies in women on these therapies.

Monitoring therapy Compliance with the therapeutic regimen is crucial in the management of this condition. Several methods of monitoring compliance have been described. The most reliable of these is the measurement of non-ceruloplasmin copper. This is a calculated figure, and is derived from the difference between the total serum copper and the copper content of ceruloplasmin (approximately three times the value of serum ceruloplasmin). In appropriately treated individuals, the non-ceruloplasmin copper should be 10 mcg/dL or less. In untreated or inadequately treated individuals, this value is often elevated above 25 mcg/dL.

The measurement of urinary copper, if properly implemented, also provides an important clue to compliance. During the early phase of treatment with chelating agents, the urinary copper excretion is often greater than 1000 mcg/dL. This declines to about 250 to 500 mcg/24 h over time. Values under 250 mcg/24 h suggest non-compliance with therapy, or an erroneous diagnosis. With zinc therapy, copper absorption is retarded and the parameters used to monitor compliance vary accordingly. A rise in the urinary copper excretion to over 150 mcg/24 h, rather than a decline, would indicate non-compliance. Plasma and urinary zinc levels may also be directly measured. With adequate therapy, urinary zinc levels should exceed 1000 mcg/24 h.

In those who are compliant with pharmacotherapy, the long-term outcome of Wilson's disease is excellent. Neurologic or psychiatric symptoms show a gradual recovery over months or years. Those with established cirrhosis or chronic hepatitis often stabilize their liver disease, with little or no progression.

Menke's disease

This is a rare X-linked disorder of copper metabolism resulting from mutations within a gene encoding a copper transporting ATPase, ATP7A, homologous to the gene defect in Wilson's disease. It is characterized by neurologic degeneration, connective tissue and vascular involvement, depigmented and brittle hair, and death in infancy and early childhood. Copper absorption from the gut is reduced with low serum copper and ceruloplasmin levels. The liver is not affected in this disorder, but it has provided some valuable insights into the pathophysiology of abnormal copper metabolism, and hence a greater understanding of Wilson's disease.

Alpha-1-antitrypsin deficiency

Alpha-1-antitrypsin deficiency is a relatively common autosomal recessive disorder characterized by hepatic involvement, pulmonary emphysema, panniculitis, and arterial aneurysms.

Alpha-1-antitrypsin deficiency and its gene

The alpha-1-antitrypsin (A1AT) deficiency gene is located on the q arm of chromosome 14. The final protein product of the A1AT gene is a 52-kDa serum glycoprotein predominantly derived from the liver. Alpha-1-antitrypsin belongs to a class of protease inhibitors known as serpins, which function mainly as serine protease inhibitors. Its plasma concentrations increase three- to fivefold during the host response to tissue injury and inflammation. Its principal physiologic function is to inhibit the destructive neutrophil proteases elastase, cathepsin G, and proteinase 3.

Variants of the alpha-1antitrypsin gene A variety of mutations within the A1AT gene can result in a deficiency or absence of the protease inhibitor in serum. Over 75 allelic variations for A1AT have been identified. In humans, these variants are classified according to the protease inhibitor phenotype system, as defined by agarose electrophoresis. The protease inhibitor classification system assigns a letter of the alphabet from A to Z, to each group of allelic variants with the same electrophoretic properties. The most common normal variant migrates to an intermediate isoelectric point, designated PiM. The PiM variant is found in 65% to 70% of caucasians in the US. It is not associated with clinical disease, as serum concentration and functional activity for A1AT is within the normal range.

Individuals with the most common severe A1AT deficiency have an A1AT allelic variant that migrates to a high isoelectric point, designated PiZ. The mutation responsible for the PiZ-type migration of A1AT is a single amino acid substitution, glu 342 to lys 342. This mutation leads to altered folding of the A1AT molecule and its selective intracellular retention within the endoplasmic reticulum. In clinical practice more than 90% of cases are caused by the PiZZ mutation.

Mechanism of hepatic disease in alpha-1-antitrypsin deficiency

Hepatic disease has been described most commonly in association with the PiZ allele. Several theories exist as to the mechanism for liver injury. The most widely accepted of these is the so-called "accumulation theory". It is believed that the PiZ mutation affects the uniquely flexible conformation of the active site loop region of A1AT. This results in abnormalities in its folding at the time of synthesis. The abnormal intermediate forms of the protein undergo polymerization and intracellular degradation with accumulation. The resultant intracellular inclusions are thought to have hepatotoxic effects. The mechanism whereby the retention of mutant A1AT leads to progressive hepatic injury is still to be elucidated. In transgenic mice expressing the human A1AT gene, nodular clusters of altered hepatocytes are seen. These progress to fibrotic dysplastic nodules, and eventually to foci of hepatocellular carcinoma.

However, difficult to reconcile with the accumulation theory is the observation that only a subset of PiZZ A1AT-deficient individuals (approximately 10% to 15%) develop significant liver damage. It is believed that additional inherited traits or environmental factors exist that exaggerate the cellular pathophysiological consequences of mutant A1AT accumulation.

Incidence and mode of inheritance

The incidence of homozygous A1AT PiZZ deficiency is highest in people of Scandinavian and northern European ancestry, affecting approximately 1 in 1600 to 1800 live births. Recent studies suggest that the incidence in the US is almost identical to that in Scandinavian populations. There are estimated to be more than 100 000 persons with A1AT deficiency in the US. Its main manifestation is the development of pulmonary emphysema by the third or fourth decade of life, but it is also associated with a lesser risk of hepatic disease. It is the most common genetic indication for liver transplantation in children, and is an important cause of chronic liver disease and hepatocellular carcinoma in adults.

Clinical manifestations of alpha-1-antitrypsin deficiency

Hepatic manifestations

Liver involvement is usually noted in the first 2 months of life, and is characterized by persistent jaundice and abnormal hepatic biochemical tests. Approximately 10% of affected individuals may present with manifestations of cirrhosis and portal hypertension in early infancy, and a smaller proportion present with fulminant hepatic failure.

In later life, the presentation of this disease may be non-specific. It should be suspected in any adult presenting with chronic hepatitis, cirrhosis, evidence of portal hypertension, or hepatocellular carcinoma.

The heterozygous A1AT MZ phenotype is not thought to cause liver disease in children by itself. Some studies in adults suggest a relationship between heterozygosity and the development of liver disease, but no convincing evidence exists to link liver injury to the heterozygous state alone.

Liver disease has been described for several other allelic variants of A1AT. Compound heterozygotes of the type PiSZ are affected by liver injury similar to PiZZ. Liver disease has also been reported with the variant PiMmalton.

Pulmonary manifestations

Chronic obstructive airway disease is seen in approximately 75% to 80% of individuals over their lifetime. Affected individuals are invariably smokers and they typically develop pulmonary emphysema in the third to fourth decade of life. Smoking has been estimated to shorten the life of these patients by approximately 20 years.

The characteristic pulmonary pathologic abnormality is diffuse panacinar emphysema. In deficiency states, the lack of A1AT in the pulmonary interstitium results in the unopposed action of proteases, the gradual destruction of pulmonary connective tissue, and the loss of alveolar units. It is thought that the oxidants associated with cigarette smoke promote lung disease by oxidatively inactivating the active site residue of the A1AT molecule, thereby resulting in a 1000-fold diminution in antiprotease activity.

Other clinical manifestations

An ulcerative neutrophilic cutaneous panniculitis associated with fever is seen in a minority of PiZZ individuals. These lesions typically occur on the trunk, and are often precipitated by minor trauma. A clinical response to exogenously administered A1AT and dapsone have been described.

An association between A1AT deficiency and renal disease in infancy has been described, although it is not well characterized. Also suggested is an association between A1AT deficiency and immune complex diseases such as rheumatoid arthritis and Wegener's granulomatosis. Certain malignancies are also reported to occur more commonly in individuals with this disorder. Whether this represents a primary protease–antiprotease imbalance or a linkage phenomenon remains to be determined.

Natural history of alpha-1-antitrypsin deficiency

Several registries of these patients have attempted to study their long-term outcome, but their data are still incomplete. The National Institutes of Health study suggests that the actuarial survival of PiZZ individuals to the age of 60 is only 16%, compared to 85% in the normal population. The Danish registry reports that the life expectancy in PiZZ individuals is 52 years in smokers, compared to 68 years in non-smokers.

The natural history of liver disease in A1AT deficiency has been studied prospectively in a Swedish nationwide screening study. Of the 127 PiZZ individuals identified by screening all newborn infants, more than 85% had persistently normal transaminases at 18 years of age. However, it is unclear as to whether occult liver disease exists in these individuals, and whether they will progress to overt liver disease in adulthood. The prognosis of hepatic disease in A1AT deficiency is difficult to predict. One study suggested that persistence of hyperbilirubinemia, hard hepatomegaly, early development of splenomegaly and prolongation of prothrombin time were all indicators of a poor prognosis. In another study, elevated transaminase levels, prolonged prothrombin time, and a lower trypsin inhibitor capacity correlated with a worse prognosis.

Diagnosis

The serum A1AT phenotype may be determined in isoelectric focusing or by agarose electrophoresis at acid pH. The serum concentrations of A1AT may be helpful when used with phenotype to distinguish individuals who are homozygous for the Z allele from SZ compound heterozygotes. This is important in genetic counseling. It should be remembered that serum A1AT levels may be misleading, as they increase in response to inflammatory states and they may be falsely elevated even in affected individuals.

The pathognomic histologic feature of homozygous PiZZ A1AT deficiency is the appearance of periodic acid Schiff-positive, diastase-resistant globules in the endoplasmic reticulum of hepatocytes. However, these are not specific for this condition and may be seen in PiMM individuals with other liver diseases. Other histologic features include variable degrees of hepatocellular necrosis, inflammatory cell infiltration, periportal fibrosis, and cirrhosis.

Treatment

Avoiding cigarette smoking, even in individuals with no definitely documented pulmonary disease, is of paramount importance. Smoking has been shown to accelerate the progression of lung involvement, and significantly truncate life expectancy in affected individuals.

No specific therapy is available for liver disease, apart from supportive care. In the decompensated cirrhotic, liver transplantation is the only corrective therapy. This has been shown to be associated with good survival rates in both children and adults, 90% at 1 year, and 80% at 5 years. A number of PiZZ individuals have relatively preserved hepatic function, and may never need liver transplantation. The etiology of hepatic involvement in A1AT deficiency is not thought to be related to deficient levels of the protein, and so replacement therapy is not indicated.

For those with pulmonary disease, replacement therapy with recombinant plasma A1AT is available, either by intravenous or intratracheal administration. It is indicated in those with established and progressive emphysema. Lung transplantation is also an option for those with severe emphysema. Data from the Lung Transplant registry show actuarial survival in this group to be similar to that in other groups.

Disorders of heme biosynthesis – the hereditary porphyrias

The hereditary porphyrias are a group of metabolic disorders caused by genetic deficiency of the enzymes involved in the formation of heme. The liver and bone marrow are major sites of heme production and, therefore, principal sites of expression of biochemical abnormalities. The first case of acute porphyria was reported in 1889 by the Dutch physician Stokvis. The term "porphyria" was first used by Waldenström to describe a disorder with episodic neurologic crises in 103 Swedish patients.

Heme biosynthetic pathway

This involves eight separate enzymatically catalyzed steps (Table 5.1). The pathway begins with the condensation of glycine and succinyl Co-A to form δ-aminolevulinic acid (ALA), mediated by the enzyme δ-aminolevulinic acid synthase (ALAS). This is followed sequentially by the condensation of ALA to porphobilinogen (PBG); the subsequent formation of a porphyrinogen macromolecule containing eight carboxyl groups; sequential decarboxylations and an oxidation step leading to the formation of the tetracarboxyl porphyrin, designated protoporphyrin-IX; and finally, the insertion of iron into the porphyrin ring forming heme. Deficiency of all but the first (i.e. the ALAS catalyzed) of the enzymatic steps in heme biosynthesis is associated with a characteristic clinical syndrome and pattern of excretion of porphyrin precursors (ALA/PBG) and/or porphyrins in the urine and/or feces. The pattern of excretion observed is a consequence of a compensatory increase in the production of compounds "up-stream" of the deficient enzymatic step.

Molecular pathogenesis of enzyme defects

Advances in molecular medicine have led to the identification of specific genetic mutations responsible for the various enzyme defects. Acute intermittent porphyria is the best studied, and has been found to be associated with as many as 70 different mutations. The prevalence of mutations varies according to the population. For example, in the US no specific mutation dominates whereas in Sweden almost half of the affected families share the same mutation. Variegate porphyria, which is common in South Africa, is unique in that 90% of affected individuals share the same mutation. However, there is no clear-cut relationship between specific mutations and the severity of clinical manifestations. Although DNA analysis has not yet been established as a method of diagnosis, it is the method of choice in screening family members if the mutation is known.

Biochemical abnormalities

Each of the eight types of porphyria is associated with a specific enzyme defect. This produces a characteristic pattern of abnormal accumulation and excretion of porphyrins and precursors. The acute porphyrias show an increase in the level of hepatic

Table 5.1 Clinical and biochemical features of the hereditary porphyrias

Glycine + Succinyl-CoA
δ-Aminolevulinate synthetase

ALA → PBG → HMB → URO'gen III → COPRO'gen III → PROTO'gen IX → PROTO IX → HEME

Type of porphyria	Enzyme deficiency	Excreted metabolites	Presentation
PBG synthase deficiency	PBG synthase	ALA	Neurovisceral
Acute intermittent porphyria	HMB synthase	PBG, ALA	Neurovisceral
Congenital erythropoietic porphyria	URO'gen III synthase	Uro; RBC uro	Cutaneous
Porphyria cutanea tarda	URO'gen decarboxylase	Uro	Cutaneous
Hereditary coproporphyria	COPRO'gen oxidase	Copro; PBG; ALA; Fecal copro	Neurovisceral and cutaneous
Variegate porphyria	PROTO'gen oxidase	Copro; PBG; ALA; Fecal proto	Neurovisceral and cutaneous
Protoporphyria	Ferrochelatase	Fecal and RBC proto	Cutaneous

*Refers to urine metabolites unless otherwise specified.
ALA = δ-aminolevulinic acid; *PBG* = porphobilinogen; *HMB* = hydroxymethylbilane; *URO'gen* = uroporphyrinogen; *COPRO'gen* = coproporphyrinogen;
PROTO'gen = protoporphyrinogen; *PROTO* = protoporphyrin; *uro* = uroporphyrin; *copro* = coproporphyrin; *proto* = protoporphyrin

ALA synthase activity during acute attacks. The increased demand for hepatic heme biosynthesis depletes the regulatory heme pool and removes the negative feedback control on ALA synthase. The acute attack abates when sufficient heme is produced to return hepatic ALA synthase activity to normal

Clinical features

The porphyrias may be classified on the basis of their clinical presentation with either neurovisceral or cutaneous manifestations. Four of the porphyrias – acute intermittent porphyria, variegate porphyria, hereditary coproporphyria, and the rare disorder of ALA dehydratase deficiency – present with episodic attacks of neurologic dysfunction. Of these, variegate porphyria and hereditary coproporphyria also have cutaneous manifestations.

The remaining four porphyrias – porphyria cutanea tarda, hepatoerythropoietic porphyria, congenital erythropoietic porphyria, and protoporphyria – have characteristic photocutaneous lesions. This discussion will focus on the acute porphyrias, and the two cutaneous porphyrias characterized by hepatic involvement, namely porphyria cutanea tarda and protoporphyria.

The acute (neurovisceral) porphyrias

The most common of these disorders is acute intermittent porphyria, with an estimated prevalence of 1 in 10 000 to 20 000 population. The clinical features of the acute porphyric attack are identical for each of the porphyrias. A number of possible precipitants have been identified. These include various medications such as the benzodiazepines, amiodarone, simvastatin, and several antibiotics. The menstrual period and the fasting state are also thought to predispose to an attack in susceptible individuals.

Abdominal pain is invariably present and is often severe enough to warrant unnecessary exploratory surgery. Symptoms of autonomic dysfunction, such as tachycardia and labile hypertension, are often present. Neurologic dysfunction may be severe, consisting of focal deficits, seizures, and bulbar involvement leading to respiratory paralysis. Depression and frank psychosis may also be encountered.

Biochemical evaluation

In the setting of a suspected porphyric attack, the urinary excretion of ALA and PBG are invariably elevated and may be used as a diagnostic test. Quantitative estimation of these compounds is indicated. While that is being processed, two quick bedside tests may provide a rapid screening – the Watson–Schwartz test and the Hoesch test both rely of the reaction of PBG with Erlich's reagent to form a red compound.

After the diagnosis of an acute porphyria has been made, the specific type may be determined by further testing. In acute intermittent porphyria, the erythrocyte PBG deaminase activity is decreased. In variegate porphyria, there is fecal excretion of protoporphyrin and a characteristic plasma porphyrin fluorescence pattern. In hereditary coproporphyria, fecal and urinary coproporphyrin excretion is increased.

Treatment of the acute porphyric attack

If this diagnosis is suspected, prompt aggressive management may often avert the more severe consequences. The patient should be admitted and the diagnostic evaluation initiated. If an incriminating medication is identified it should be discontinued, and other porphyrinogenic drugs should be avoided. Infections should be treated expeditiously, and an adequate caloric intake provided. At least 400 grams of glucose should be administered as a carbohydrate load has been found to suppress hepatic ALA synthase activity.

If no improvement is noted within 24 to 48 hours on the above regimen, hematin should be administered. This has been found to suppress ALA synthase activity, and to cause a rapid decline in serum and urine levels of ALA and PBG. However, its clinical benefits are not well defined. There are no randomized controlled trials attesting to its utility, and many of the data supporting its use are derived from small case series.

The dose of hematin is 3 to 4 mg/kg body weight once daily for 4 days, or twice daily for 3 days. Its most common complication is the development of thrombophlebitis which may be prevented by a slow infusion of the medication.

Symptomatic treatment of the acute attack with analgesics, anxiolytics, antihypertensives, and antiseizure medications, form an important part of the overall therapeutic plan.

With careful counseling aimed at avoiding common precipitants, most patients have very few porphyric attacks during their lifetime. However, the small minority with recurrent attacks present a management challenge. There is no evidence that long-term hematin treatment is of any benefit. In the absence of any form of effective therapy, most of these individuals are managed by narcotics, and potential addiction is a significant concern. Adequate and thoughtful pain management is crucial in the long-term care of these individuals.

Differential diagnosis

Several non-hereditary disorders can be associated with an increase in the urinary excretion of porphyrins, especially coproporphyrin. These include the poorly understood condition of multiple chemical sensitivity syndrome, as well as lead poisoning and hereditary tyrosinemia. Patients with these disorders often have chronic abdominal pain and subjective neurologic symptoms, leading to a diagnostic dilemma. Measurement of the urinary excretion of the porphyrin precursor PBG, and to a lesser extent, ALA, are the most useful tests in differentiating these patients from those with a true porphyria. All the conditions associated with a secondary porphyrinuria, with the exception of lead poisoning and hereditary tyrosinemia, have normal urinary levels of ALA and PBG. Lead poisoning is associated with several abnormalities in porphyrin metabolism. Erythrocyte levels of zinc protoporphyrin are elevated in this condition, and form the basis for a diagnostic test. Tyrosinemia is characterized by the development of hepatic failure and hepatocellular carcinoma in early childhood, and is readily distinguishable on clinical grounds from the porphyrias.

Cutaneous porphyrias

A detailed discussion of these disorders is beyond the scope of this text. An approach to their diagnosis is summarized in Figure 5.3. The urine talc and amyl alcohol tests provide for a rapid screening examination, but require confirmation by measurement of urinary PBG and ALA.

The focus of this discussion will be the two cutaneous porphyrias associated with liver involvement, namely the common condition of porphyria cutanea tarda and the uncommon condition of protoporphyria.

Porphyria cutanea tarda

This is the most common of the clinically expressed porphyrias in the US. It is also common among the Bantu of South Africa and is attributed to the ingestion of a local beer brewed in iron pots.

Pathogenesis and classification There is a complex but incompletely understood interplay between alcohol, the heme synthetic pathway, and iron accumulation in the liver. Porphyria cutanea tarda is a known association of alcoholic liver disease and requires the presence of both alcohol and iron for its manifestation. Porphyria cutanea tarda results from the absence or functional deficiency of uroporphyrinogen decarboxylase, an enzyme responsible for decarboxylation of the intermediate porphyrinogens. As a result, there is accumulation in blood, and excretion in urine, of uroporphyrins, hepta-, hexa- and pentacarboxylic porphyrin, and coproporphryin. The porphyrins are also deposited in the skin, where they undergo photoactivation resulting in a photosensitive dermatitis characterized by the presence of vesiculo-erosive lesions and fragility of sun-exposed skin (Figure 5.4), which may be followed by hyperpigmentation, hirsutism, and atrophy.

Porphyria cutanea tarda occurs in two forms.

1. Sporadic (type I) porphyria cutanea tarda is the most common form. It is characterized by decreased uroporphyrinogen decarboxylase activity restricted to the liver, suggesting that the liver-specific inactivation of uroporphyrinogen decarboxylase is triggered directly or indirectly by an exogenous agent.
2. Familial (type II) porphyria cutanea tarda affects families in an autosomal dominant pattern with variable penetrance. It accounts for 20% of patients with porphyria cutanea tarda. It differs from sporadic porphyria cutanea tarda in that the uroporphyrinogen decarboxylase enzyme deficiency is present in all tissues, especially erythrocytes. The onset of this disease is in childhood with characteristic skin manifestations.

The mere presence of a uroporphyrinogen decarboxylase gene defect is not sufficient for clinical expression of the disease, requiring an additional insult in the liver, which is usually provided by alcohol, estrogen, or viral infections such as the hepatitis C virus. Eighty to ninety percent of patients with porphyria cutanea tarda have a history of alcohol intake, and 90% have iron overload in the liver.

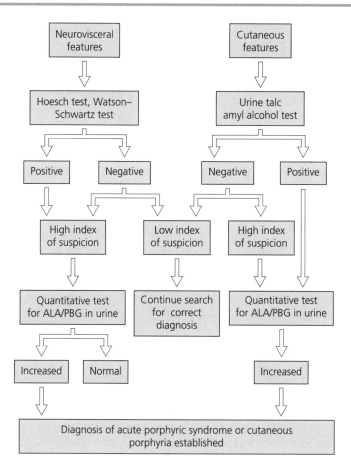

ALA = δ-aminolevulinic acid
PBG = Porphobilinogen

Figure 5.3 Laboratory evaluation of patients with suspected porphyric syndromes.

Further evidence for the role of iron in the manifestation of porphyria cutanea tarda is provided by the clinical and biochemical improvement following

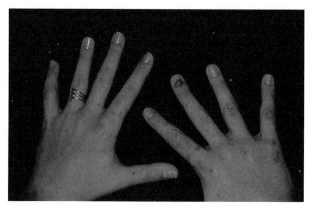

Figure 5.4 Porphyria cutanea tarda. The lesions of porphyria cutanea tarda, characterized as chronic blistering lesions, are found on sun-exposed parts of the body as on the hands *(see plate section for color)*.

iron-chelating therapy. Some studies consider the inheritance of the hemochromatosis mutation (C282Y) an important susceptibility factor for the manifestation of porphyria cutanea tarda. Others do not see an association between hemochromatosis and porphyria cutanea tarda. However, when compared to the amount of iron deposition in hemochromatosis, rather modest amounts of iron are required to set off porphyria cutanea tarda in a susceptible individual. Similarly, clinical inactivity can be achieved by modest venesection, making the effect of iron disproportionate to the degree of accumulation.

It has been suggested that the ferrous iron may directly damage uroporphyrinogen decarboxylase, but the bulk of evidence suggests that the damage by iron is more indirect and may be mediated by the formation of reactive oxygen molecules

Iron-dependent hydroxyl-generating systems assist the p450 microsomal enzymes in oxidizing uroporphyrinogen to uroporphyrin and other non-porphyrin compounds, that inhibit uroporphyrinogen decarboxylase *in vitro*. Alcohol, by inducing the p450 enzyme systems, increases the formation of uroporphyrin. A second inactivator of uroporphyrinogen decarboxylase is ALA. Alcohol increases the concentration of ALA as it is shown to decrease the activity of PBG synthase. Irrespective of the mechanisms involved, it is clear that alcohol and iron have a self-perpetuating and synergistic effect in the genesis of sporadic porphyria cutanea tarda.

Hepatic pathology Liver injury is almost universal in those with clinically overt porphyria cutanea tarda. On gross examination, the liver is found to have a patchy gray discoloration, and exhibits a red fluorescence when exposed to ultraviolet light. Hepatic iron overload is common, as is fatty infiltration of the liver. The extent of hepatic damage is variable, and is partly related to the duration of porphyria cutanea tarda. Hepatocellular carcinoma development has been linked to porphyria cutanea tarda. Autopsy series have reported rates of cirrhosis of 64%, and rates of hepatocellular carcinoma of 47% in those with documented porphyria cutanea tarda. It is recommended that those with long-standing porphyria cutanea tarda undergo standard surveillance practices for hepatocellular carcinoma.

Clinical features The most prominent manifestation of porphyria cutanea tarda is the appearance of photosensitive lesions in sun-exposed areas of the skin. These lesions initially present with superficial erosions and bullae which heal with scarring and hyperpigmentation. Less commonly, sclerodermatous plaques, scarring alopecia, and conjunctival damage are also seen. Similar cutaneous manifestations are noted in the other cutaneous porphyrias, namely variegate porphyria, hepatoerythropoietic porphyria, and hereditary coproporphyria.

Several disorders are associated with the development of porphyria cutanea tarda. These include hepatitis C infection, autoimmune disorders, synthetic estrogen use, and human immunodeficiency virus (HIV) infection.

Treatment An important component of management of this condition is withdrawal of the precipitant, if identifiable (e.g. alcohol and estrogens), and avoidance of light wavelengths that stimulate porphyrins (400 to 410 nm). The mainstay of therapy is depletion of iron stores by repeated venesection. In general, 4 to 8 liters of blood will need to be

removed. Urine levels of uroporphyrin are seen to decline with adequate iron depletion, and resolution of skin fragility usually accompanies this biochemical improvement. In those in whom phlebotomy is either ineffective or poorly tolerated, chloroquine or related compounds may be administered. Chloroquine is thought to complex with uroporphyrin and promote its release from the liver. It is used in doses of 125 mg twice weekly, and produces a clinical improvement in about 4 months.

Protoporphyria

Protoporphyria is the only other porphyria characterized by liver involvement. It occurs in all ethnic groups and is thought to be a relatively common disorder (1 in 5000 to 10 000). It is inherited in an autosomal dominant pattern with variable penetrance

Its biochemical hallmark is an increased level of protoporphyrin in feces and red blood cells. It manifests with skin lesions that are different from other cutaneous porphyrias and consist mainly of edema and itching on exposure to sunlight. Approximately 10% of patients develop a sub-fulminant liver failure. Autopsy studies show a black liver due to massive deposits of protoporphyrin pigment. These deposits are birefringent under polarization microscopy. Liver damage is thought to be caused by the progressive accumulation of protoporphyrin in the liver.

Management Most patients only require treatment for photosensitivity. In those with liver disease, oral administration of chenodeoxycholic acid has been found to reduce protoporphyrin levels. Oral administration of cholestyramine and activated charcoal is also used to interrupt the enterohepatic circulation of protoporphyrin. If the liver disease is advanced, a combination of hematin administration and plasmapheresis may be used for stabilization. Liver transplantation is often the only real option in those with end-stage liver disease. Anecdotally, it appears to have a successful outcome. It is important to keep several unique aspects of this disease in mind while planning transplantation or any form of surgery. These patients are prone to photodamage and it is important to use filters over operating-room lights in order to minimize tissue injury. It should be remembered that liver transplantation does not correct the basic ferrochelatase defect in the bone marrow. Bone marrow transplantation is a theoretical option should liver disease recur in the transplanted liver. However, there is limited clinical experience in the combined procedure for this particular indication.

Sphingolipidoses

These are a group of metabolic disorders characterized by both hepatic and neurologic defects. The most commonly encountered of these diseases in adult practice is Gaucher's disease which will be discussed here.

Gaucher's disease

This is an autosomal recessive disorder resulting from mutations of the gene encoding β-glucosidase (glucocerebrosidase), an enzyme which catalyzes the breakdown of the cerebrosides. This results in the accumulation of cerebrosides, specifically glucosylceramide, in lysosomes of reticuloendothelial cells. These reticuloendothelial cells enlarge and develop a characteristic appearance with an eccentric nucleus and fibrillar or "wrinkled tissue paper" cytoplasm, to form the pathognomic Gaucher cells.

Clinical features

Gaucher's disease exists in three clinical forms.

1. Type 1 is the most common, and is also called the adult or non-neuronopathic type. Onset may be at any age, including infancy, but neurologic involvement does not occur. The main clinical features are hepatosplenomegaly, thrombocytopenia, pathologic bone fractures, and pinguecula. These patients are often referred to hepatologists because of hepatomegaly and abnormal hepatic biochemical tests. However, the phenotypic manifestations of this form of Gaucher's disease vary widely, with some patients having minimal disease. Portal hypertension, and ascites have been described but are rare. Recent studies suggest that a plexogenic pulmonary vasculopathy causing pulmonary hypertension may occur in a proportion (5%) of affected individuals.
2. Patients with type 2 disease (infantile or acute neuronopathic disease) develop hepatosplenomegaly and progressive neurologic deterioration. Death within the first year of life is the usual course.
3. Type 3 (juvenile or subacute neuronopathic form) is a less severe form of the disease, and characteristically affects children with multiple neurologic defects. Gaucher's cells are demonstrated in visceral organs, and survival is prolonged compared to type 2 disease.

Liver histology is similar in all three types and consists of infiltration by Gaucher's cells with varying degrees of fibrosis.

Treatment

Enzymatic replacement therapy is the mainstay of treatment for type 1 disease. It cannot be used for types 2 and 3 as it does not cross the blood–brain barrier. Since placental mannose-terminated glucocerebrosidase (alglucerase, Genzyme Corp., Cambridge MA, US) and the carbohydrate-expressed enzyme (imiglucerase, Genzyme Corp.), were approved by the Food and Drug Administration, over 2000 patients have received replacement therapy. This treatment has been shown to be remarkably effective in ameliorating visceral, hematologic, and skeletal manifestations of type 1 Gaucher's disease, and is also very safe. In the future, it is hoped that gene therapy will become a viable option.

In summary, the inherited metabolic disorders of the liver offer an intriguing glimpse into the many complex pathophysiological mechanisms mediated by the liver, and its associated organs. With the exciting new advances in molecular medicine, our understanding of these disorders is increasing exponentially, and with these greater insights comes the hope of new and more effective therapies.

Further reading

Bacon BR, Powell LW, Adams PC, *et al*. Molecular medicine and hemochromatosis: at the crossroads. *Gastroenterology* 1999; 116: 193–207.

Bonkovsky HL, Barnard GF. Diagnosis of porphyric syndromes: a practical approach in the era of molecular biology. *Semin Liver Dis* 1998; 18: 57–65.

Coakley RJ, Taggart C, O'Neill S, McElvaney NG. Alpha–1-antitrypsin deficiency: biological answers to clinical questions. *Am J Med Sci* 2001; 321(1): 33–41.

Khanna A. Liver transplantation for metabolic liver diseases. *Surg Clin N. Am* 1999; 79(1): 153–162.

Meyer UA, Schuurmans MM, Lindberg RLP. Acute porphyrias: pathogenesis of neurological manifestations. *Semin Liver Dis* 1998; 18: 43–52.

Perlmutter DH. Liver injury in alpha–1 antitrypsin deficiency. *Clin Liv Dis* 2000; 4(1): 220–229.

Powell LW. Hemochromatosis. *Clin Liv Dis* 2000; 4(1): 211–228.

Schilsky ML. Treatment for Wilson's disease: what are the relative roles of penicillamine, trientine, and zinc supplementation. *Curr Gastro Reports* 2001; 3: 54–59.

Sternlieb I. Wilson's Disease. *Clin Liver Dis* 2000; 4(1): 229–239.

Tavill AS. Diagnosis and management of hemochromatosis. (AASLD Practice Guidelines). *Hepatology* 2001; 33: 1321–1328.

Chapter 6

Primary Biliary Cirrhosis, Primary Sclerosing Cholangitis, and Autoimmune Hepatitis

Thomas W. Faust and Stanley Martin Cohen

CHAPTER OUTLINE

Introduction

Primary biliary cirrhosis is thought to be a disorder of immune regulation. Antimitochondrial antibodies against a family of inner mitochondrial antigens are found in the majority of patients. Humoral and cell-mediated injury to interlobular and septal bile ducts within the liver results in progressive cholestasis, fibrosis, and the development of cirrhosis. Patients with long-standing primary biliary cirrhosis ultimately develop liver failure and complications of portal hypertension and cholestasis. Ursodeoxycholic acid (UDCA) has been shown to improve cholestatic liver function tests, whereas its effect on hepatic histology and transplant-free survival is less certain. In addition to the treatment of the underlying pathophysiologic process, therapies should also be directed toward complications of portal hypertension and prolonged cholestasis. Orthotopic liver transplantation is the treatment of choice for patients with advanced primary biliary cirrhosis.

Primary sclerosing cholangitis is also thought to be a disease of disordered immune regulation. Clinical, biochemical, cholangiographic, and histologic criteria are important for the diagnosis of patients with primary sclerosing cholangitis. Inflammatory and fibrotic destruction of intrahepatic and extrahepatic bile ducts results in progressive cholestasis and the development of cirrhosis. Primary sclerosing cholangitis is also a risk factor for cholangiocarcinoma, especially for patients with coexistent inflammatory bowel disease. There is no proven therapy for patients with primary sclerosing cholangitis that halts or reverses the underlying pathophysiologic process. Medical therapies should be directed towards complications of portal hypertension and progressive cholestasis. Orthotopic liver transplantation is the only definitive option that has been clearly shown to improve patient survival.

As with the biliary tract disorders, autoimmune hepatitis may be a disease of altered immune regulation. Aberrant human leukocyte antigen (HLA) expression on hepatocytes leads to activation and proliferation of lymphocytes and production of proinflammatory cytokines followed by the development of hepatocellular necrosis. Antinuclear, antismooth muscle, and liver-kidney-microsomal (LKM1) antibodies with elevated aminotransferases and hypergammaglobulinemia are typically seen. Interface hepatitis and lobular necrosis on liver biopsy are also important for the diagnosis of autoimmune hepatitis. Corticosteroids and azathioprine have been shown to improve symptoms, biochemical liver tests, histology, and survival. Orthotopic liver transplantation is reserved for patients with impaired hepatic reserve and portal hypertensive complications.

The purpose of this review is to highlight the epidemiology, pathogenesis, and clinical features of primary biliary cirrhosis, primary sclerosing cholangitis, and autoimmune hepatitis. Diagnostic, medical, and surgical options will also be addressed. The chapter will conclude with an overview of the natural history and prognosis for patients with autoimmune liver diseases.

Primary biliary cirrhosis

Key features

- Primary biliary cirrhosis is a chronic cholestatic liver disease that predominantly affects middle-aged females.
- Humoral and cellular immune mechanisms may be important in the pathogenesis of primary biliary cirrhosis.
- Patients with progressive disease develop complications attributable to liver failure, portal hypertension, and chronic cholestasis.
- Granulomatous destruction of interlobular and septal bile ducts within the liver is characteristic of primary biliary cirrhosis.
- Ursodeoxycholic acid has been shown to improve liver function tests, and may also have a positive effect on hepatic histology and patient survival.
- Liver transplantation is recommended for patients with marginal hepatic reserve and complications of portal hypertension or cholestasis.

History and overview

Primary biliary cirrhosis was rarely reported before the 1950s. However, with current advances in immunology and hepatobiliary imaging, much progress has been made in the understanding of this disorder. Addison was the first person to provide a clinical description of the disease, Ahrens and colleagues were the first to use the term "primary biliary cirrhosis", and Rubin and Scheuer were the first to provide a pathologic description of primary biliary cirrhosis. Primary biliary cirrhosis is a chronic cholestatic liver disease that is presumed to have an autoimmune basis. Patients with primary biliary cirrhosis are typically middle-aged females. It is also frequently associated with a variety of extrahepatic autoimmune disorders that may account for significant morbidity. Cholestatic complications include osteoporosis, fat-soluble vitamin deficiency, pruritus, hypercholesterolemia, and malabsorption.

Characteristic histopathology includes granulomatous destruction of interlobular and septal bile ducts within the liver. Portal and periportal inflammation may also be present. Ductopenia, fibrosis, cirrhosis with portal hypertensive complications, and liver failure develop in patients with progressive disease.

Most patients with primary biliary cirrhosis are asymptomatic at the time of diagnosis. Typically cholestatic liver function indices and antimitochondrial antibodies are found during routine health maintenance examinations, evaluation for other suspected causes of liver disease, or surveillance of relatives of patients with primary biliary cirrhosis.

Ursodeoxycholic acid is standard therapy for patients with early or advanced disease. Even though UDCA may improve transplant-free survival and delay or prevent the need for orthotopic liver transplantation, progressive disease usually develops in the majority of cases. Other immunmodulators have not been shown to consistently improve liver function tests, histology, or alter the natural course of primary biliary cirrhosis.

Orthotopic liver transplantation is reserved for patients with decompensated cirrhosis, with or without complications of portal hypertension including refractory variceal bleeding, intractable ascites, or severe encephalopathy. Patients with poor quality of life indicators, such as severe osteoporosis or intractable pruritus, may also be candidates for liver replacement. Prognostic models aid the clinician in terms of timing the orthotopic liver transplantation and evaluating the efficacy of medical therapies for primary biliary cirrhosis. Primary biliary cirrhosis can recur after orthotopic liver transplantation, but overall patient and graft survival is excellent over the medium term.

Epidemiology

The incidence in females outnumbers that in males by a ratio of 9:1. Primary biliary cirrhosis can be seen in patients between 30 and 70 years of age, but most patients present during middle age. The clinical presentation is similar between genders and races, and is present throughout the world. The highest prevalence and incidence have been reported from northern Europe. The prevalence and incidence of primary biliary cirrhosis are 19 to 150 cases per million, and 4 to 15 cases per million per year respectively. Primary biliary cirrhosis also accounts for 2% of deaths worldwide from chronic liver disease. Familial clustering of primary biliary cirrhosis has been reported even though the disease is not inherited in a strictly recessive or dominant fashion. There may be a weak association between HLA-DR8 and the predisposition to develop primary biliary cirrhosis. First-degree relatives of patients have a 570-fold increase in developing antimitochondrial antibodies and clinical disease when compared to individuals without a family history of primary biliary cirrhosis.

Pathogenesis

Primary biliary cirrhosis is presumed to have an autoimmune basis. Humoral and cellular immune mechanisms may be important. Antimitochondrial antibodies are present in the majority of patients with primary biliary cirrhosis, but there is no correlation between antibody titer and the severity of primary biliary cirrhosis. Antimitochondrial antibodies are directed to a family of autoantigens expressed on inner mitochondrial membranes that include pyruvate dehydrogenase, branched chain oxoacid dehydrogenase, and oxaloglutarate dehydrogenase of the 2 oxoacid dehydrogenase complex. Antibodies directed to the E2 subunit of these enzymes, particularly pyruvate dehydrogenase, are present in over 90% of patients with primary biliary cirrhosis.

Molecular mimicry has been suggested as possibly important in the pathogenesis of primary biliary cirrhosis. The E2 subunit of pyruvate dehydrogenase is highly conserved in bacteria, yeast, and xenobiotics, but the antigen is also expressed on the inner mitochondrial membranes of humans. With molecular mimicry, alloantigens or autoantigens on the biliary epithelial cell share epitopes (E2 subunit of pyruvate dehydrogenase) with that of the inner mitochondrial membrane and possibly an exogenous agent. *Escherichia coli*, *Klebsiella pneumonia*, *Proteus mirabilis*, *Staphylococcus aureus*, *Salmonella minnesota*, and *Mycobacterium gordonae* have been evaluated, but no organism has been conclusively shown to induce primary biliary cirrhosis. With molecular mimicry, the genetically predisposed host elicits a B and T lymphocyte response to a presumed exogenous agent that shares the E2 epitope with the biliary epithelial cell and the inner mitochondrial membrane. Production of autoreactive antimitochondrial antibodies to the E2 subunit on the biliary epithelial cell similar to that of an exogenous agent may subsequently result in immune-mediated injury to the interlobular and septal bile ducts. Furthermore, presentation of E2 antigen with upregulation of HLA-I and aberrant HLA-I production on the biliary epithelial cell may result in cell-mediated destruction of the intrahepatic bile ducts by autoreactive T lymphocytes. Induction of intracellular adhesion molecule (ICAM-1) and vascular cell adhesion molecule (VCAM) may play an accessory role in promoting cell-mediated injury. Circulating T lymphocytes are decreased, whereas CD4 and CD8 lymphocytes are increased within the liver of patients with primary biliary cirrhosis. T helper 2 cells within portal zones induce mast cell and eosinophil activation and are most commonly associated with early disease, whereas T helper 1 cells are more commonly seen in patients with advanced primary biliary cirrhosis. Cytotoxic CD8 cells are the primary cells responsible for cell-mediated injury to the interlobular and septal bile ducts. Proinflammatory cytokines may also be important in the pathogenesis of injury. Retention of hydrophobic bile acids leads to progressive hepatocellular injury followed by the development of fibrosis and cirrhosis. Patients with end-stage disease develop hepatic failure with complications of portal hypertension and progressive cholestasis.

Clinical features

Patients with primary biliary cirrhosis can present in a variety of ways (Box 6.1). Asymptomatic disease is diagnosed in 48% to 60% of patients during routine health maintenance examinations, evaluation for other diseases, or when screening the relatives of patients with primary biliary cirrhosis. The asymptomatic or presymptomatic phase may last for 20 years before symptoms and complications develop. Patients with asymptomatic disease typically have elevated antimitochondrial antibodies and liver histology consistent with primary biliary cirrhosis; liver function tests can be either normal or primarily cholestatic.

Most patients with asymptomatic disease ultimately develop symptoms. The symptomatic phase can last for 5 to 10 years and is associated with a variety of symptoms and signs that are typical of patients with cholestatic liver disease. Fatigue (in 65% to 70% of patients) is usually a non-specific and persistent complaint that does not correlate with disease severity. Pruritus (in 55% of patients) may occur as a result of upregulation of central opioid receptors and/or accumulation of endogenous opioid agonists, and is more frequently seen with early disease. Jaundice (in 10% to 30% of patients) is a poor prognostic indicator and indicates progressive destruction of the interlobular and septal bile ducts. Patients who develop jaundice, progressive hepatic synthetic dysfunction, and complications of portal hypertension or cholestasis should be considered for orthotopic liver transplantation. Hepatosplenomegaly, right upper quadrant pain, and hyperpigmentation are present in 15% to 70% of patients. Xanthelasmas and xanthomas are not uncommon and may or may not be associated with hypercholesterolemia. Xanthomas may spontaneously disappear as the disease progresses. Primary biliary cirrhosis is also associated with many extrahepatic, primarily autoimmune diseases.

Complications of primary biliary cirrhosis may be attributable to progressive cholestasis or portal hypertension (Box 6.2). Prolonged cholestasis is commonly associated with hepatic osteodystrophy and malabsorption. Osteoporosis, present in 25% of patients, is more common than osteoma-

---

Box 6.1   Features of primary biliary cirrhosis

Symptoms
fatigue
pruritus
jaundice
right upper quadrant pain

Physical findings
hepatomegaly
splenomegaly
jaundice
hyperpigmentation
xanthomas and/or xanthelasmas

Box 6.2   Complications of primary biliary cirrhosis

Steatorrhea and malabsorption
Hepatic osteodystrophy
Ascites
Variceal bleeding
Hepatic encephalopathy
Hypercholesterolemia
Hepatocellular carcinoma

lacia and may account for an increased risk of vertebral and rib fractures before and after orthotopic liver transplantation. Malabsorption can occur as a consequence of reduced bile-acid delivery to the small intestine leading to a significant reduction in the micellar concentration of bile acids. Coexistent pancreatic insufficiency and celiac disease may also be responsible for malabsorption and steatorrhea. Patients with steatorrhea are susceptible to deficiencies of vitamins A, D, E, and K. The preterminal phase of primary biliary cirrhosis lasts approximately 2 years and is associated with hepatic synthetic dysfunction and complications of portal hypertension. Bleeding from esophageal or gastric varices, intractable ascites, refractory encephalopathy, and malnutrition subsequently develop and are indications for orthotopic liver transplantation. Patients with advanced disease are at risk for hepatobiliary malignancies. Hepatocellular carcinoma can develop in 6% of patients with stage III or IV primary biliary cirrhosis, and may be more prevalent in males. Cholangiocarcinoma has also been reported but is rare. At the present time, primary biliary cirrhosis is not thought to be a risk factor for breast cancer.

Patients with primary biliary cirrhosis can develop a variety of extrahepatic, primarily autoimmune disorders. Thyroid disease is present in 15% to 20% of patients. Hashimoto's thyroiditis is more common than Grave's disease. Autoimmune thyroid disorders often predate primary biliary cirrhosis and are frequently associated with the production of antithyroid antibodies. Thyroid function tests should be checked in all patients with primary biliary cirrhosis. Connective tissue disorders often coexist with primary biliary cirrhosis. CREST (calcinosis, Raynaud's phenomenon, esophageal dysfunction, sclerodactyly, telangiectasia) syndrome, scleroderma, systemic lupus erythematosus, and rheumatoid arthritis are present in 5%, 15%, 5%, and 10% of patients respectively. Raynaud's phenomenon and polymyositis may also develop in 10% of patients. Seventy percent of patients with primary biliary cirrhosis complain of xerophthalmia, xerostomia, dysphagia, and dyspareunia consistent with the sicca syndrome. Proximal or distal renal tubular acidosis and membranous or focal proliferative glomerulonephritis can develop in 50% and 5% of patients respectively. Other rare extrahepatic manifestations of primary biliary cirrhosis include celiac disease, gallstones, autoimmune warm and cold hemolytic anemia, immune thrombocytopenia, inflammatory bowel disease, fibrosing alveolitis, pulmonary interstitial fibrosis, myasthenia gravis, vitiligo, and hypertrophic pulmonary osteoarthropathy.

Diagnosis

The diagnosis of primary biliary cirrhosis is based upon clinical, biochemical, serologic, and histologic criteria. No one test should be used alone to make a diagnosis of primary biliary cirrhosis.

Biochemical tests

In most patients with primary biliary cirrhosis the alkaline phosphatase level is greater than three to four times the upper limits of normal, however, values may be normal in patients with antimitochondrial antibodies and biopsies consistent with primary biliary cirrhosis. Alkaline phosphatase levels do not correlate with disease severity and are not prognostically important. Other cholestatic indices include gamma glutamyl transpeptidase and 5' nucleotidase. Like alkaline phosphatase, they are also not prognostically important. Most patients with primary biliary cirrhosis have elevations in the aminotransferases usually below three times the upper limits of normal. Markedly elevated values in patients with primary biliary cirrhosis suggest other coexistent conditions including viral hepatitis, drug-induced hepatotoxicity, or an overlap syndrome with autoimmune hepatitis. The bilirubin of patients with early primary biliary cirrhosis is usually normal. With significant destruction of the intrahepatic bile ducts, values will rise over time and are usually suggestive of progressive disease and hepatic synthetic dysfunction. The rise in serum bilirubin is prognostically important and is a useful biochemical marker when determining the need for orthotopic liver transplantation. Prolongation of the prothrombin time and hypoalbuminemia are also suggestive of impaired hepatic reserve. Patients with significant cholestasis typically have hypercholesterolemia but are not at increased risk for ischemic heart disease.

Serology

Antimitochondrial antibodies are the serologic hallmark of primary biliary cirrhosis. Antimitochondrial antibodies are directed to the 2-oxo-acid dehydrogenase complex of the inner mitochondrial membrane, principally the E2 subunit of pyruvate dehydrogenase as described above. Titers equal to or above 1:40 are significant and are present in 90% to 95% of patients with primary biliary cirrhosis. The sensitivity and specificity of antimitochondrial antibodies for diagnosis approaches 95%. Titers below 1:40 are not specific for primary biliary cirrhosis but may be found in patients with autoimmune hepatitis, primary sclerosing cholangitis, myocarditis, syphilis, and drug-induced liver disease. For patients with significant antimitochondrial antibody titers and normal liver function tests, annual biochemical liver tests should be performed; most patients have histologic injury compatible with primary biliary cirrhosis, and develop symptomatic disease over time. Antinuclear and/or anti-smooth muscle antibodies are present in low titer in one third of patients. Antithyroid, antiacetylcholine receptor, antiplatelet, antihistone, and anticentromere antibodies have also been identified with primary biliary cirrhosis in isolated cases. Patients with primary biliary cirrhosis typically have elevated immunoglobulin M (IgM) in serum. Antimitochondrial antibody-negative primary biliary cirrhosis or autoimmune cholangiopathy is associated with clinical, biochemical, and histologic features compatible with a diagnosis of primary biliary cirrhosis in patients who do not develop antimitochondrial antibodies. Patients with antimitochondrial antibody-negative primary biliary cirrhosis may have high titers of either antinuclear or antismooth muscle antibodies and elevated IgG in serum. The natural history for patients with antibody negative disease is similar to that of classic primary biliary cirrhosis.

Medical imaging

Medical imaging does not serve an important role in the diagnosis of primary biliary cirrhosis. Ultrasound, CT, and MRI are primarily used to exclude biliary obstruction or malignancy and to assess the degree of portal hypertension. Typical findings on helical CT include a normal or large liver with early disease, a small heterogenous liver with intra-abdominal collaterals and splenomegaly with advanced disease, ascites, and portacaval or portahepatic adenopathy. Hepatocellular carcinoma can also be readily detected in patients with advanced disease by CT. As with CT, MRI is useful in the assessment of advance disease with complications of portal hypertension and hepatocellular carcinoma. The "periportal halo sign" may be a specific MRI sign of primary biliary cirrhosis. Low-intensity signals around enhancing intrahepatic portal branches represent cellular drop out and fibrosis, and may affect all hepatic segments in patients

with primary biliary cirrhosis. Additional studies will be required to confirm these findings. Cholangiography is generally not required in the evaluation of patients with suspected primary biliary cirrhosis. However, if clinical, biochemical, or non-invasive radiologic studies suggest extrahepatic disease, a cholangiogram is required.

Pathology

The livers of patients with early primary biliary cirrhosis are usually large, smooth, and bile stained. Nodular regenerative hyperplasia can also be seen with early disease and may account for portal hypertension in patients without obvious cirrhosis. Cirrhosis is associated with advanced disease. Other gross findings include pigment or cholesterol gallstones and enlarged portacaval or portahepatic nodes secondary to benign reactive hyperplasia.

Liver biopsy may not be necessary for diagnosis in patients with antimitochondrial antibody titers equal to or above 1:40, typical symptoms and signs of primary biliary cirrhosis, and markedly cholestatic liver indices. However, biopsy is useful for staging and determining prognosis.

Four stages of primary biliary cirrhosis have been described.

- Stage I (portal stage) is represented by segmental and patchy granulomatous destruction of interlobular and septal bile ducts (the florid duct lesion) (see Figure 6.1). Infiltration of portal tracts with lymphocytes, plasma cells, and histiocytes is typical. Rare

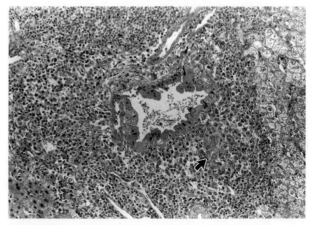

Figure 6.1 Primary biliary cirrhosis. Liver biopsy specimen showing an interlobular bile duct with marked mononuclear inflammation and destruction. An early granuloma (arrow) is present (hematoxylin and eosin × 200) (reproduced with permission of Dr Sugantha Govindarajan).

neutrophils and eosinophils may also be present. The florid duct lesion is identified in only 10% of liver biopsies.

- Bile-duct loss in association with ductular proliferation and portal tract expansion with chronic inflammatory cells represents stage II or the periportal stage. Interface hepatitis is present with extension of the lymphocytic infiltrate into the hepatic parenchyma.
- Stage III is associated with portal and periportal inflammation, bridging necrosis, septal fibrosis between adjacent portal tracts, bile-duct loss, and cholestasis.
- Established cirrhosis with regenerative nodule formation represents stage IV.

Granulomatous destruction of bile ducts is pathognomonic, whereas breaks in the biliary epithelial basement membrane, portal and periportal inflammatory infiltrates, non-caseating granulomas, loss of biliary epithelial cells, lymphocytic bile-duct destruction, and ductopenia are suggestive, but not diagnostic. Staging of primary biliary cirrhosis is subject to sampling error, as different stages may be present within different hepatic segments. Staging is based upon the most advanced lesion.

Differential diagnosis

Many diseases associated with intrahepatic and extrahepatic cholestasis require exclusion before a diagnosis of primary biliary cirrhosis can be made (Box 6.3). Choledocholithiasis, isolated biliary strictures, and pancreaticobiliary neoplasms can produce extrahepatic obstruction with cholestasis. Non-invasive imaging and cholangiography are usually required to exclude these conditions. Primary sclerosing cholangitis is an inflammatory

Box 6.3 Differential diagnosis of primary biliary cirrhosis

Choledocholithiasis
Biliary strictures
Pancreaticobiliary malignances
Medications
   estrogens
   androgenic steroids
   phenothiazines
Sarcoidosis
Granulomatous hepatitis

and fibrotic disease of the intrahepatic and extrahepatic bile ducts that results in the development of progressive cholestasis and biliary cirrhosis. Most patients with primary sclerosing cholangitis have coexistent inflammatory bowel disease. Antimitochondrial antibody titers are usually negative and liver biopsy reveals typical features of fibrous cholangitis or concentric fibrosis and fibro-obliterative lesions involving the intrahepatic bile ducts. Cholangiography is the gold standard for diagnosis. Many medications (e.g. estrogens, androgenic steroids, and phenothiazines) can produce intrahepatic cholestasis. Autoimmune hepatitis can occasionally be confused with primary biliary cirrhosis, especially if an overlap syndrome exists. Low antimitochondrial antibody titer is present in 25% of patients with autoimmune hepatitis. Patients with autoimmune hepatitis and primary biliary cirrhosis overlap have high titer antimitochondrial antibodies and antinuclear or antismooth muscle antibodies, with histology consistent with autoimmune hepatitis and primary biliary cirrhosis. Granulomatous destruction of bile ducts is associated with hepatitis C. However, antimitochondrial antibody titers are usually negative and antibody or polymerase chain reaction testing for hepatitis C is usually positive. Sarcoidosis is associated with granulomatous portal inflammation and intrahepatic cholestasis. Ninety percent of patients with sarcoidosis have abnormal chest radiographs. Occasionally sarcoidosis and primary biliary cirrhosis may coexist in the same patient. Autoimmune cholangiopathy or antimitochondrial antibody-negative primary biliary cirrhosis is associated with cholestasis, negative antimitochondrial antibodies, positive antinuclear and/or antismooth muscle antibodies, and histology consistent with primary biliary cirrhosis. Prolonged intrahepatic cholestasis has also been associated with alcoholic and granulomatous hepatitis, but the history, physical examination, and appropriate laboratory testing usually exclude these disorders.

Treatment

Survival of patients with asymptomatic and symptomatic primary biliary cirrhosis is inferior to that of a healthy control population. Consequently, medical or surgical treatment is warranted in all patients. Unfortunately, no medical treatment has been shown conclusively to alter the natural course of primary biliary cirrhosis or obviate orthotopic liver transplantation. The overall goals of treatment are to slow disease progression and to treat symptoms of cholestasis or complications of portal hypertension.

Medical therapy of primary biliary cirrhosis

As primary biliary cirrhosis was thought to be an autoimmune disease, trials with immunosuppressive medications were initiated with the hope of improving clinical symptoms and signs of cholestasis, improving biochemical indices of cholestasis, reducing or eliminating bile-duct injury and fibrosis, and improving overall survival. Unfortunately, none of the immunmodulatory agents has been uniformly effective. Systemic corticosteroids may improve symptoms, cholestatic liver function tests, and histology in some patients, but there is no improvement in overall survival. Furthermore, corticosteroids may worsen osteopenia frequently present in patients with prolonged cholestasis. The efficacy of budesonide has also been studied in small trials and has not been shown to be effective. Likewise, azathioprine and penicillamine are not effective at improving symptoms, biochemical liver indices, histology, or survival. Liver function improves with the administration of cyclosporine and colchicine, but histology and patient survival are not favorably affected. Biochemical indices and hepatic inflammation may also improve with chlorambucil, but its toxicity and lack of efficacy regarding fibrosis and survival limit its use. Pilot studies suggest a possible improvement in clinical symptoms, cholestatic liver indices, hepatic inflammation, and fibrosis in primary biliary cirrhosis patients who receive methotrexate. However, patients with advanced cirrhosis do not benefit. Additional studies are warranted before methotrexate can be uniformly recommended. Mycophenolate mofetil inhibits lymphocyte proliferative responses, induces apoptosis of activated T lymphocytes, inhibits antibody responses by B lymphocytes, and has antiviral properties. Combination therapy with mycophenolate and UDCA may reduce alkaline phosphatase levels and hepatic inflammation after 12 to 24 months of treatment. Mycophenolate is safe for long-term administration and may be useful to treat patients with either asymptomatic or symptomatic disease. At the present time, none of the above immunosuppressive agents can be considered standard therapy for patients with primary biliary cirrhosis. Combination therapy with immunosuppressive medications and UDCA will require additional studies to assess safety and efficacy for patients with early or advanced disease.

Ursodeoxycholic acid is the most effective medication for patients with primary biliary cirrhosis. At dosages of 13 to 15 mg kg^{-1} day^{-1} it leads to an improvement in clinical parameters, cholestatic liver indices, and hepatic inflammation in patients with either asymptomatic or symptomatic disease. It may also benefit patients with early (stage I or II) or late (stage III or IV) disease. Studies differ regarding the benefit of UDCA on hepatic fibrosis and transplant-free survival. Transplant-free survival may be modestly improved for patients with moderate-to-severe disease (stage III or IV) who receive UDCA at the above dose for over 4 years. Even though UDCA may delay the need for orthotopic liver transplantation, most patients will ultimately progress to end-stage disease, despite medical therapy, and require liver replacement. A recent meta-analysis on the benefit of UDCA for the treatment of patients with primary biliary cirrhosis suggests that liver function tests, portal, periportal, and bile-duct inflammation, and ductopenia improve with prolonged treatment, but fibrosis, the need for orthotopic liver transplantation, overall death, and liver-related death do not improve. Ursodeoxycholic acid may also reduce the severity of portal hypertension and the rate of variceal development. It has a variable effect on pruritus but does not favorably affect fatigue or osteopenia. The hepatoprotective effect of UDCA is not entirely clear but may include stabilization of cell membranes, choleretic effects through increased transport of bile acids into the biliary canaliculus, and alteration of the bile-acid pool with an increased hydrophilic to hydrophobic bile acid ratio. Reduced HLA-I and HLA-II expression on biliary epithelial cells, reduced production of cytokines, and anti-apoptotic effects may also be important.

Liver transplantation

Orthotopic liver transplantation is indicated for patients with advanced primary biliary cirrhosis and evidence of impaired hepatic reserve. Progressive hyperbilirubinemia and a Mayo risk score between 7.5 and 8 are poor prognostic signs and important indicators of decompensated disease and the need to consider orthotopic liver transplantation. Refractory variceal bleeding or encephalopathy, intractable ascites, spontaneous bacterial peritonitis, hepatorenal syndrome, hepatopulmonary syndrome, and early hepatocellular carcinoma are other indicators of marginal hepatic function for which transplantation is indicated. Patients with intractable pruritus and severe osteopenia may also benefit from liver replacement.

Cadaveric transplantation is the standard of care for patients with decompensated cirrhosis, but adult-to-adult living donor transplantation is another option for carefully selected patients. Patients considered for live donation should be reasonably well compensated and have a low Mayo risk score. Living donor grafts should be equal to or greater than 40% of the patient's standard liver volume for optimal results, but smaller grafts can be used under ideal circumstances in low-risk patients. The patient and graft survival at 1 and 5 years after transplantation are over 90% and 70% respectively. Even though UDCA has been shown to delay the need for orthotopic liver transplantation for patients with early or late disease, the outcome after transplantation for patients on UDCA is not negatively affected. Patients who receive allografts for primary biliary cirrhosis are at higher risk for acute and chronic rejection. Between 15% and 25% of patients transplanted for primary biliary cirrhosis can develop recurrence of the disease within the graft. Antimitochondrial antibodies persist after transplantation, but there is no correlation between antimitochondrial antibody titers and the risk of histologic recurrence. Liver biopsy is the gold standard and should reveal granulomatous bile-duct destruction before a diagnosis of recurrent primary biliary cirrhosis can be made. Moreover, exclusion of acute and chronic rejection, medication effects, viral hepatitis, and graft-versus-host disease is important. Patients who receive tacrolimus may be at higher risk for recurrence when compared to patients who receive cyclosporine. Most recurrences are asymptomatic, and patient and graft survival are not affected over the medium term.

Complications

Patients with primary biliary cirrhosis are susceptible to complications of portal hypertension and chronic cholestasis. Therapeutic strategies should focus not only on medical and surgical therapies to retard the progression of primary biliary cirrhosis, but also on alleviating the complications associated with progressive disease.

Portal hypertension

Portal hypertension can develop either as a consequence of progressive liver disease and the development of cirrhosis or as a result of nodular regenerative hyperplasia in patients without hepatic decompensation. Endoscopy is recommended for patients with newly diagnosed primary biliary cirrhosis to screen for esophagogastric varices. The examination should be repeated every 3 years to assess for the development of new varices or enlargement of previously detected varices. Non-selective beta-blockers are recommended for patients without a history of variceal bleeding and for those who have previously bled. Endoscopic sclerotherapy and band ligation of varices are appropriate for patients with a history of variceal bleeding. For patients with variceal bleeding refractory to endoscopic therapy and beta-blockers, distal splenorenal shunts are appropriate for patients with well-preserved hepatic synthetic function, whereas transjugular intrahepatic portosystemic shunts are advised for patients with decompensated liver disease awaiting orthotopic liver transplantation. Sodium-restricted diets, spironolactone, and furosemide are recommended for patients with volume overload and ascites. Therapeutic paracentesis and transjugular intrahepatic portosystemic shunts are appropriate for patients with ascites refractory to sodium restriction and diuretics. Lactulose, neomycin, and diets enriched with branched-chain amino acids are standard therapies for patients with hepatic encephalopathy.

Chronic cholestasis

Most studies suggest that metabolic bone disease is present in 30% to 50% of patients with primary biliary cirrhosis. Osteoporosis (a T score more than 2.5 standard deviations below the mean for normal young adults) is more common than osteomalacia. After a diagnosis of primary biliary cirrhosis has been made, dual energy X-ray absorptiometry should be performed with a repeat examination every 2 years. One third of patients with primary biliary cirrhosis have bone densities below the fracture threshold, and are at risk for progressive osteopenia during the first 6 months after orthotopic liver transplantation. The pathogenesis of osteoporosis associated with primary biliary cirrhosis is poorly understood, but it may develop as a consequence of reduced bone formation or increased bone resorption in the setting of progressive cholestasis.

No medical therapies have been uniformly effective at preventing and treating osteoporosis. Patients with significant steatorrhea are at risk for calcium and vitamin D malabsorption. All patients with normal serum calcium and vitamin D levels should receive 1500 mg of calcium and 1000 IU of vitamin D daily, whereas patients with significant vitamin D deficiency require 25 000 to 50 000 units of vitamin D, two to three times per week. Furthermore, all patients are encouraged to stop smoking and exercise in moderation. Estrogen replacement may be beneficial in postmenopausal patients and does not appear to worsen cholestasis, especially if the transdermal preparation is used. The role of biphosphonates (alendronate and etidronate) for patients with osteopenia is not clear, but early studies appear promising. Calcitonin has not been shown to improve osteoporosis associated with cholestatic liver disease. Orthotopic liver transplantation is recommended for primary biliary cirrhosis patients with progressive osteopenia. Even though bone density decreases shortly after orthotopic liver transplantation, T scores approach those of healthy controls approximately 2 years after transplantation as a result of improved hepatic function, corticosteroid reduction, and increased mobility.

Pruritus is a significant problem in many patients with primary biliary cirrhosis. Antihistamines, phenobarbital, and UDCA are not uniformly effective. Pruritus improves in 90% of patients who receive either cholestyramine or colestipol. Bile-acid binding agents are preferably taken before and after breakfast for best results. For patients who do not respond to bile-acid binders, rifampin (300–600 mg/day) has been shown to be effective within 1 month of administration. Endogenous opioid antagonists (naloxone, nalmaphene, and naltrexone) may also be effective in selected patients with primary biliary cirrhosis and disabling pruritus who do not respond to the above measures. Plasmapheresis may help some patients with disabling pruritus. Orthotopic liver transplantation is reserved for patients with intractable pruritus and evidence of impaired hepatic reserve.

Fat-soluble vitamin deficiency is seen in 20% of patients and is proportional to the degree of cholestasis and hepatic synthetic dysfunction. Lower vitamin levels are associated with stage III or IV disease and Mayo risk scores above 5. Reduced bile-acid delivery to the small intestine is the primary mechanism responsible for the malabsorption of fat-soluble vitamins. Twenty percent of patients with primary biliary cirrhosis have vitamin A deficiency, but most patients are asymptomatic and do not have night blindness. Vitamin A replacement (10 000 to 25 000 units daily or 25 000 to 50 000 units, two to three times weekly) is recommended and follow-up of serum levels is required. Vitamin D deficiency is seen in 13% of patients with primary biliary cirrhosis, but osteomalacia is rare. Patients with a significant deficiency require replacement with vitamin D plus supplemental calcium and close follow-up of serum vitamin D levels. Vitamin E deficiency is rarely seen in the adult population, but a significant deficiency is associated with reduced proprioception and gait disturbance. Daily doses between 400 and 1000 units are usually sufficient to replace losses. Prolongation of the prothrombin time in patients without cirrhosis is usually the result of vitamin K malabsorption, which corrects after parenteral vitamin K administration.

Eighty-five percent of patients with primary biliary cirrhosis have hypercholesterolemia. Stage I or II disease is associated with elevated HDL cholesterol, whereas advanced disease is associated with a fall in HDL cholesterol and a rise in the LDL fraction. Patients with hyperlipidemia are not at increased risk for cardiovascular events. Ursodeoxycholic acid has been shown to reduce and increase LDL and HDL cholesterol levels respectively.

Steatorrhea is not uncommon in patients with advanced primary biliary cirrhosis. Decreased bile-acid delivery, pancreatic insufficiency, celiac disease, and bacterial overgrowth, either alone or in combination, play a role in fat malabsorption. Low-fat diets with or without medium chain triglyceride supplementation is recommended for patients with luminal bile-acid deficiency, whereas pancreatic enzyme supplementation is appropriate for patients with impaired pancreatic function. Gluten-free diets and antibiotic therapy are recommended for primary biliary cirrhosis patients with celiac disease and bacterial overgrowth respectively.

Natural history and prognosis

Primary biliary cirrhosis usually progresses over 15 to 20 years. Survival of patients with asymptomatic disease is less than that of controls matched for age, race, and gender, however, asymptomatic patients live longer than patients with symptomatic disease. Median survival for patients with asymptomatic and symptomatic primary biliary cirrhosis is 10 to 16 years and 7.5 to 10 years respectively. Between 40% and 100% of asymptomatic patients develop symptoms within 2 to 4 years of diagnosis. No variables have been definitively associated with the progression from asymptomatic to symptomatic primary biliary cirrhosis. Numerous prognostic models have been developed which aid the clinician in terms of predicting patient survival without orthotopic liver transplantation and timing of orthotopic liver transplantation. The most popular model is the Mayo model which uses five variables – age, total bilirubin, albumin, prothrombin time, and edema. Bilirubin is the most important variable in predicting disease severity and the need to consider orthotopic liver transplantation. Unfortunately, the Mayo model does not take into account intercurrent events such as variceal hemorrhage, the development of hepatocellular carcinoma, or quality of life parameters.

Primary sclerosing cholangitis

Key features

- Primary sclerosing cholangitis is a chronic cholestatic liver disease that primarily affects young to middle aged males.
- Immunologic mechanisms may be important in the pathogenesis of primary sclerosing cholangitis.
- Patients are at risk for bacterial cholangitis, cholangiocarcinoma, and complications attributable to liver failure, portal hypertension or chronic cholestasis.
- Fibrous cholangitis and fibro-obliterative lesions are characteristic of primary sclerosing cholangitis.
- Medical therapies are not effective in preventing progression of the disease.
- Liver transplantation is recommended for patients with marginal hepatic reserve and complications of portal hypertension or chronic cholestasis.

History and overview

Primary sclerosing cholangitis was rarely reported before 1980. Delbet was credited with the first description of the disease and increased recognition of primary sclerosing cholangitis has been primarily attributable to advances in cholangiography. Primary sclerosing cholangitis is a progressive chronic cholestatic liver disease that primarily affects young to middle aged males. Genetic, environmental, immunologic, and non-immunologic mechanisms may be important in disease pathogenesis. Primary sclerosing cholangitis is frequently associated with inflammatory bowel disease, especially ulcerative colitis. Diffuse fibrosing inflammatory destruction of the intrahepatic and/or extrahepatic bile ducts

eventually results in progressive cholestasis, secondary biliary cirrhosis, and complications related to liver failure, portal hypertension, or chronic cholestasis. Cholangiocarcinoma is an ever-present risk for patients with long-standing primary sclerosing cholangitis. A diagnosis of primary sclerosing cholangitis is based on clinical, biochemical, cholangiographic, and histologic criteria; secondary causes of sclerosing cholangitis require exclusion before a diagnosis of primary sclerosing cholangitis can be made confidently. As for patients with primary biliary cirrhosis, prognostic models can assist the clinician in defining the natural history of the disease, predicting patient survival, evaluating the efficacy of treatment protocols, and determining the appropriate time for orthotopic liver transplantation evaluation. Medical therapy is generally ineffective in preventing progression of the disease. Orthotopic liver transplantation is the standard of care for patients with decompensated liver disease and associated complications.

Epidemiology

Males with primary sclerosing cholangitis outnumber females by a ratio of 2:1. The median age of patients is 40 years, and the clinical presentation is similar between genders and races. An incidence of 2 to 7 cases of primary sclerosing cholangitis per 100 000 population is commonly quoted, but this may be an underestimate as not all patients with primary sclerosing cholangitis have abnormal liver function tests or present with symptomatic disease.

Pathogenesis

The pathogenesis of primary sclerosing cholangitis is not entirely clear. Genetic, immune, and non-immune factors have been evaluated and these will be discussed individually.

Even though the pathogenesis of primary sclerosing cholangitis is unknown, genetic and immune factors are thought to play an important role. Primary sclerosing cholangitis can develop in multiple family members. As for patients with primary biliary cirrhosis, molecular mimicry may also be important. Viruses or xenobiotics are thought to present antigens similar to those on the biliary epithelial cell followed by autoimmune destruction of the intrahepatic and extrahepatic bile ducts of genetically predisposed individuals.

Abnormalities in the cellular immune response are commonly seen in patients with primary sclerosing cholangitis. A low number of circulating T cells caused by a disproportionate decrease in CD8 suppressor/cytotoxic cells with an increase in the CD4:CD8 ratio is commonly observed in patients with sclerosing cholangitis. Furthermore, an increase in the absolute number and percentage of circulating B cells is observed. CD4 cells are the predominant lymphocytes within the portal tracts, but CD8 cells can also be seen. Normal bile ducts express HLA class I antigen but do not express HLA class II antigen; increased expression of HLA class I antigens and aberrant expression of HLA class II antigens and ICAM-1 on biliary epithelial cells are found in patients with primary sclerosing cholangitis. Presentation of alloantigens or autoantigens to class II restricted T lymphocytes followed by immune-mediated destruction of the intrahepatic and extrahepatic bile ducts is thought to be important in the pathogenesis of primary sclerosing cholangitis.

In addition to abnormalities in the cellular immune response, patients with primary sclerosing cholangitis frequently have a variety of autoantibodies, but their relevance to disease pathogenesis is not clear. Antinuclear antibodies and antismooth muscle antibodies are present in 30% to 70% and 15% to 75% of patients respectively. Over 70% of patients with primary sclerosing cholangitis have elevated perinuclear antineutrophil cytoplasmic antibody (pANCA) titers; unfortunately, elevated titers can also be seen in patients with autoimmune hepatitis and primary biliary cirrhosis. Mitochondrial antibodies are usually not detectable in patients with sclerosing cholangitis. Increased serum IgM and circulating immune complexes, reduced hepatic clearance of immune complexes, and activation of the complement system are also observed. Human leukocyte antigens A1, B8, DR2, DR3, DRw52a, and DR4 have been associated with primary sclerosing cholangitis, and HLA-DR4 may be associated with more aggressive disease.

In addition to genetic and immune hypotheses, non-immune theories have also been suggested. Bacteria and endotoxins released into the portal circulation from the inflamed colon of patients with inflammatory bowel disease were originally thought to be important; however, significant bacteremia and endotoxemia were not present in patients presenting with chronic ulcerative colitis. Since primary sclerosing cholangitis may exist without inflammatory bowel disease, or years before the development of inflammatory bowel disease, and sclerosing cholangitis may also occur years after colectomy for ulcerative colitis, it is thought that portal infection is not important in the pathogenesis of primary sclerosing cholangitis. Cytomegalovirus and reoviral infections have also been proposed as causes of sclerosing cholangitis, but no study has fully supported this theory. Hepatotoxic bile acids (e.g. lithocholic acid) have also been evaluated, but no study supports a role for bile salts in the pathogenesis of biliary tract injury. Finally, as the biliary tree receives its blood supply from branches off the hepatic artery, ischemic injury has also been suggested as a cause of primary sclerosing cholangitis; however, no studies have fully supported this concept.

Clinical features

The clinical presentation of patients with primary sclerosing cholangitis is highly variable (Box 6.4). Between 15% and 45% of patients are asymptomatic and present with cholestatic liver indices during health maintenance examinations or during evaluation for other diseases; however, most patients will ultimately develop symptoms associated with progressive disease. Fatigue, jaundice, pruritus, and abdominal pain are present in 75%, 30% to 65%, 25% to 70%, and 16% to 37% of patients respectively. Less frequent manifestations include fever (35%), ascites (2% to 10%), gastrointestinal bleeding from esophagogastric varices (2% to 14%), bacterial cholangitis (5% to 28%), hyperpigmentation (25%), xanthomas and xanthelasma (4%), weight loss (10% to 40%), hepatosplenomegaly (30% to 55%), gallbladder and common bile-duct

---

Box 6.4 Clinical features of primary sclerosing cholangitis

Symptoms
  fatigue
  jaundice
  pruritus
  abdominal pain
  fever
  weight loss

Physical findings
  hepatomegaly
  splenomegaly
  jaundice
  hyperpigmentation

cholesterol and pigment stones (25% to 30%), and hepatocellular carcinoma (rare). As for patients with primary biliary cirrhosis, complications of cholestasis can develop (Box 6.5), these include fat-soluble vitamin deficiency, hypercholesterolemia, and steatorrhea. Patients with primary sclerosing cholangitis are also susceptible to either osteoporosis or osteomalacia. Even though osteodystrophy is more commonly seen in patients with primary biliary cirrhosis, 50% of patients with end-stage primary sclerosing cholangitis are below the fracture threshold at the time of transplantation, and one third of patients with significant osteopenia will develop fractures after orthotopic liver transplantation. Dual energy X-ray absorptiometry should be performed in all patients with primary sclerosing cholangitis and evidence of significant cholestasis. Patients with decompensated cirrhosis are at risk for portal hypertensive complications that include bleeding from esophageal or gastric varices, ascites, encephalopathy, and bleeding from peristomal varices after colectomy for inflammatory bowel disease.

Between 4% and 20% of patients with primary sclerosing cholangitis will develop cholangiocarcinoma. Patients with malignancy can present with progressive jaundice, anorexia, weight loss, and abdominal pain. The common hepatic duct and its bifurcation are most commonly involved. Risk factors for cholangiocarcinoma include older age, the duration and stage of liver disease, the duration of inflammatory bowel disease and associated dysplasia, smoking, alcohol use, and a carbohydrate antigen (CA 19–9) greater than 100 U/mL. A variety of tests have been employed in the evaluation of patients with suspected cholangiocarcinoma, but unfortunately no test is truly reliable. Ultrasound and CT scanning are insensitive non-invasive tests for early disease. Furthermore, biliary brush cytology is only 50% sensitive for cholangiocarcinoma. An index that uses CA 19–9 and carcinoembryonic antigen has been shown to be 67% sensitive and 100% specific for malignancy when the value

exceeds 400 units. More recently, a CA 19–9 threshold of 100 U/mL has been shown to be 89% sensitive and 86% specific for diagnosing cholangiocarcinoma. At the present time, tumor markers have limited utility in diagnosing cholangiocarcinoma at an early, potentially treatable stage. The role of positron emission tomography (PET) in the evaluation of patients with suspected cholangiocarcinoma is not clear and will require additional studies. Therapeutic options for patients with cholangiocarcinoma are limited but include resection, systemic chemotherapy, and radiation. Novel protocols using 5-fluorouracil, external beam radiation, brachytherapy, staging laparotomy, followed by orthotopic liver transplantation are currently underway and may be effective in carefully selected patients, however, long-term results will need to be carefully evaluated. Long-term survival is poor after orthotopic liver transplantation for patients with primary sclerosing cholangitis and cholangiocarcinoma. Consequently, cholangiocarcinoma is a relative or absolute contraindication to liver replacement.

Primary sclerosing cholangitis can coexist with other autoimmune liver diseases. Autoimmune hepatitis and primary sclerosing cholangitis overlap is predominantly seen in children and young adults. Patients with an overlap syndrome typically have cholangiographic and histologic findings consistent with primary sclerosing cholangitis and necroinflammatory activity within portal tracts and bridging necrosis consistent with autoimmune hepatitis. Other features of autoimmune hepatitis include elevated gamma globulins, IgG, antinuclear antibodies, antismooth muscle antibodies, and aminotransferases.

Patients with primary sclerosing cholangitis frequently have other diseases that may have an autoimmune basis. Inflammatory bowel disease is present in 75% to 90% of patients with primary sclerosing cholangitis, and primary sclerosing cholangitis is present in 2% to 7% of patients with inflammatory bowel disease. Eighty-seven percent of patients with primary sclerosing cholangitis and inflammatory bowel disease have ulcerative colitis, and 13% of patients have Crohn's colitis. Small-bowel Crohn's disease alone has not been associated with primary sclerosing cholangitis. Inflammatory bowel disease in primary sclerosing cholangitis patients is usually a quiescent, pancolitis. Patients with primary sclerosing cholangitis and ulcerative colitis have a greater risk of developing cholangiocarcinoma and adenocarcinoma of the colon when compared to patients who have either biliary tract disease or colitis alone. There is no

---

Box 6.5 Complications of primary sclerosing cholangitis

Steatorrhea and malabsorption
Hepatic osteodystrophy
Ascites
Variceal bleeding
Hepatic encephalopathy
Cholangiocarcinoma

relationship between the clinical course of inflammatory bowel disease and that of primary sclerosing cholangitis. Proctocolectomy should not be performed with the intent of altering the natural course of biliary tract disease. If a colectomy is required for inflammatory bowel disease refractory to medical therapy, the ileoanal pouch procedure is preferred to avoid the risk of peristomal variceal formation associated with a conventional ileostomy. Acute and chronic pancreatitis, diabetes mellitus, the sicca syndrome, autoimmune thyroid disease, retroperitoneal fibrosis, celiac sprue, autoimmune hemolytic anemia, immune thrombocytopenic purpura, systemic lupus erythematosus, rheumatoid arthritis, vasculitis, and systemic sclerosis can also be seen. Polymyositis, ankylosing spondylitis, myasthenia gravis, angioimmunoblastic lymphadenopathy, and membranous glomerulonephritis are rarely observed.

Diagnosis

The diagnosis of primary sclerosing cholangitis is based on clinical, biochemical, cholangiographic, and histologic criteria. As with primary biliary cirrhosis, no one test should be used alone to make a diagnosis.

Biochemical and serologic tests

Liver function tests reveal a typical cholestatic pattern. As in primary biliary cirrhosis, the alkaline phosphatase is usually greater than three to five times the upper limit of normal, whereas the aminotransferases are more commonly less than three times the upper normal limit. The serum bilirubin may be normal or elevated with early disease, but it usually rises steadily with disease progression. A sudden rise in the bilirubin suggests biliary obstruction with inspissated bile, common bile-duct stones, a dominant stricture, or cholangiocarcinoma. A variety of autoantibodies are commonly observed in primary sclerosing cholangitis patients, but they serve no role in diagnosis. Antineutrophil cytoplasmic antibodies are present in 80% of patients, whereas antinuclear and antismooth muscle antibodies can be seen in low titer in 20% of patients. Low titer antimitochondrial antibodies may also be seen in 5% of patients. As in other patients with chronic liver disease, impaired hepatic reserve is associated with a fall in albumin and prolongation of the prothrombin time.

Medical imaging

Cholangiography remains the gold standard for diagnosis of primary sclerosing cholangitis. Endoscopic retrograde cholangiopancreatography (ERCP) is the initial procedure of choice. Percutaneous transhepatic cholangiography should be reserved for patients in whom ERCP cannot be successfully accomplished. At the time of cholangiography, brushings for cytology, and balloon dilation with stenting of dominant strictures can also be performed. Magnetic resonance cholangiography (MRC) is a non-invasive imaging test that is 88% sensitive and 97% specific for detecting primary sclerosing cholangitis involving larger order bile ducts. Even though MRC is not as effective as ERCP in evaluating disease of smaller, third and forth order bile ducts, MRC is superior to ERCP for assessing disease proximal to a dominant stricture. The accuracy of MRC for detecting cholangiocarcinoma has not been determined. Distinguishing benign from malignant strictures can be difficult, but PET scanning may be useful. As with MRC, additional studies will be necessary to assess the utility of PET in the armamentarium of diagnostic tests.

Diffuse multifocal strictures of the intrahepatic and/or extrahepatic bile ducts are seen in approximately 90% of patients (see Figure 6.2). Short segments of normal-appearing bile ducts or diver-

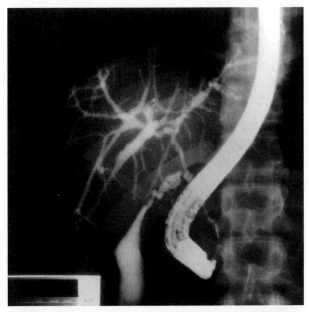

Figure 6.2 Primary sclerosing cholangitis. Endoscopic retrograde cholangiopancreatography demonstrating diffuse intra- and extrahepatic strictures (reproduced with permission of Dr Irving Waxman).

ticulum-like outpouchings can be seen between biliary strictures giving the classic beaded appearance on cholangiography. The gallbladder and cystic duct are also involved in 15% of patients. Markedly dilated bile ducts in the presence of a dominant stricture or mass suggest cholangiocarcinoma. Before a diagnosis of primary sclerosing cholangitis can be made, secondary causes of biliary strictures require exclusion; hepatic metastases, cirrhosis, polycystic liver disease, and lymphoma can produce strictures that resemble primary sclerosing cholangitis. Ten percent of patients will have disease limited to the interlobular and septal bile ducts within the liver. Normal cholangiograms and liver biopsies consistent with sclerosing cholangitis are typical of patients with small-duct primary sclerosing cholangitis. As with primary biliary cirrhosis, ultrasonography, CT, and MRI are used primarily to assess for other causes of cholestasis such as gallstones or pancreaticobiliary malignancies.

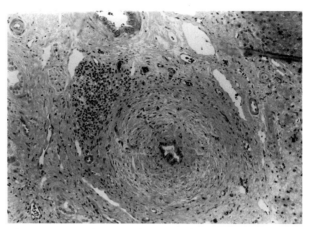

Figure 6.3 Primary sclerosing cholangitis. Liver biopsy specimen showing an interlobular bile duct with concentric fibrosis and focal chronic inflammation (hematoxylin and eosin × 150). (Photograph courtesy of Dr Sugantha Govindarajan.)

Pathology

On gross inspection, the explants of patients transplanted for primary sclerosing cholangitis are bile stained and cirrhotic. Thickening and luminal narrowing of bile ducts and intrahepatic cholangiectases can also be appreciated.

Liver biopsy is complementary to cholangiography in the evaluation of patients with suspected primary sclerosing cholangitis. Even though cholangiography is the gold standard for diagnosis, biopsy is useful for determining the stage of disease and patient prognosis. As with primary biliary cirrhosis, four histologic stages have been described.

- Stage I (portal stage) is associated with portal hepatitis and edema. Fibrosis does not extend beyond the limiting plate. Lymphocytes, plasma cells, and neutrophils surround the interlobular and septal bile ducts. Concentric (periductal) fibrosis can also be seen with stage I disease (see Figure 6.3).
- Periportal inflammation extending beyond the limiting plate with piecemeal necrosis, ductular proliferation, ductopenia, and mild portal fibrosis with thin radiating septa is characteristic of stage II (periportal stage).
- Portal-to-portal septal fibrosis, bridging necrosis, and prominent cholestasis define Stage III (septal stage).
- Stage IV (cirrhotic stage) is associated with regenerative nodules and biliary cirrhosis.

Liver biopsies are subject to sampling error and are not generally required for a diagnosis of primary sclerosing cholangitis. Fibrous cholangitis and fibro-obliterative lesions of the interlobular and septal bile ducts are characteristically seen in less than one third of patients. Whereas CD4-positive T cells are prominently seen within the portal area, CD8-positive cells are more commonly seen in areas of piecemeal necrosis.

Differential diagnosis

Many other diseases can produce findings similar to those of primary sclerosing cholangitis (Box 6.6). AIDS cholangiopathy, choledocholithiasis, congenital biliary tract disease, previous biliary tract surgery, biliary malignancy (unless a previous diagnosis of primary sclerosing cholangitis has been established), and ischemic bile-duct injury can produce cholangiographic findings similar to those of primary sclerosing cholangitis. Hepatic arterial chemotherapy with fluoxuridine, cirrhosis not related to primary sclerosing cholangitis, submassive hepatic necrosis, amyloidosis, metastatic carcinoma, and hepatic infiltration with leukemia or lymphoma can also resemble primary sclerosing cholangitis. Secondary causes of sclerosing cholangitis produce intrahepatic and/or extrahepatic strictures on cholangiography similar to those of patients with primary sclerosing cholangitis.

Box 6.6 Differential diagnosis of primary sclerosing cholangitis

Choledocholithiasis
AIDS cholangiopathy
Congenital biliary tract disease
Previous biliary surgery
Biliary malignancy
Ischemic biliary injury
Metastatic carcinoma
Hepatic infiltrative diseases

Treatment

As for patients with primary biliary cirrhosis, survival of patients with asymptomatic and symptomatic primary sclerosing cholangitis is inferior to that of healthy controls. Consequently, medical or surgical treatment is warranted for all patients with sclerosing cholangitis. Unfortunately, no medical treatment has been shown conclusively to alter the natural course of primary sclerosing cholangitis. The overall goals of treatment are to slow progression of primary sclerosing cholangitis and to treat symptoms of cholestasis or complications of portal hypertension.

Medical therapy of primary sclerosing cholangitis

As with primary biliary cirrhosis, the goal of medical treatment for patients with primary sclerosing cholangitis is to treat both the underlying disease and complications associated with cholestasis and portal hypertension. Many different medications have been tried without clear benefit on the clinical expression of primary sclerosing cholangitis, liver function tests, cholangiographic or histologic parameters, or time to liver failure. Colchicine, cyclosporine, methotrexate, penicillamine, tacrolimus, corticosteroids, azathioprine, pentoxifylline, nicotine, and budesonide are not uniformly effective in halting or reversing the underlying process. Most patients with primary sclerosing cholangitis are diagnosed at a later fibrotic stage. Consequently, one would expect that medical therapies would not be effective in this population. Future studies should address risk factors for primary sclerosing cholangitis, screen for early inflammatory disease, and enroll patients early in controlled clinical trials with prolonged follow-up.

Ursodeoxycholic acid is effective therapy for patients with primary biliary cirrhosis, but unfortunately most trials to date have shown limited efficacy for patients with primary sclerosing cholangitis. Ursodeoxycholic acid at a dose of 13 to 15 mg kg^{-1} day^{-1} for 6 years led to an improvement in biochemical parameters, but there was no improvement in either histology, or time to death or transplantation when compared to placebo. In a small controlled trial, UDCA at 20 mg kg^{-1} day^{-1} also led to an improvement in biochemical liver indices, but, unlike the Lindor study, histologic inflammatory parameters, cholangiographic appearance, and stage also improved with 2 years of follow-up. Ursodeoxycholic acid at 25 to 30 mg kg^{-1} day^{-1} was also shown to be more effective than 13 to 15 mg kg^{-1} day^{-1} with regards to improvement in liver function tests and the Mayo risk score. Projected survival at 4 years for patients on high-dose UDCA was superior to that of the low-dose regimen. Larger randomized controlled trials are warranted to see if the above findings translate into improved survival free of transplantation. Furthermore, future trials should address combination drug therapy with UDCA, methotrexate, antibiotics, and other immunmodulatory agents for patients with primary sclerosing cholangitis.

Medical treatment of complications

Patients with cholestasis may have dominant strictures of the common bile and common hepatic ducts that are amenable to endoscopic or radiologic dilation and stenting. Patients with dominant strictures require careful assessment to exclude cholangiocarcinoma. Surgical revision of the bile duct is generally not recommended for patients who are transplant candidates. Patients with primary sclerosing cholangitis and symptomatic cholelithiasis and choledocholithiasis may require cholecystectomy and sphincterotomy with stone extraction respectively. Patients who present with symptoms and signs consistent with bacterial cholangitis require either endoscopic or radiologic biliary drainage in conjunction with broad-spectrum antibiotics (e.g. ciprofloxacin, amoxicillin, or trimethoprim and sulfamethoxazole). Long-term antibiotic prophylaxis is justified for patients with recurrent bacterial infections. Low-fat diets and medium-chain triglycerides are appropriate for patients with significant steatorrhea secondary to reduced delivery of bile acids to the gut. Pancreatic enzyme supplements and gluten-free diets are recommended for patients with coexistent pancreatic insufficiency and celiac disease respectively. Vitamin A deficiency is seen in approximately 80% of patients with advanced disease and requires replacement as for patients with primary biliary cirrhosis. Vitamin D deficiency is present in 40% to 50% of patients with end-stage primary sclerosing cholangitis, but there is little data to support the routine use of vitamin D in patients with hepatic osteodystrophy who do not have osteomalacia. For patients with osteomalacia, 50 000 to 100 000 IU of vitamin D weekly is recommended with calcium supplementation. There is no data to recommend the routine use of calcitonin or biphosphonates outside controlled clinical trials. Estrogen replacement therapy should be given to postmenopausal females with primary sclerosing cholangitis. Vitamin E deficiency is rarely seen, but any deficiency should be corrected as appropriate. The prothrombin time will correct with parenteral vitamin K in patients with malabsorption. As for patients with primary biliary cirrhosis, a variety of agents have been used to treat pruritus associated with primary sclerosing cholangitis. Antihistamines are rarely helpful, but bile-acid binding agents are effective for most patients. Rifampin, methyltestosterone, phenobarbital, UDCA, S-adenosylmethionine, ondansetron, ultraviolet light, large-volume plasmapheresis, and opiate receptor antagonists have also been effective in selected patients.

The treatment of portal hypertensive complications in patients with decompensated primary sclerosing cholangitis is the same as for cirrhotic patients without sclerosing cholangitis. Encephalopathy is treated with lactulose and/or neomycin. Treatment of ascites includes sodium restriction, diuretics, large-volume paracentesis, and/or transjugular intrahepatic portosystemic shunts. Broad-spectrum antibiotics to cover both gram-positive and gram-negative organisms are required for patients with spontaneous bacterial peritonitis. Non-selective beta-blockers, endoscopic sclerotherapy or ligation, and transjugular intrahepatic portosystemic shunts are useful for the prevention and treatment of hemorrhage from esophageal or gastric varices. Transjugular intrahepatic portosystemic shunts and decompressive surgical shunts are also useful in patients who bleed from peristomal varices.

Biliary reconstruction

Surgical repair of dominant biliary strictures is generally not recommended for patients who are transplant candidates; longer operative times and greater intraoperative blood loss at transplantation are more commonly seen in patients who have undergone prior biliary surgery. In addition, patients are at increased risk for bacterial cholangitis after undergoing biliary reconstruction. For selected patients with stage I or II disease complicated by progressive cholestasis, recurrent bacterial cholangitis, jaundice, and pruritus not amenable to endoscopic or radiologic intervention, resection of dominant extrahepatic biliary strictures with hepaticojejunostomy and transhepatic stenting may be appropriate. The impact of biliary reconstruction on transplant-free survival and the development of cholangiocarcinoma is not clear.

Liver transplantation

Liver transplantation with Roux-en-Y choledochojejunostomy is the standard of care for primary sclerosing cholangitis patients with decompensated cirrhosis, complications of portal hypertension or cholestasis, and recurrent bacterial cholangitis. Patient survival at 1 and 5 years is 97% and 88% respectively. Patients should be considered for transplantation early in their course, preferably with a Mayo risk score below 4.4. Patients who are transplanted for primary sclerosing cholangitis are at increased risk for non-anastomotic biliary strictures, and acute and chronic rejection when compared to patients transplanted for other diseases. Primary sclerosing cholangitis may recur in the allograft in 20% of patients based upon clinical, biochemical, cholangiographic, and histologic criteria, but medium-term patient and graft survival are excellent. Before a diagnosis of recurrent primary sclerosing cholangitis can be made, other causes for post-transplant biliary strictures must be excluded, including hepatic arterial occlusion, ABO incompatibility between donor and recipient, prolonged cold ischemia time, chronic rejection, and infections. Annual colonoscopy with random biopsies is recommended for patients with ulcerative or Crohn's colitis after transplantation.

Natural history and prognosis

As with primary biliary cirrhosis, primary sclerosing cholangitis is a slowly progressive cholestatic liver disease. Over 75% of asymptomatic patients develop symptoms. Survival of patients with asymptomatic and symptomatic disease is shorter than that of healthy controls matched for age, gender, and race. The median survival of patients with primary sclerosing cholangitis from the time of diagnosis is 10 to 12 years without transplantation. Age, bilirubin, albumin, aspartate aminotransferase, and variceal bleeding are independent predictors of survival for patients with primary sclerosing cholangitis. The Child-Pugh classification appears to be as accurate as the Mayo primary sclerosing cholangitis model in predicting survival before transplantation. Prognostic models may assist the clinician in determining the need to consider orthotopic liver transplantation. Unfortunately, no prognostic model takes into account quality of life indicators or the development of cholangiocarcinoma.

Autoimmune hepatitis

Key features

- Autoimmune hepatitis primarily affects young women.
- Elevated liver function tests and hypergammaglobulinemia characterize autoimmune hepatitis.
- Active periportal inflammation, predominance of plasma cells, and varying degrees of fibrosis are typically seen.
- Three distinct subtypes of autoimmune hepatitis are based on autoantibody patterns.
- Autoimmune hepatitis is associated with other extrahepatic autoimmune diseases.
- Most patients respond to immunosuppressive medications with improvement in clinical symptoms, biochemical liver tests, hepatic histology, and patient survival.
- Liver transplantation is recommended for patients with decompensated liver disease with or without complications of portal hypertension.

History and overview

Kunkel and associates first described hepatitis of unclear etiology associated with hypergammaglobulinemia in 1951. Mackay, Taft, and Cowling further characterized the disease in 1956. The disorder was initially termed chronic active liver disease, autoimmune chronic active hepatitis, or lupoid hepatitis because of its association with the lupus erythematosus prep test. Autoantibodies were initially linked to autoimmune hepatitis in the mid-1960s, and immunosuppressive agents were used to treat the condition at that time. Prednisone was also shown to improve patient survival in two controlled studies in the early 1970s.

Autoimmune hepatitis is an inflammatory condition of the liver associated with altered immune regulation. Piecemeal necrosis and portal plasma cell infiltrates on liver biopsy, hypergammaglobulinemia, and the presence of autoantibodies are typically seen. The disease is also characterized by steroid responsiveness in most patients.

Epidemiology

Autoimmune hepatitis affects 100 000 to 200 000 people in the US. The mean annual incidence is 1.9 per 100 000, and the point prevalence is 16.9 per 100 000. Caucasian northern Europeans are more susceptible to autoimmune hepatitis than other patient groups. Women account for 70% of the cases, and 50% of the affected women are 40 years of age or younger.

Autoimmune hepatitis can occasionally occur in multiple family members. Relatives can also demonstrate hypergammaglobulinemia and the presence of autoantibodies.

Pathogenesis

Despite extensive research into autoimmune hepatitis, the exact cellular and humoral mechanisms involved in initiating and propagating liver-cell damage remain speculative. Presumably a genetically predisposed individual is exposed to a stimulus which triggers an autoimmune process directed towards the liver.

Genetic predisposition focuses on the major histocompatibility complex class II genes in the HLA-DR locus. Type 1 autoimmune hepatitis is associated with HLA-DR3 (DRB1˙0301) and HLA-DR4 (DRB1˙0401). Eighty-five percent of patients with type 1 autoimmune hepatitis have either HLA-DR3, HLA-DR4, or both. Patients with HLA-DR3 are younger, have a higher rate of treatment failure, are more likely to relapse after drug withdrawal, and are more likely to need liver transplantation. Patients with HLA-DR4 are typically older, have other concurrent autoimmune disorders, and respond better to steroid therapy. Type 2 autoimmune hepatitis has been associated with HLA-B14, HLA-DR3, HLA-DRB1˙0701, and HLA-C4A-QO. Human leukocyte antigen associations have not yet been established for type 3 autoimmune hepatitis.

Exogenous agents in genetically predisposed hosts may be important in the pathogenesis of disease. Hepatitis A, Epstein–Barr virus, and rubella have been implicated as triggering stimuli in susceptible patients. Furthermore, medications such as interferon may also initiate the autoimmune response.

Cell-mediated, antibody-dependent cytotoxicity and cytotoxic T lymphocytes are thought to be important in the pathogenesis of hepatic injury. T-lymphocyte regulatory disturbances exist which result in abnormal antigen-induced antibody production by B cells. Immunoglobulin G production by plasma cells leads to the formation of antigen–antibody complexes on the hepatocyte membranes. These immune complexes are subsequently targeted by natural killer cells and destroyed. The above process appears to be under the regulation of cytokines, especially interleukin-10 (IL-10). The specific antigens that are targeted vary by the subtype of autoimmune hepatitis. The autoantigen for type 1 autoimmune hepatitis has not yet been established. The target autoantigen in type 2 autoimmune hepatitis is cytochrome P450 IID6 (CYP2D6), and the autoantigen in type 3 autoimmune hepatitis appears to be a 50 kDa cytosolic protein. In addition to the above, cytokine-mediated differentiation of T helper cells into cytotoxic T lymphocytes can lead to cellular injury.

Clinical features

Subclassification

Three subtypes of autoimmune hepatitis have been proposed based on different autoantibody patterns (Table 6.1). Approximately 13% of cases can not be classified because of lack of typical autoantibodies. Type 1 (classic or lupoid) autoimmune hepatitis is the most common form of the disease. It represents approximately 80% of all cases of autoimmune hepatitis. Seventy percent of patients are women less than 40 years of age, and 15% to 30% have other autoimmune diseases. Type 2 autoimmune hepatitis (4% of cases) is much less common and affects mostly children. Patients with the type 2 variant frequently present with severe acute or fulminant disease. Type 2 autoimmune hepatitis also tends to progress more commonly to cirrhosis despite medical therapy. Approximately 40% of patients have other extrahepatic autoimmune diseases. Type 3 autoimmune hepatitis (3% of cases) is the least understood form of the disease. The frequency of extrahepatic autoimmune diseases is uncertain in this group of patients.

Clinical presentation

The clinical presentation of autoimmune hepatitis is extremely variable. Although generally a disease of insidious onset in young women, autoimmune hepatitis can present as a spectrum ranging from an asymptomatic condition to acute fulminant hepatitis. Approximately 25% of patients have cirrhosis at the time of diagnosis.

The common symptoms and physical findings at initial presentation are outlined in Box 6.7. Fatigue is the most common symptom and affects 85% of patients. Jaundice can also be seen in 77% of patients. Approximately 50% of patients report some degree of right upper quadrant pain. Other complaints include pruritus (36%), polymyalgias (30%), anorexia (30%), and diarrhea (28%). Amenorrhea occurs frequently in young women, mostly in association with severe disease.

Physical findings include hepatomegaly and splenomegaly in 78% and 45% of patients respectively. Spider angiomata (58%), jaundice (50%), ascites (20%), and hepatic encephalopathy (14%) are seen in patients with severe or long-standing disease.

Autoimmune hepatitis can present with concurrent autoimmune disorders in up to 40% of cases. Autoimmune thyroid disease, rheumatoid arthritis, and chronic ulcerative colitis are frequently seen. Thyroid disorders are the most common affecting 57% of patients (43% with Hashimoto's thyroiditis and 14% with Grave's disease). Of the different subtypes, type 2 autoimmune hepatitis is most commonly identified with extrahepatic autoimmune disorders. Moreover, patients with HLA-DR4 have concurrent autoimmune diseases more frequently than patients who lack this genetic marker.

Diagnosis

The diagnosis of autoimmune hepatitis is based upon clinical, biochemical, serologic, and histologic criteria. A definitive diagnosis requires the exclusion of other types of liver disease that can mimic autoimmune hepatitis. Criteria for diagnosing autoimmune hepatitis were established by the International Autoimmune Hepatitis Group in 1993, and subsequently revised in 1999 (Table 6.2). These diagnostic criteria allow for the classification of autoimmune hepatitis as "probable" or "definite" based on objective information. The scoring system can also be used to diagnose autoimmune hepatitis after treatment with immunosuppressive medications.

Table 6.1   Subclassification of autoimmune hepatitis

Features	Type 1	Type 2	Type 3
Autoantibodies	ANA[1], SMA[2]	Anti-LKM[3]-1	Anti-SLA/LP[4]
Age onset (mean)	40 years	25 years	35 years
Proportion of patients who are women	70%	90%	90%
Extrahepatic immune disorders	15%–30%	40%	?
Autoantigen	?	Cytochrome P450 IID6	50 kDa protein
Steroid response	70%	40%–70%	90%–100%
Progression to cirrhosis	40%	80%	?

[1] *antinuclear antibodies.*
[2] *smooth muscle antibodies.*
[3] *liver-kidney-microsomal antibodies.*
[4] *antibodies to soluble liver antigen/liver-pancreas.*

Box 6.7   Clinical features of autoimmune hepatitis

Symptoms
  fatigue
  amenorrhea
  jaundice
  right upper quadrant pain
  polymyalgia
  anorexia

Physical findings
  hepatomegaly
  splenomegaly
  jaundice
  ascites
  encephalopathy

A pretreatment score of more than 15 is defined as definite and a score of 10 to 15 is defined as probable for autoimmune hepatitis. A post-treatment score of more than 17 is defined as definite, whereas a score of 12 to 17 is defined as probable for autoimmune hepatitis.

The diagnostic scoring system has been validated and shown to have a sensitivity of 98% and a specificity of 97% for patients with definite autoimmune hepatitis. The scoring system is not as accurate for patients with probable autoimmune hepatitis or overlap syndromes (autoimmune hepatitis in the presence of primary biliary cirrhosis or primary sclerosing cholangitis).

Biochemical tests

The principal biochemical abnormalities at presentation are elevations of the aminotransferases and hypergammaglobulinemia. Up to 16% of patients will have aspartate aminotransferase and/or alanine aminotransferase levels exceeding 1000 U/L. More than 85% of patients will also have a polyclonal hypergammaglobulinemia. Hyperbilirubinemia is extremely common but only exceeds 3 mg/dL in 46% of patients with autoimmune hepatitis. Elevations in alkaline phosphatase are also common, but values exceeding two times and ten times the upper limit of normal are seen in only 33% and 10% of patients respectively.

Serology

Many autoantibodies are identified with autoimmune hepatitis. These autoantibodies define the various types of autoimmune hepatitis, but are not disease or liver specific, and do not appear to be directly pathogenic.

Type 1 autoimmune hepatitis is identified by elevated titers of antinuclear antibodies, antismooth muscle antibodies, and pANCA. Antinuclear antibodies (median titer of 1:320) are found in 74% of patients with type 1 autoimmune hepatitis. Immunofluorescence can demonstrate either a homogeneous or speckled pattern; the speckled pattern occurs in younger patients and is associated with higher aminotransferase levels. Antinuclear antibodies can also be seen with primary biliary cirrhosis, primary sclerosing cholangitis, viral hepatitis, and drug-induced hepatitis, but titers are generally lower with these disorders. Antismooth muscle antibodies are the principal autoantibodies in type 1 autoimmune hepatitis. They occur alone or with antinuclear antibodies in 25% to 35% and 86% to 91% of cases respectively. The median titer at presentation is 1:160. Antiactin antibodies (a subset of smooth muscle antibodies) have been

Table 6.2 Scoring criteria for autoimmune hepatitis

Female sex	+ 2
Alk phos – AST (ALT) ratio	
> 3	− 2
< 1.5	+ 2
Gamma globulin or immunoglobulin G levels	
> 2	+ 3
1.5–2	+ 2
1–1.4	+ 1
Antimitochondrial antibodies	− 4
Antinuclear antibodies, smooth muscle antibodies, or anti-liver-kidney-microsomal 1	
> 1:80	+ 3
1:80	+ 2
1:40	+ 1
< 1:40	0
Viral serologies	
positive	− 3
negative	+ 3
Hepatotoxic drugs	
yes	− 4
no	+ 1
Alcohol use	
< 25 g/day	+ 2
> 60 g/day	− 2
Human leukocyte antigen DR3 or human leukocyte antigen DR4	+ 1
Concurrent autoimmune disease	+ 2
Other liver-related autoantibodies	+ 2
Interface hepatitis	+ 3
Plasmacytic infiltrate	+ 1
Rosettes	+ 1
No characteristic biopsy features	− 5
Biliary changes on biopsy	− 3
Other biopsy features (e.g. fat, etc.)	− 3
Treatment response	+ 2
Treatment relapse	+ 3

associated with a poorer prognosis. Perinuclear anti-neutrophil cytoplasmic antibodies are present in 50% to 92% of patients with type 1 autoimmune hepatitis.

Type 2 autoimmune hepatitis is associated with antibodies to LKM1. The target autoantigen for LKM1 is cytochrome P450 IID6 (CYP2D6). Only 4% of adults with autoimmune hepatitis in the US have anti-LKM; however, this antibody is seen in up to 20% of cases of autoimmune hepatitis in Europe. Anti-LKM is not specific to autoimmune hepatitis, as 10% of patients with hepatitis C have anti-LKM1. Anti-LKM2 is associated with drug-induced hepatitis, and anti-LKM3 is associated with hepatitis D.

Type 3 autoimmune hepatitis is identified by antibodies to soluble liver antigen (anti-SLA). Anti-SLA are identical to antibodies to liver-pancreas (anti-LP). Consequently, antibodies in patients with type 3 autoimmune hepatitis are now referred to as anti-SLA/LP. The target autoantigen for anti-SLA/LP is a 50-kDa cytosolic protein. Though mostly associated with type 3 autoimmune hepatitis, anti-SLA/LP can be seen in 11% of patients with type 1 autoimmune hepatitis. Anti-SLA/LP may also be seen in patients previously diagnosed with cryptogenic hepatitis, as 26% of them will be anti-SLA/LP positive.

Antibodies to asialoglycoprotein receptors (anti-ASGPR) are present in all types of autoimmune hepatitis. Over 80% of patients with type 1 autoimmune hepatitis are anti-ASGPR positive. Titers correlate with activity and may rise in the face of impending relapse.

Medical imaging

Medical imaging does not play a significant role in the diagnosis of autoimmune hepatitis. Ultrasound, CT, or MRI can suggest the presence of portal hypertension or cirrhosis, based on findings of a small and nodular liver, venous collaterals, ascites, or splenomegaly. As in other patients with chronic liver disease complicated by cirrhosis, non-invasive imaging is recommended to screen for the development of hepatocellular carcinoma.

Pathology

The hallmark pathologic findings of autoimmune hepatitis are piecemeal necrosis or interface hepatitis, plasma cell infiltrates, and lobular inflammation (see Figure 6.4). Various stages of fibrosis can also be seen. Up to 25% of patients have cirrhosis at the time of diagnosis. The above findings can be seen with hepatitis C but they are more common and more specific for autoimmune hepatitis. Piecemeal necrosis is seen in 84% and 77%, moderate-to-severe lobular activity in 47% and 16%, and plasma cells in 66% and 21% of patients with autoimmune hepatitis and hepatitis C respectively. Overall, biopsy specimens are 81% specific with a positive predictive value of 68% for autoimmune hepatitis.

Bile-duct abnormalities can be seen in autoimmune hepatitis. Up to 26% of patients exhibit evidence of cholangitis and/or ductopenia. However, these features are more often associated with overlap syndromes between autoimmune hepatitis and primary biliary cirrhosis, or autoimmune hepatitis and primary sclerosing cholangitis.

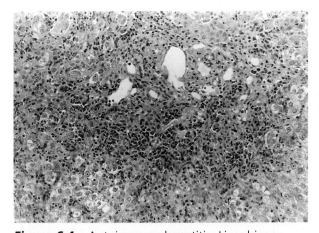

Figure 6.4 Autoimmune hepatitis. Liver biopsy specimen showing a portal tract with inflammation and piecemeal necrosis. Significant numbers of plasma cells are seen (hematoxylin and eosin × 100) (reproduced with permission of Dr Sugantha Govindarajan).

Differential diagnosis

Many diseases associated with hepatocellular inflammation need to be excluded prior to establishing the diagnosis of autoimmune hepatitis (Box 6.8). Historical features, biochemical liver indices, serology, and possibly liver biopsy are required. Furthermore, overlap syndromes between autoimmune hepatitis and primary sclerosing cholangitis or primary biliary cirrhosis exist which can be extremely difficult to separate from autoimmune hepatitis alone.

Treatment

The indications for treatment of autoimmune hepatitis are sustained abnormalities in the amino-transferases (at least five times the upper limit of normal), elevations of serum gamma globulin (at least two times the upper limit of normal), significant fatigue, arthralgias, jaundice, or the presence of active bridging necrosis on liver biopsy. The treatment of patients with mild histologic abnormalities, a mild aberration in liver function tests, or inactive cirrhosis is controversial. The goal of treatment is to slow disease progression, prevent complications of cirrhosis, and postpone liver transplantation.

Medical therapy of autoimmune hepatitis

The mainstays of therapy are corticosteroids and azathioprine. Corticosteroids have been shown to improve clinical symptoms and signs of disease,

Box 6.8 Differential diagnosis of autoimmune hepatitis
Acute and chronic viral hepatitis
Medication-induced hepatitis
methyldopa
nitrofurantoin
oxyphenistatin
propylthiouracil
Alcoholic liver disease
Alpha-1-antitrypsin deficiency
Hemochromatosis
Non-alcoholic steatohepatitis
Primary biliary cirrhosis
Wilson's disease

hepatic inflammation, and survival in patients with significant autoimmune hepatitis. Life expectancy in treated patients is equivalent to age- and sex-matched controls. Patients with cirrhosis and active inflammation on biopsy respond as well to therapy as those without cirrhosis, but they have a higher risk of relapse. Patients with inactive cirrhosis do not respond well to immunosuppressive medications.

Prednisone, with or without azathioprine, should be used as first-line therapy. Various dosing regimens have been proposed. Generally prednisone monotherapy is initiated at 40 to 60 mg daily and tapered over a 4 to 6 week period to a maintenance dose of 15 to 20 mg daily. Combination regimens use 20 to 30 mg of prednisone with 0.5 to 1 mg/kg of azathioprine daily. Prednisone is withdrawn over 1 to 3 months or tapered to 5 to 10 mg daily. Azathioprine is increased to a maintenance dose of 1 to 2 mg/kg daily during this period. Regimens using only high-dose prednisone are appropriate if a short course of therapy is contemplated, the patient is or may become pregnant, or the patient has contraindications to azathioprine. However, high-dose prednisone alone is associated with a higher risk of complications when compared to combination therapy.

Side effects necessitating dose reduction or discontinuation occur in about 13% of patients. Patients with cirrhosis (25%) are more susceptible to complications when compared to those without (8%). Significant complications of steroid use, including osteoporosis, diabetes, hypertension, and psychosis, generally occur in patients on prolonged courses at doses exceeding 10 mg/day.

Prednisone and azathioprine can induce clinical, biochemical, and histologic remission in 70% to 80% of patients with classic autoimmune hepatitis within 2 years. The response rate for patients with type 2 autoimmune hepatitis is inferior to that of the classic variant. Despite rapid improvement in aminotransferase levels, histologic improvement may take up to 3 to 6 months. Consequently, therapy must be continued for at least 3 months beyond the time of biochemical remission in order to minimize the chance of relapse when the drug is withdrawn.

Treatment is continued until remission of the disease, deterioration despite therapy, development of drug toxicity, or failure to induce remission despite a long-term course of treatment. If remission is achieved, drug withdrawal should be considered after 12 to 24 months of therapy.

Unfortunately, complete and sustained remission of autoimmune hepatitis is uncommon, and occurs in only 17% of patients. The major problem is relapse following withdrawal of therapy. Fifty percent of patients will develop recurrent disease within 6 months of stopping therapy, and 70% will recur within 36 months of cessation of immunosuppression. Re-institution of therapy generally induces another remission, but relapse is common in patients who subsequently discontinue treatment. Patients who relapse should probably be maintained on the lowest dose of prednisone alone, azathioprine alone, or combination therapy necessary to keep biochemical and clinical parameters in the normal to near normal range. Any of the above regimens will be expected to give an 80% to 90% remission rate. Attempts to discontinue immunosuppressive medications should be considered for every patient after a long treatment course.

A liver biopsy should be considered prior to withdrawing medication, as histology may be helpful in predicting the risk of recurrent autoimmune hepatitis. The discontinuation of medication after resolution of inflammation is associated with a 20% risk of recurrence, whereas cessation of immunosuppression in patients with portal inflammation is associated with a 50% risk of recurrent disease. Patients who enter therapy with cirrhosis, or develop it during therapy, have an 87% to 100% risk of autoimmune hepatitis recurrence after medications are discontinued.

Incomplete response, defined as improvement in biochemical and clinical parameters without histologic improvement, occurs in approximately 13% of patients. A longer treatment schedule generally does not increase the rate of remission, but should probably be used to control the clinical and biochemical features of the disease. Use of the lowest possible doses is prudent to minimize side effects associated with corticosteroids and azathioprine over the long term.

Treatment failures despite therapy with conventional doses of corticosteroids, or corticosteroids with azathioprine, occur in 10% to 15% of patients. High-dose prednisone (30 to 60 mg/day) with or without azathioprine (2 mg kg^{-1} day^{-1}) can induce biochemical remission in more than 60% of patients within 2 years; however, histologic remission occurs in only 20% of patients. The benefit of increased immunosuppression must be weighed against the risk of significant side effects. The goal of therapy is to taper medications to the lowest doses needed to maintain biochemical and clinical improvement.

Several medications have been evaluated for patients who fail standard therapies. Cyclosporine, 6-mercaptopurine, cyclophosphamide, methotrexate,

UDCA, budesonide, mycophenolate mofetil, and tacrolimus are intuitively appealing but none of these agents has been proven conclusively to be effective in controlled clinical trials.

Despite therapy, patients with autoimmune hepatitis can progress to cirrhosis. Up to 40% of patients develop cirrhosis within 10 years of diagnosis. Cirrhosis most commonly occurs in patients with multiple relapses requiring retreatment. Patients who exhibit sustained remission after withdrawal of therapy have a 5% chance of developing cirrhosis. As for any patient with chronic liver disease and cirrhosis, periodic screening for hepatocellular carcinoma is recommended.

Liver transplantation

Orthotopic liver transplantation is recommended for patients who develop end-stage liver disease despite medical therapy. End-stage liver disease due to autoimmune hepatitis accounts for approximately 6% of liver transplants in the US. The 5-year patient and graft survival exceeds 90% in many centers. Indications for orthotopic liver transplantation include refractory variceal bleeding or encephalopathy, intractable ascites, spontaneous bacterial peritonitis, hepatorenal or hepatopulmonary syndromes, and localized hepatocellular carcinoma.

Approximately 30% of patients transplanted for autoimmune hepatitis will develop recurrent disease within the graft. Most recurrences are generally mild, but patients can present with aggressive disease. A diagnosis of recurrent disease is based on typical histology and exclusion of other conditions that can mimic autoimmune hepatitis. Patient and graft survival are not affected over the medium term in patients who develop recurrent disease. Patients transplanted for autoimmune hepatitis may benefit from a more intensive immunosuppressive regimen. Switching from cyclosporine to tacrolimus, or adding additional agents such as mycophenolate mofetil may be appropriate strategies for patients transplanted for autoimmune hepatitis.

Complications

Patients with autoimmune hepatitis are susceptible to complications of cirrhosis and portal hypertension. Patients with autoimmune hepatitis and cirrhosis who receive immunosuppressive therapy have fewer portal hypertensive complications and enjoy better long-term survival when compared to patients with other causes of cirrhosis. Treatment strategies for portal hypertensive complications are the same as those for other causes of end-stage liver disease. The presence of esophageal varices is less common in cirrhotic patients with autoimmune hepatitis who receive immunosuppression, and the probability of variceal hemorrhage in this cohort is below 10%. A patient survival rate at 5 and 10 years of 90% is quoted in most long-term studies.

Hepatocellular carcinoma develops in 7% of autoimmune hepatitis patients with cirrhosis. The risk is 311 times higher than that of an age- and sex-matched control group. Patients with at least 5 years of cirrhosis are most susceptible to malignant degeneration.

Complications of long-term corticosteroids include weight gain, diabetes mellitus, hypertension, and osteopenia. Azathioprine has been associated with bone marrow suppression, liver function test abnormalities, and, rarely, malignancy.

Natural history and prognosis

The 3-year survival of patients with untreated, severe autoimmune hepatitis is 50%, whereas the 10-year survival is approximately 10% to 30%. The prognosis is much better for patients with mild histologic disease. Five-year survival in this subset is comparable to that of age- and sex-matched controls. The rate of progression for patients with mild disease is less than 20%. The natural history of autoimmune hepatitis can be altered in patients who respond to therapy. Life expectancy in treated patients approximates that of age- and sex-matched controls; however, 40% of patients will progress to cirrhosis despite receiving appropriate treatment.

The prognosis of autoimmune hepatitis depends on the severity of inflammation at the time of presentation, the presence or absence of cirrhosis, underlying medical conditions, and the patient's HLA haplotype. Patients with aminotransferases more than ten times the upper limit of normal, or more than five times the upper limit of normal plus gamma globulin levels more than two times the upper limit of normal have a worse prognosis. Furthermore, patients with active bridging necrosis, cirrhosis, or HLA-DR3 have an inferior outcome when compared to patients without these parameters.

Summary

Primary biliary cirrhosis, primary sclerosing cholangitis, and autoimmune hepatitis are thought to be disorders of immune regulation. Cellular and humoral injury to the biliary tree and hepatocytes lead to progressive liver injury, cirrhosis, and complications of portal hypertension.

The diagnosis of primary biliary cirrhosis is based on typical symptoms and signs, cholestatic liver indices, antimitochondrial antibodies, and granulomatous bile-duct injury. Progressive cholestasis ultimately results in the development of cirrhosis with portal hypertensive complications or problems related to prolonged cholestasis. Ursodeoxycholic acid is recommended for all patients with primary biliary cirrhosis; improvement in hepatic biochemical parameters is typical, whereas the effects of bile-acid therapy on liver histology and transplant-free survival are less certain. Medical therapies should also focus on complications of portal hypertension or chronic cholestasis. Orthotopic liver transplantation is reserved for patients with advanced primary biliary cirrhosis and hepatic decompensation.

Clinical, biochemical, cholangiographic, and histologic criteria are important in the diagnosis of primary sclerosing cholangitis. As with primary biliary cirrhosis, primary sclerosing cholangitis is associated with progressive cholestasis and the development of cirrhosis in most patients. Primary sclerosing cholangitis is also a risk factor for cholangiocarcinoma. There are no effective medical therapies that alter the natural course of primary sclerosing cholangitis. Medical treatment should be directed towards complications of portal hypertension or progressive cholestasis. Orthotopic liver transplantation is the only remedy that has been shown to improve patient survival.

The diagnosis of autoimmune hepatitis is based on typical clinical, biochemical, serologic, and histologic criteria. Corticosteroids with or without azathioprine result in improvement in biochemical liver tests, histology, and survival in most patients with autoimmune hepatitis. Orthotopic liver transplantation is reserved for patients with severe disease that does not respond to conventional medical therapies.

We have come a long way in the diagnosis and treatment of patients with autoimmune liver diseases. Much work remains to be done to better understand the pathogenesis of primary biliary cirrhosis, primary sclerosing cholangitis, and autoimmune hepatitis in order to provide more effective medical and surgical therapies for our patients with these disorders.

Further reading

Al-Khalidi JA, Czaja AJ. Current concepts in the diagnosis, pathogenesis, and treatment of autoimmune hepatitis. *Mayo Clin Proc* 2001; 76(12): 1237–1252.

Angulo P, Lindor KD. Primary biliary cirrhosis and primary sclerosing cholangitis. *Clin Liver Dis* 1999; 3(3): 529–570.

Angulo P, Lindor KD. Primary sclerosing cholangitis. *Hepatology* 1999; 30(1): 325–332.

Heathcote EJ. Management of primary biliary cirrhosis. *Hepatology* 2000; 31(4): 1005–1013.

Heneghan MA, McFarlane IG. Current and novel immunosuppressive therapy for autoimmune hepatitis. *Hepatology* 2002; 35(1): 7–13.

Holtmeier J, Leuschner U. Medical treatment of primary biliary cirrhosis and primary sclerosing cholangitis. *Digestion* 2001; 64(3): 137–150.

Johnson PJ, McFarlane IG. Meeting report: international autoimmune hepatitis group. *Hepatology* 1993; 18(4): 998–1005.

Lazaridis KN, Wiesner RH, Porayko MK, *et al.* Primary sclerosing cholangitis. In: Schiff ER, Sorrell MF, Maddrey WC (eds) *Schiff's Diseases of the Liver* 8th edn, vol. I. Lippincott-Raven, Philadelphia, 1999; p. 649.

Lee YM, Kaplan MM. Management of primary sclerosing cholangitis. *Am J Gastroenterol* 2002; 97(3): 528–534.

Lindor KD, Dickson ER. Primary biliary cirrhosis. In: Schiff ER, Sorrell MF, Maddrey WC (eds) *Schiff's Diseases of the Liver* 8th edn, vol. I. Lippincott-Raven, Philadelphia, 1999; p. 679.

Ponsioen CIJ, Tytgat GNJ. Primary sclerosing cholangitis: a clinical review. *Am J Gastroenterol* 1998; 93(4): 515–523.

Sherlock S. Primary biliary cirrhosis, primary sclerosing cholangitis, and autoimmune cholangitis. *Clin Liver Dis* 2000; 4(1): 97–113.

Chapter 7

Vascular Disorders of the Liver

Barbara Piasecki and Linda Greenbaum

CHAPTER OUTLINE

Normal vascular anatomy of the liver

It is important to have a basic knowledge of the anatomy of the great blood vessels of the liver in order to understand the pathophysiology underlying certain vascular disorders of the liver. Disease processes affecting the pre-hepatic (inflowing), the intrahepatic, and the post-hepatic (outflowing) vessels may result in portal hypertension and other potential complications.

Blood vessels flowing into the liver

Blood is delivered to the liver by the hepatic artery and the portal vein. The hepatic artery delivers 30% of the liver's blood supply while the portal vein delivers the remaining 70%. The hepatic artery is a branch of the celiac axis and carries oxygenated blood to the liver. At the porta hepatis the hepatic artery divides into the right and left hepatic arteries that serve their respective lobes of the liver. Anomalies of the hepatic artery are quite common and may occur in up to 50% of individuals.

The portal vein carries most of the inflow of blood to the liver (70%). The definition of a portal system is a series of blood vessels in which two different capillary beds lie between the arterial supply and the final venous drainage back into the inferior vena cava. The portal vein fits this definition as it lies between the capillary beds of the gastrointestinal tract, gallbladder, pancreas, and spleen and the capillary beds of the liver. It is formed by the confluence of the superior mesenteric and splenic veins and drains the digestive tract, spleen, pancreas, and gallbladder. At the porta hepatis the portal vein divides into the right and left portal veins. As the branches become smaller the terminal twigs give way to the microcirculation of the liver which consists of the sinusoids. The sinusoidal bed supplies the hepatocytes directly. Anomalies of the portal venous system and the hepatic microcirculation are quite rare.

Blood vessels flowing out of the liver

The liver itself is drained by the hepatic veins. There are three main hepatic veins, the right, middle, and left veins. The hepatic veins drain blood from the myriad of central veins that are the terminal areas of the hepatic lobules. The hepatic veins drain into the inferior vena cava. The veins have variable branching patterns and anatomic differences in hepatic veins are quite common.

Hepatic outflow obstruction

Veno-occlusive disease

Introduction

Hepatic veno-occlusive disease is characterized by hepatomegaly, right upper quadrant pain, jaundice, and ascites. It was first identified as a disorder of vascular origin in South Africa. The term veno-occlusive disease was coined by investigators in Jamaica in order to describe the obliterative fibrosis within small hepatic venules that appears to be characteristic of this disease. There are multiple risk factors and theorized causes of veno-occlusive disease. Fundamentally it appears that the development of veno-occlusive disease involves toxic injury to sinusoidal hepatic endothelial cells, which leads to fibrosis and obstruction of blood flow at the level of terminal hepatic venules.

Epidemiology

The incidence and recognition of veno-occlusive disease has increased since the 1950s with the increasing use of radiation and chemotherapy. Certain alkaloid toxins and chemotherapeutic agents have been identified as important risk factors for veno-occlusive disease. Prior to the 1950s veno-

occlusive disease was most often associated with the ingestion of herbal teas or food sources containing pyrrolizidine alkaloids. This compound is found in certain plant species including *Crotalaria* spp., *Heliotropium* spp., *Senecio* spp. and *Symphytum* spp. Epidemics of veno-occlusive disease in less-developed nations have been associated with the ingestion of bread contaminated with seeds from these plants. Today veno-occlusive disease is most commonly seen in patients who have undergone bone-marrow ablative chemotherapy conditioning regimens prior to receiving a hematopoietic cell transplantation.

The incidence of veno-occlusive disease appears to be quite variable. The reported rates range from 5% to 50% depending on the transplant center and the marrow ablative conditioning regimen used. Before the risk factors for veno-occlusive disease were identified, the incidence of veno-occlusive disease increased over the last 20 years as higher doses of cytoreductive therapy were employed in evolving bone-marrow transplantation protocols. In more recent years, as knowledge about the risk factors leading to veno-occlusive disease has increased, the incidence has been dramatically reduced as transplantation centers have made an effort to minimize the risk for developing veno-occlusive disease. Specific changes in practice have included decreasing chemotherapeutic doses, using non-myeloablative regimens, avoiding cyclophosphamide-based regimens, tailoring regimens in the context of individual risk factors for veno-occlusive disease, and limiting exposures to other drugs that may increase the risk of veno-occlusive disease.

Pathogenesis and etiology

The development of veno-occlusive disease appears to be related to injury to the hepatic sinusoid endothelium. In zone three of the liver acinus, the causative toxin damages the endothelial cells. This leads to venule dilation and congestion by erythrocytes thus initiating the cascade leading to portal hypertension. This most commonly occurs after hematopoietic cell transplantation conditioning regimens, particularly those containing cyclophosphamide. Veno-occlusive disease is also associated with the ingestion of pyrrolizidine alkaloids as in herbal sources (bush tea, other herbal teas), high-dose radiation therapy (without chemotherapy and usually exceeding 30 Gy), female gender, immunosuppression using azathioprine, and pre-existing liver disease such as chronic hepatitis or non-alcoholic steatohepatitis.

Diagnosis

Veno-occlusive disease is usually diagnosed clinically. The constellation of tender hepatomegaly, jaundice, and fluid retention in a person at risk for the disorder should raise suspicion for this diagnosis. It is important to remember that there can be many causes of jaundice in post-bone marrow transplant patients. Common causes of hyperbilirubinemia and jaundice in this group include sepsis, renal insufficiency, hemolysis, and hyperacute graft-versus-host disease. In this group of patients a thorough investigation into the potential etiologies of jaundice is warranted even if veno-occlusive disease is the most likely explanation. In cases of veno-occlusive disease there may be abnormalities in serum blood tests, imaging studies such as ultrasound, and liver biopsy.

Serum biochemical markers The serum profile of veno-occlusive disease is characterized by hyperbilirubinemia (above 2 mg/dL) as well as elevation in aspartate aminotransferase (AST) and alanine aminotransferase (ALT). Hepatomegaly and fluid retention typically precede the development of hyperbilirubinemia. There are other plasma proteins that have been found to be abnormal in patients with veno-occlusive disease, although these findings have been based on relatively small series of patients. Serum procollagen type III has been shown to be increased in individuals with veno-occlusive disease. Levels of antithrombin III and protein C have been found to be lower in patients with veno-occlusive disease. While laboratory tests for serum procollagen, antithrombin III, and protein C may be available in some medical centers, the more commonly used tests for diagnosing veno-occlusive disease are serum bilirubin, AST, and ALT.

Ascitic fluid analysis Ascites may develop in veno-occlusive disease and is characteristically distinguished from ascites that is caused by cirrhosis from viral hepatitis or alcoholic liver injury. In ascites that is secondary to post-sinusoidal obstruction, as in veno-occlusive disease, the ascitic fluid typically has a high serum albumin to ascitic fluid gradient (SAAG above 1.1) as well as a high total protein content (usually greater than 2.5 gm/dL) whereas in cirrhosis due to viral infections or alcohol the total protein content tends to be low (less than 2.5 gm/dL).

Ultrasonography In cases of veno-occlusive disease, imaging studies of the liver may reveal hepatomegaly, ascites, and attenuated hepatic venous flow. Typically, imaging studies may be useful in demonstrating an absence of biliary ductal dilatation and other causes of obstruction. It is important to realize that many patients undergoing hematopoietic cell transplantation are seriously ill and may have abnormal imaging studies that are characteristic of, but not specific for, veno-occlusive disease. As veno-occlusive disease progresses ultrasonography may be useful for demonstrating altered liver blood flow, particularly reversal of portal flow and portal vein thrombosis.

Liver biopsy In most cases the diagnosis of veno-occlusive disease is made without the use of invasive tests such as liver biopsy. Patients at risk for veno-occlusive disease, such as bone-marrow transplant patients, often have comorbidities including thrombocytopenia and coagulopathies that increase the risk of complications from a liver biopsy. A liver biopsy may be informative in cases where the diagnosis is less certain. In such patients the transjugular rather than the percutaneous approach for the liver biopsy may be preferable. The transjugular approach is considered safer in terms of bleeding complications and would allow for the measurement of the hepatic–portal venous gradient at the time of the liver biopsy. A hepatic–portal venous gradient, that is increased (above 10 mmHg) is highly specific for veno-occlusive disease, under the appropriate clinical circumstances.

Early histologic abnormalities that may be detected on liver biopsy specimens include venular changes of a widened subendothelial zone between the basement membrane and the adventitia of central veins and sublobular veins. In addition early changes include dilation and engorgement of sinusoids and necrosis of perivenular hepatocytes. Later histologic changes include deposits of extracellular matrix in subendothelial spaces and in sinusoids (Figure 7.1). Special staining will reveal increased collagen lining the sinusoids and venules.

Clinical features

In the most common scenario the clinical picture of veno-occlusive disease develops within the first 3 weeks after hematopoietic cell transplantation. Less commonly, a late-onset form of veno-occlusive disease has been described occurring more than 30 days after bonemarrow transplant and which may be associated with busulfan-containing regimens. The presentation of veno-occlusive disease may vary from mild to very severe. The clinical features may include tender hepatomegaly, weight gain due

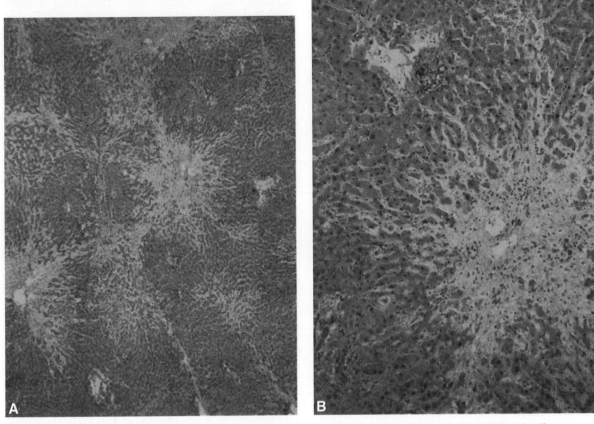

Figure 7.1 Veno-occlusive disease (VOD). Histopathology demonstrating stagnant red blood cells and intimal change with narrowing. There is intrahepatic hemorrhage and zone necrosis. A. Low power. B. Higher power *(see plate section for color)*.

to ascites, abdominal pain, and jaundice. Patients may demonstrate abnormalities in hepatic biochemical tests. Typically, there is elevation in serum aminotransferases and serum bilirubin. In more severe cases patients may demonstrate elevation of prothrombin time. Patients with severe disease may progress to develop hepatic encephalopathy, bleeding, and renal and cardiopulmonary failure.

Prognosis

In severe cases, veno-occlusive disease can be an important cause of mortality related to bone-marrow transplants. It is estimated that approximately 25% to 30% of cases of veno-occlusive disease are severe. In these cases veno-occlusive disease may lead to acute liver failure, coagulopathy, hepatic encephalopathy, hepatorenal syndrome, and multiorgan failure. The mortality rate among these patients may be very high. It is estimated that 70% to 85% of patients with veno-occlusive disease will

recover spontaneously. In those patients who recover from veno-occlusive disease there is not usually any lasting liver damage or evident liver dysfunction.

A prognostic model for the outcome of veno-occlusive disease has been developed. The model was developed in a cohort of 355 patients undergoing bone-marrow transplantation by measuring risk factors at certain points in time. The model was then validated in a separate cohort of 392 patients planning to undergo bone-marrow transplantation, and was found to have high specificity and moderate sensitivity. The most predictive factors in this model were serum bilirubin and percentage weight gain in the first 1 to 2 weeks following transplantation. In other studies renal function has been suggested as an important predictor of veno-occlusive disease outcome. Worsened renal function was correlated with increased mortality. Other studies have suggested that D-dimer levels may be higher in more severe cases of veno-occlusive disease. D-dimer may be an early marker for the severity of the disease.

Treatment

There are no randomized controlled clinical trials demonstrating a clearly efficacious therapy for veno-occlusive disease. Treatment for veno-occlusive disease is mainly supportive. The two main treatments that have been investigated include the use of human tissue-type plasminogen activator and defibrotide. Other treatments tried in small studies include antithrombin III concentrate, prostaglandin E1, antioxidants such as glutathione, transjugular intrahepatic portosystemic shunt, and liver transplantation.

Prevention

Since no optimal therapy exists yet, efforts to prevent the development of veno-occlusive disease play an important role in decreasing the incidence of this disease. In addition to decreasing the use of conditioning regimens known to increase risk for veno-occlusive disease, preventive measures may include the use of a synthetic bile acid (UDCA), heparin, and peripheral blood progenitor cells as a stem cell source.

Budd–Chiari syndrome and obliterative hepatocavopathy

Introduction

Budd–Chiari syndrome is the partial or complete obstruction of blood flow out of the liver usually involving the hepatic veins. The name is derived from the researchers who characterized the syndrome. In 1857 Budd described the pathologic features of hepatic vein thrombosis. In 1899 Chiari described the clinical picture that typically accompanies hepatic vein obstruction. Budd–Chiari may be due to occlusion of one, two, or all three of the major hepatic veins (right, middle, left) and/or complete or partial occlusion of the inferior vena cava. Traditionally the term Budd–Chiari syndrome has encompassed those disorders involving occlusion of the hepatic veins and/or occlusion of the inferior vena cava at its hepatic portion. More recently it has been suggested that primary hepatic vein obstruction and primary hepatic inferior vena cava obstruction represent quite distinct disease processes. In order to clarify this, it has been proposed that obstructive processes involving mainly the vena cava should be considered as a separate

disorder called obliterative hepatocavopathy. Since most of the clinical experience and case series to date have not made this distinction our clinical knowledge is based on these groups combined. For the purposes of this chapter the term Budd–Chiari syndrome will refer to the clinical entity that may result from hepatic vein and/or inferior vena cava obstruction.

Blood flows into the liver via the hepatic artery and portal veins. Blood flows out of the liver via the hepatic veins. When there is an obstruction at the level of the hepatic veins which drain the liver the result is outflow obstruction and congestion. Patients develop hepatomegaly, ascites, and abdominal pain. Most patients who present with Budd–Chiari syndrome have an underlying hypercoagulable state, although the specific causes of the hypercoagulable state may vary broadly.

Epidemiology

Budd–Chiari syndrome occurs more commonly in women than in men. Typically the syndrome is diagnosed in individuals in their third or fourth decade of life.

Pathogenesis and etiology

The development of Budd–Chiari syndrome depends on the partial or complete occlusion of the hepatic veins. In approximately 80% of cases an explanation for the occlusion can be found, the remaining 20% of cases of Budd–Chiari syndrome are labeled idiopathic. Thrombosis is the main mechanism leading to hepatic venous obstruction. As our knowledge about hypercoagulable states increases, the percentage of "idiopathic" cases of Budd–Chiari is likely to decrease. By far the most common cause of Budd–Chiari is a known (or previously unidentified) underlying myeloproliferative disorder. It is estimated that myeloproliferative disorders that lead to hypercoagulable states may underlie up to 50% of the cases of Budd–Chiari syndrome. The four major myeloproliferative disorders implicated as leading to Budd–Chiari syndrome are polycythemia rubra vera, chronic myelogenous leukemia, essential thrombocythemia, and agnogenic myeloid metaplasia. An underlying myeloproliferative disorder may be diagnosed in the work-up of Budd–Chiari syndrome. Other important causes of Budd–Chiari syndrome include malignancy, infections of the liver, benign lesions of the liver, oral contraceptives, pregnancy, Behçet's disease, membranous webs of the inferior vena cava, collagen vascular disorders, and hypercoagulable states such as factor V Leiden mutation (see Box 7.1). It has been theorized that the interaction of one or more predisposing conditions may lead to the development of the syndrome. For example an individual may have Factor V Leiden mutation but will not develop Budd–Chiari until a malignancy or myeloproliferative disorder develops and increases the hypercoagulable state further.

Diagnosis

The Budd–Chiari syndrome should be considered in the differential diagnosis of acute and chronic

---

Box 7.1 Causes of Budd–Chiari syndrome

Myeloproliferative disorders
  polycythemia rubra vera
  chronic myelogenous leukemia
  essential thrombocythemia
  agnogenic myeloid metaplasia
Malignancy
Infections of the liver
  hepatic abscess
  syphilitic gumma
  invasive aspergillosis
  mucormycosis
Benign lesions of and around the liver
  hepatic cysts
  hepatic adenoma and cystadenoma
  aortic aneurysm
Oral contraceptives and pregnancy
Hypercoagulable states
  G1691A factor V Leiden gene mutation
  G20210A factor II gene mutation
  antiphospholipid antibodies
  antithrombin deficiency
  protein C deficiency
  protein S deficiency
  paroxysmal nocturnal hemoglobinuria
Behçet's disease
Membranous webs causing obstruction of
  the inferior vena cava
Collagen vascular and inflammatory diseases
  systemic lupus erythematosus
  Sjögren's syndrome
  inflammatory bowel disease
  hypereosinophilic syndrome
  sarcoidosis
Trauma to the liver
Idiopathic causes

---

liver failure as it can present in both these ways. Typically ascites is a prominent feature of Budd–Chiari syndrome. Budd–Chiari syndrome may be distinguished from congestive hepatopathy due to right-sided heart failure, by the absence of jugular venous distension. This may be an important distinction to make as right-sided heart failure may present with similar features of hepatic outflow obstruction.

Serum biochemical markers The serum profile of patients with Budd–Chiari syndrome may vary. There are no classic diagnostic laboratory tests for Budd–Chiari syndrome. In the acute setting there may be marked elevation of the aminotransferases (AST and ALT). In acute fulminant failure there will also be a disruption in liver synthetic function including elevation of prothrombin time, decrease in albumin, and other derangements of electrolytes and renal function. In subacute and chronic Budd–Chiari syndrome the serum biochemical profile will be consistent with chronic-appearing liver disease including elevation of prothrombin time and decreased albumin levels. In addition, analysis of ascitic fluid will be consistent with a high serum albumin to ascites gradient (SAAG >1.1) indicative of portal hypertension.

Imaging studies Imaging studies play an important role in the diagnosis and work-up of Budd–Chiari syndrome as they can demonstrate the obstructing thrombosis, characterize its extent, and identify any other concomitant thromboses in other blood vessels that may impact the prognosis and therapeutic options.

Appropriate non-invasive studies for identifying thromboses of the hepatic and other vasculature include ultrasonography with Doppler studies, CT, and magnetic resonance angiography (MRA). The accuracy of these studies for diagnosing Budd–Chiari syndrome may be influenced by the size, location, and clinical characteristics of the obstruction. Importantly, at the time of these non-invasive studies, it is important to evaluate the portal and splenic circulations as well since this will have important prognostic and therapeutic implications. The characteristic findings on non-invasive imaging studies such as ultrasound, CT, and MRI include an inability to visualize normal hepatic venous connections to the vena cava, comma-shaped intrahepatic collateral vessels and the absence of waveforms in the hepatic veins.

Hepatic system venography is considered the gold standard for establishing the diagnosis of

Budd–Chiari syndrome. This is an invasive test whereby the hepatic venous circulation is accessed percutaneously (Figure 7.2). Venous pressure measurements are taken above and below their entrance into the inferior vena cava in order to identify whether a pressure gradient exists. With the injection of contrast the hepatic venous vasculature can be visualized. In cases of Budd–Chiari syndrome, a characteristic "spider-web" pattern is seen on contrast venography which is made up of collateral blood vessels that develop to bypass the obstructed hepatic vein(s) (Figure 7.3). Because hepatic venography is an invasive test it is usually reserved for cases in which non-invasive tests are not able to provide adequate or complete information.

In addition to venography, arteriography is used in cases of Budd–Chiari syndrome. Arteriography is an important part of the work-up when a surgical shunt procedure is planned to bypass the obstructed area. Delineating the arterial anatomy can be very important in planning the surgery and this allows further investigation of the anatomy in order to exclude occult tumors involving the liver, inferior vena cava, or hepatic and portal veins,

which may have contributed to the development of Budd–Chiari syndrome.

Liver biopsy The liver biopsy may play a very important role in establishing the diagnosis of Budd–Chiari syndrome as well as assisting in ascertaining a prognosis for planning treatment. Typically, if the liver biopsy shows only severe congestion then the condition is likely to be reversible with the removal of the outflow obstruction via a radiologic or surgical procedure. If the liver biopsy shows that fibrosis is present then it is likely that orthotopic liver transplantation will be needed. This may be especially important in the more acute presentations of the syndrome. Specific histological features reflect the venous outflow obstruction and include centrizonal congestion, hepatocellular necrosis, and fibrosis in more chronic cases (Figure 7.4).

Clinical picture

The clinical presentation of Budd–Chiari syndrome may be acute, subacute, or chronic. The rapidity

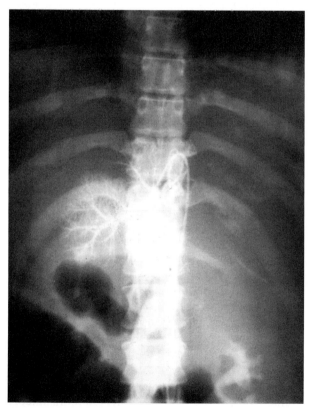

Figure 7.2 Normal venogram. In normal outflow of the liver a venogram will show clear opacification of the right and left hepatic veins and their smaller branches.

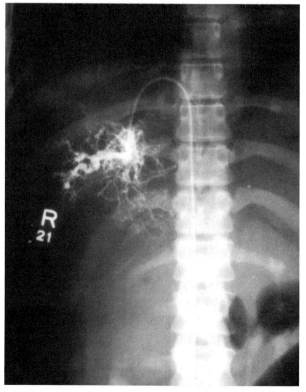

Figure 7.3 Venogram in Budd–Chiari syndrome. In a patient with Budd–Chiari syndrome this venogram fails to show the left hepatic venous system and thus confirms obstruction in hepatic outflow. A "spider web" pattern is seen.

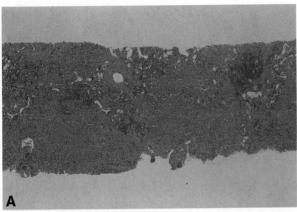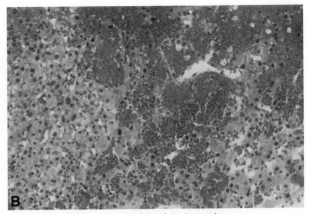

Figure 7.4 Budd–Chiari syndrome. Histology of the liver in a patient with Budd–Chiari syndrome shows centrizonal congestion, hemorrhage, and liver cell loss. A. Low power. B. Higher power *(see plate section for color)*.

with which Budd–Chiari syndrome presents is mainly dependent on how quickly the hepatic veins occlude and how complete the occlusion is. The faster and more complete the obstruction, the more acutely the clinical syndrome will present. In the acute presentation liver dysfunction and symptoms develop over days to weeks. While the acute presentation of Budd–Chiari tends to be more dramatic and life threatening, the subacute and chronic presentations are more common. In the subacute and chronic forms of Budd–Chiari the clinical picture evolves over weeks to months.

In its acute presentation Budd–Chiari syndrome presents with severe right upper quadrant pain, hepatomegaly, and evidence of liver dysfunction. Jaundice and ascites may develop shortly afterwards. Although ascites may not be an initial symptom it usually develops and is estimated to occur in 90% of such cases. The acute presentation of Budd–Chiari is typically seen more often in women. A common scenario for acute Budd–Chiari would be in a pregnant female when the physiologic and hormonal changes of pregnancy in combination with an underlying clotting disorder lead to hepatic vein thrombosis and occlusion. In the acute presentation there may be associated abnormalities in the serum biochemical markers of liver function. These changes may vary markedly and may include elevation in the aminotransferases (ALT and AST to greater than 600 IU/), elevation of alkaline phosphatase (in the range of 300 to 400 mg/dL), and elevation of serum bilirubin (usually less than 7 mg/dL at presentation but may rise further later). It is important to make the diagnosis early as liver function may deteriorate rapidly leading to complications such as variceal bleeding and acute fulminant

hepatic failure. In the subacute presentation of Budd–Chiari clinical manifestations due to portal hypertension and cirrhosis may not be evident for several weeks to several months. The clinical manifestations as well as the time to diagnosis may vary and may depend on the degree of occlusion as more severe or complete occlusion will become clinically evident sooner than partial occlusion. If only one or two of the hepatic veins are involved in the obstruction then there may even be a good chance for spontaneous recovery without complications such as ascites, cirrhosis, or portal hypertension.

In the chronic presentation of Budd–Chiari patients may present just as any other patient with chronic liver disease. In chronic Budd–Chiari syndrome patients may develop hypertrophy of the caudate lobe. Interestingly this enlarged caudate lobe may lead to compression of the intrahepatic portion of the inferior vena cava which may cause further hepatic outflow obstruction. One of the characteristic features of chronic Budd–Chiari syndrome associated with inferior vena cava thrombosis is the development of collaterals on the abdominal wall and the back, draining blood from the infrahepatic portion of the cava into the suprahepatic portion.

With long-standing hepatic vein obstruction patients may go on to develop cirrhosis due to the persistent intrahepatic congestion. With the development of cirrhosis and portal hypertension these patients are at risk for variceal bleeding and massive ascites. While in the acute form of Budd–Chiari syndrome hepatic encephalopathy may quickly develop as part of acute fulminant hepatic failure, in chronic Budd–Chiari syndrome hepatic encephalopathy is far less common. Patients with subacute or chronic Budd–Chiari may have abnormalities in liver function tests but the severity of these abnormalities may vary a great deal.

Prognosis

Most patients who are diagnosed with Budd–Chiari syndrome undergo some form of therapy for the disorder. A study was performed in order to identify factors that may influence prognosis. The factors associated with a good prognosis included younger age, better liver function by Child–Pugh score, diuretic-responsive ascites, and lower serum creatinine. The presence of concomitant portal vein thrombosis is known to be associated with a significantly worse prognosis. Just as the clinical picture may vary with the level and completeness of vascular occlusions, the prognosis may be influenced by the degree of vascular occlusion. Thrombosis of one or two hepatic veins alone may not have the feature of ascites and may have a very good prognosis with a high probability of spontaneous recovery.

Treatment

There are multiple therapeutic options for managing Budd–Chiari syndrome. These options include medical therapy, interventional radiologic therapy, and surgical therapy. The focus of therapy is to manage the clinical symptoms of hepatic outflow obstruction, to identify and treat the underlying hypercoagulable states, to prevent propagation of the thrombosis, and to decompress the congested liver either by radiologic or surgical procedures.

Medical therapy

The management of the clinical syndrome of hepatic vein obstruction includes management of fluid retention and ascites. This may include the use of diuretics, therapeutic paracenteses, and counseling on low-sodium dietary intake. In addition, medical management includes identifying and treating the underlying hypercoagulable disorder with anticoagulation. Most patients with an underlying hypercoagulable disorder will require chronic anticoagulation. In cases of acute and subacute Budd–Chiari syndrome thrombolytic therapy may be considered. Patients with chronic Budd–Chiari are not typically considered good candidates for thrombolytic therapy as their thromboses are mature and unlikely to respond to thrombolytics and the risk of bleeding complications is high if the patient has developed portal hypertension. It is important to weigh the risks and benefits of thrombolytic therapy since the complications can be sig-

nificant and alternative therapies exist. The cases of Budd–Chiari syndrome that do not require anticoagulation are those that are caused by anatomic abnormalities such as inferior vena cava webs which will require radiologic or surgical correction alone.

Interventional radiologic therapy

Interventional radiologic techniques have contributed tremendously to the management of portal hypertension. In the case of Budd–Chiari syndrome management may include angioplasty with or without stent placement and transjugular intrahepatic portosystemic shunt placement. Angioplasty can be used for the treatment of membranous webs in the inferior vena cava and in combination with thrombolytics in the management of thrombotic occlusions. A stent can be placed at the time of angioplasty in order to minimize the risk of re-occlusion. Importantly, stents should be avoided in patients awaiting cadaveric liver transplantation as the placement of a stent can greatly complicate the ability to create the necessary anastomosis between the donor graft and the recipient's inferior vena cava. A transjugular intrahepatic portosystemic shunt is sometimes offered to patients in cases of Budd–Chiari syndrome as a means to decompress the liver. It is not a perfect therapy in these cases as it may not be technically feasible in certain patients, there is a high rate of re-occlusion, and it may only drain a small part of the liver.

Surgical therapy

Surgical therapy includes the creation of shunts to decompress the liver which essentially creates a new drainage route for the blood flowing out of the liver, as well as orthotopic liver transplantation. Surgical shunting is a good option for patients with Budd–Chiari syndrome that is not very long-standing. The type of shunt created depends on the extent of thrombosis and the extent to which the hypertrophied caudate lobe is obstructing the inferior vena cava. The possible types of shunts include side-to-side, mesocaval, or mesoatrial. In a side-to-side shunt an anastamosis is created between the portal vein and the intrahepatic inverior vena cava. This type of shunt has the highest patency rate. The mesocaval shunt procedure is a less complicated operation but may suffer from re-occlusion in a significant number of cases. A mesoatrial shunt returns blood from the splanchnic circulation directly to the heart. The survival after shunt surgery depends on the degree of liver damage sustained before the operation. Survival in patients without cirrhosis with a persistently patent shunt can be excellent. In cases of long-standing Budd–Chiari syndrome, cirrhosis of the liver may already be present and overall these patients would be high risk for surgery and would benefit more from liver transplantation.

In addition to patients with long-standing disease, orthotopic liver transplantation may be the best possible therapy for patients who do not qualify for radiologic or shunt procedures for other reasons. It is important to consider both the short-term management for decompressing the liver and how therapeutic options will affect the long-term options.

Prevention

The prevention of *de novo* or recurrent Budd–Chiari syndrome rests on treating the underlying hypercoagulable disorder. This may be anticoagulation as well as treating the cause of the hypercoagulability such as a myeloproliferative disorder. In cases of Budd–Chiari syndrome that are attributed to anatomic abnormalities in the region of the hepatic vein, correction of the abnormality and surgical connection to the inferior vena cava will be important for preventing re-obstruction.

Cardiac failure and the liver

Introduction

Cardiac failure involving the right side of the heart leads to systemic congestion including functional hepatic outflow obstruction. The clinical picture of right-sided heart failure may share features similar to that of Budd–Chiari syndrome. Liver congestion caused by cardiac failure may be referred to as congestive hepatopathy. The liver dysfunction associated with congestive heart failure is characterized by both outflow obstruction as well as poor inflow due to poor cardiac output. If it is long-standing, congestive hepatopathy can lead to fibrosis and permanent liver injury.

Epidemiology

Over the last several decades the medical management of cardiac disease has improved tremendously. New medications and procedures have become available to help patients with failing hearts achieve improved overall cardiac and systemic sta-

tus. As a result, long-standing congestive hepatopathy due to right-sided cardiac failure is becoming less common than it once was.

Pathogenesis and etiology

The systemic congestion caused by poor forward flow into the heart is responsible for the congestion that occurs in the liver.

Diagnosis

The diagnosis of cardiac-related congestive hepatopathy depends on the clinical findings and physical examination findings of right-sided heart failure and the exclusion of other causes of liver injury. There are certainly systemic diseases, such as hemochromatosis, that may affect both the heart and the liver; therefore, congestive hepatopathy should be approached as a diagnosis of exclusion. It is appropriate to perform investigations to exclude other causes of liver injury, including infectious, toxic, and hereditary causes, at the time of initial presentation. Work-up may include laboratory studies and imaging, for example ultrasonography. If there is no evidence of other causes of liver disease and right-sided heart failure is present the diagnosis of congestive hepatopathy can be made. Liver biopsy may also be informative.

Liver biopsy

On gross examination the liver appears enlarged. Classically, after long-standing chronic congestive heart failure the liver has been described as having a "nutmeg" appearance. In a patient with long-standing cardiac failure the liver tissue will show dilated central veins with centrilobular congestion. The degree of injury and fibrosis may vary depending on the severity and duration of congestive heart failure.

Clinical picture

The clinical picture of cardiac failure-induced congestive hepatopathy may include right upper quadrant pain due to hepatomegaly with liver capsule distension, ascites, and jaundice. Jaundice may be mild to moderate and is caused by a combination of hepatocyte injury and hemolysis in poorly perfused tissues. A useful way to distinguish hepatic congestion due to cardiac failure from congestion due to Budd–Chiari syndrome is to test for the hepatojugular reflux. In cardiac-induced hepatic congestion placing pressure on the liver may give a visible pulse in the neck veins. In Budd–Chiari syndrome such a maneuver will not induce a wave in the neck veins since the outflow obstruction is fixed.

Prognosis

Over time chronic cardiac failure may lead to frank cirrhosis. The overall prognosis depends on how quickly and how successfully the cardiac failure is treated. The typical complications of portal hypertension may develop, although often the patient's mortality may be affected by the cardiac disease when it is severe. A poor prognostic sign may be a consistently rising bilirubin level.

Treatment

The treatment of cardiac-related hepatopathy depends on the management of the cardiac failure in order to reduce the hepatic congestion.

Constrictive pericarditis and the liver

Introduction

Constrictive pericarditis may cause outflow obstruction to the liver. In constrictive pericarditis there is a limitation of blood flow through the right side of the heart and therefore systemic congestion, including hepatic congestion, can develop. The overall clinical picture may be similar to that seen in Budd–Chiari syndrome or in congestive hepatopathy caused by right-sided cardiac failure due to other causes.

Diagnosis

A certain level of suspicion for underlying pericarditis is essential to accurately making this diagnosis. Right and left-sided cardiac catheterization may help to clarify the diagnosis.

Clinical picture

The clinical picture is characterized by tender hepatomegaly, a prominent hepatojugular reflex, and possibly distended neck veins in the upright position. Patients may develop ascites but tend to have less peripheral edema than patients with right-sided cardiac failure.

Prognosis

The hepatic congestion due to constrictive pericarditis is usually largely reversible. The exception would be in cases of long-standing outflow obstruction when permanent damage to the liver has occurred.

Treatment

Treatment consists of surgical removal of the scarred and fibrosed pericardium. With the removal of the pericardium the forward flow obstruction is essentially removed. Hepatic congestion should then reverse and cardiac function becomes more normal.

Hepatic inflow obstruction

Portal vein thrombosis

Introduction

Thrombosis or obstruction of the portal vein is a major cause of non-cirrhotic portal hypertension. Recall that the definition of a portal system is a series of blood vessels in which two different capillary beds lie between the arterial supply and the final venous drainage back into the inferior vena cava. The hepatic portal vein fits this definition as it lies between the capillary beds of the gastrointestinal tract, gallbladder, pancreas and spleen, and the capillary beds of the liver. The portal vein is formed by the confluence of the superior mesenteric vein, the splenic vein, and the inferior mesenteric vein. The main portal vein divides into left and right branches that empty into the sinusoids of the liver. When flow through the portal vein is impeded this causes hepatic inflow obstruction and increased pressure in the splanchnic bed. Portal hypertension develops and potentially any of the complications therein.

Epidemiology

Portal vein thrombosis occurs in both children and adults. It is a very important cause of non-cirrhotic portal hypertension, particularly in under-developed countries.

Pathogenesis and etiology

There are many potential risk factors for the development of portal vein thrombosis (see Box 7.2). Generally, the specific etiology varies with age and the clinical circumstances. In children the most common cause of portal vein thrombosis is thrombophlebitis of the umbilical vein. Presumably infec-

---

Box 7.2   Causes of portal vein thrombosis

Hypercoagulable disorders
Cirrhosis
Neoplasia causing compression of the portal
  vein – pancreatic cancer, hepatocellular cancer
Myeloproliferative disorders
Hormonal level changes – use of oral
  contraceptives and pregnancy
Collagen vascular diseases
Pancreatitis
Umbilical sepsis
Intra-abdominal sepsis
Umbilical catheterization
Trauma

---

tion occurs in the umbilical vein before the vein obliterates and proceeds proximally to the portal vein. The infection serves as the nidus for thrombus formation. In adults the causes of portal vein thrombosis may vary, and approximately 25% of adult patients with portal vein thrombosis will have underlying cirrhosis. The likelihood of portal vein thrombosis against the backdrop of cirrhosis appears to be related to the severity of the liver disease. Those individuals having worse liver disease are more likely to develop thrombosis. The reason why more advanced cirrhosis may be a risk factor for portal vein thrombosis may be because of the higher intrahepatic resistance to blood flow and the relative stasis or reversal of blood flow in the portal vein which drains into the liver. In one third to one half of adults with portal vein thrombosis the etiology is unknown. It is very likely that many of these individuals may have an occult underlying hypercoagulable state. This hypercoagulable state may be due to genetic abnormalities in coagulation factors, medications, medical procedures, or may be related to underlying neoplastic, infectious, or inflammatory conditions.

Diagnosis

It is important to consider portal vein thrombosis as a cause of gastrointestinal variceal bleeding both in a patient without evidence of liver disease and in patients with known cirrhosis. Acute portal vein thrombosis should always be considered in a patient who has variceal bleeding but no history or evidence to suggest intrinsic liver disease. Similarly, in a patient known to have cirrhosis the development of portal vein thrombosis may be the explanation for sudden decompensation with variceal bleeding.

Patients in whom portal vein thrombosis is suspected should undergo radiologic testing in order to identify and characterize the extent of the clot. The imaging studies that are available and appropriate for evaluating a portal vein thrombosis include ultrasonography with Doppler flow studies, CT, and MRA. The gold standard for diagnosing this condition is venous phase angiography. The main disadvantage of this modality is that it is invasive. Angiography is reserved for patients with a clinical picture consistent with portal vein thrombosis but in whom non-invasive imaging tests have been not been definitive. In addition to the identification and characterization of the thrombosis it is important to perform upper endoscopy to characterize and treat the varices. If a portal vein thrombus is identified then a hypercoagulability work-up may be indicated.

Clinical picture

Portal vein thrombosis leads to portal hypertension and therefore can lead to complications that include variceal bleeding, hepatic encephalopathy, and ascites. However, the manifestations of ascites and hepatic encephalopathy are likely to occur in cases where there is underlying cirrhosis and with a superimposed thrombosis of the portal vein. It is important to remember, however, that portal vein thrombosis alone causes non-cirrhotic portal hypertension and the primary manifestation is of variceal hemorrhage. Non-cirrhotic cases of portal hypertension due to portal vein thrombosis have a better prognosis. In most cases of portal vein thrombosis without cirrhosis this means that the actual function of the liver beyond the portal obstruction is intact. The exception is when portal vein thrombosis develops in an individual whose cirrhosis was present prior to the development of the portal vein thrombosis. The synthetic function of the liver is disrupted exclusively by the inflow obstruction. The most common clinical manifestation of chronic portal vein thrombosis is variceal hemorrhage. The risk for developing liver failure, hepatic encephalopathy, and death are much lower in portal vein thrombosis without cirrhosis than by other causes of liver disease. In addition ascites is far less common. On physical examination patients with portal vein thrombosis can have splenomegaly which may become quite massive. The splenomegaly may be associated with thrombocytopenia and anemia. In cases where the underlying liver is not cirrhotic, patients should not have the peripheral stigmata of liver disease such as palmar erythema and spider angiomata. Jaundice is rare unless there is an underlying hepatic or biliary process.

Prognosis

The overall prognosis for portal vein thrombosis may be quite good in those patients who do not have cirrhosis or a malignancy as an etiologic factor. In those patients in whom there is cirrhosis or a malignancy the prognosis is significantly affected by the stage of disease at the time of portal vein thrombosis.

Treatment

The specific management plan chosen will depend on the clinical picture and the likely duration of the portal vein thrombosis. The treatment options for acute portal vein thrombosis may vary somewhat from the options for chronic portal vein thrombosis. In all cases where portal vein thrombosis is suspected an imaging study such as ultrasound with Doppler flow studies, CT scanning, or MRA should be obtained to confirm the diagnosis. If these studies are unrevealing but the diagnosis is still suspected then venous phase angiography should be performed. In addition, individuals diagnosed with portal vein thrombosis should undergo upper endoscopy in order to evaluate for esophageal varices. An investigation for an underlying hypercoagulable disorder should also be undertaken.

Acute portal vein thrombosis There has been some experience using thrombolytics such as streptokinase and tissue plasminogen activator to treat portal vein thrombosis by delivering the thrombolytic agent directly into the portal vein. The experience with thrombolytics as a treatment is not extensive and it is important to weigh the benefits of such a treatment with the risk of life-threatening bleeding in a patient with portal hypertension.

Chronic portal vein thrombosis The management of chronic portal vein thrombosis may be medical or surgical. Medical management would include screening for varices and use of a non-selective beta-blocker for variceal bleed prophylaxis. The use of anticoagulation may be of use in a subset of patients in whom there is no other underlying liver disease, in whom the thrombus is subacute, and in whom recanalization has not yet occurred. In the majority of cases of chronic portal vein thrombosis in which recanalization has occurred there is no

role for anticoagulation. There is inherent risk in giving anticoagulants to a patient at significant risk for a variceal bleed. If a patient with chronic portal vein thrombosis presents with an active variceal bleed they should undergo emergent endoscopy with banding and/or sclerotherapy to control the bleeding. In most cases bleeding from varices can be handled with endoscopic therapy and if patients do not have underlying cirrhosis, they respond well to endoscopic therapy and have good outcomes. However, if bleeding is recurrent and cannot be adequately managed using endoscopic techniques then surgical therapy may be required.

The surgical therapies available include splenectomy and devascularization, and shunt operation. Transjugular intrahepatic portosystemic shunting can be considered but the shunt will have to extend beyond the clot in the portal vein which also requires declotting and technically may not be possible. The specific surgical intervention chosen depends on the location and associated anatomy of the portal flow obstruction.

Prevention

Portal vein thrombosis may be avoided by using anticoagulation in patients without a history of such thrombosis but with a known hypercoagulable disorder. The complications of portal vein thrombosis can be prevented by aggressive investigation for and treatment of portal vein thrombosis.

Splenic vein thrombosis

Splenic vein occlusions or thrombosis is most commonly caused by pancreatic inflammation or tumors within or near the pancreas. Occlusion of the splenic vein may lead to extrahepatic portal hypertension with the possible complications of splenomegaly and variceal bleeding. The classic finding in cases of splenic vein thrombosis is the presence of gastric varices without esophageal varices. It should be noted, however, that splenic vein thrombosis has been associated with the development of varices in the esophagus, stomach, duodenum and colon. Because the development of splenic vein thrombosis is often associated with a pancreatic or peripancreatic processes it is important to consider this diagnosis in any patient who is found to have isolated gastric varices and a history of pancreatic disease. Accurate diagnosis of this condition is important since splenectomy is the surgical procedure of choice rather than portosystemic shunting or liver transplantation. In cases of advanced liver injury liver transplantation may be required. The diagnosis may be made using dynamic CT, ultrasonography, and 3D MR venography. In cases where these non-invasive tests are inconclusive celiac or splenic arteriogram may be performed. The angiographic findings may include the presence of splenoportal collaterals and non-opacification of the splenic vein during the venous phase. The treatment for splenic vein thrombosis may include splenectomy or splenic artery embolization if the patient is not an optimal surgical candidate.

Vascular tumors of the liver

Hepatic hemangiomas

Introduction

A hemangioma is defined as a benign tumor of blood vessels. Hemangiomas are the most common benign mesenchymal lesions found in the liver. Typically hemangiomas are solitary but may also be multiple. Hemangiomas may involve the right or left hepatic lobes. Hemangiomas may be detected incidentally in asymptomatic persons who undergoing cross-sectional imaging for other reasons or they may be quite symptomatic. Hemangiomas may range in size from a few millimeters to 20 cm. Most hemangiomas are smaller than 5 cm. Larger hemangiomas may be referred to as giant hemangiomas and are more likely to be symptomatic.

Epidemiology

The prevalence of hemangiomas is reported to range between 0.4% to 20%. Overall hepatic hemangiomas appear to be common in the general population. Hemangiomas may occur in children and adults although most are diagnosed in adulthood between the ages of 30 and 50 years. This may partly be because individuals of this age group are more likely to undergo imaging studies of the abdomen for other reasons. During these tests hemangiomas are incidentally diagnosed. In addition, it has been postulated that hemangiomas are actually congenital hamartomas or tissue malformations present from birth that grow over time. Based on this theory, hemangiomas would reach a more appreciable size as individuals grows older. Hemangiomas occur in both men and women but

in adults they are more common in women with a male to female ratio of 3:1.

Pathogenesis and etiology

The etiology of hepatic hemangiomas is not completely understood. It has been suggested that hemangiomas are in fact congenital hamartomas or vascular malformations that grow slowly from birth. This growth in size is attributed to ectasia rather than hypertrophy or hyperplasia. Based on clinical observation it appears that exposure to hormones may influence the growth of some hepatic hemangiomas. It has been observed that pregnancy and exogenous estrogen and progesterone administration have been associated with enlargement of hepatic hemangiomas. The withdrawal of exogenous hormones may be associated with regression of the hemangiomas. Not all hepatic hemangiomas may be hormonally responsive, however, since these tumors do not always express estrogen receptors and certainly can grow in size without an increase or alteration in hormone levels. By the same token, not all hemangiomas will regress with the withdrawal of supplemental hormones or the end of a pregnancy.

Diagnosis

The diagnosis of hepatic hemangiomas is typically made on cross-sectional imaging studies. Often hemangiomas are discovered incidentally. The imaging studies that frequently identify hemangiomas include ultrasonography, CT, and MRI. Occasionally more than one imaging study is required in order to fully characterize the lesion.

Ultrasonography On ultrasound a hepatic hemangioma will appear as a well-demarcated homogeneous hyperechoic mass. If the liver is infiltrated with fat the lesion may appear hypoechoic. It is possible to use color Doppler to characterize the lesion as a hemangioma by demonstrating blood flow through it although it should be noted that this is not always a reliable test. The Doppler flow study may be falsely negative. The character of the sonographic image may also depend on the size of the hemangioma.

Computed tomography Hemangiomas may be detected on non-contrast enhanced CT scans. In a small percentage of cases calcifications will be visible in the hemangioma. If contrast is used initially the lesion will look like a peripheral nodule. After a delay of 3 or more minutes the hemangioma will fill with blood and the lesion will appear isodense or hyperdense on the delayed scans. If the lesion is particularly large the center may remain unopacified.

Magnetic resonance imaging Magnetic resonance imaging may be a very accurate modality for characterizing lesions as hemangiomas. On MRI hemangiomas will appear smooth, well-demarcated, and homogeneous with a low signal intensity on T1-weighted images and hyperintense on T2-weighted images.

Angiography Angiography is not typically required to make the diagnosis of a hepatic hemangioma. Occasionally, angiography may be used to help characterize a lesion, particularly when an atypical tumor is a possible diagnosis.

Serum biochemical markers Serum laboratory tests are usually within normal limits unless the hemangioma has been complicated by thrombosis or rarely causes biliary obstruction.

Liver biopsy Liver biopsy is not routinely used to make the diagnosis of a hepatic hemangioma. The risk of inducing serious hemorrhage exists and for this reason lesions that have the appearance of a hemangioma on cross-sectional imaging studies are not routinely biopsied. Biopsy may play a role in cases of liver lesions where the lesion is not clearly vascular and the question of neoplasia needs to be investigated.

Clinical picture

Most commonly, hepatic hemangiomas are discovered incidentally in asymptomatic individuals. They may be discovered in imaging studies performed for unrelated reasons or during laparotomy or autopsy. Symptoms are more likely from larger lesions such as those exceeding 4 cm in size. Symptoms may include abdominal pain and right upper quadrant fullness. Patients may present with acute abdominal pain if bleeding or thrombosis occurs within the hemangioma leading to inflammation or stretching of the liver capsule. In addition, although rarely, hemangiomas may spontaneously rupture and this is manifest as hemobilia. In children giant hemangiomas have been associated with high output cardiac failure and hypothyroidism. The hypothyroidism is explained by the presence of 3 iodothyronine deiodinase in the hemangioma tissue which leads to conversion of triiodothyronine to biologically inactive hormones, triiodothyronine, and 3, 3'-diiodothyronine. In addition, the Kasabach–Merritt syndrome refers to a consumptive coagulopathy that has been described in children with giant hemangiomas. It has been called into question whether the coagulopathy is related to giant hemangiomas or to kaposiform hemangioendotheliomas which may resemble hemangiomas.

Prognosis

The natural history of hepatic hemangiomas has not been completely studied. Since these lesions are so common and so often asymptomatic it is difficult to estimate with confidence the overall prevalence and the incidence of complications. In general the prognosis for these lesions appears very favorable. Intervention is usually not required. The development of complications such as spontaneous rupture or rupture secondary to blunt abdominal trauma is quite rare.

Treatment

If hepatic hemangiomas are relatively small (less than 1.5 cm) and asymptomatic there is no need for specific management. Larger hemangiomas are at greater risk for symptoms and complications. For a large hemangioma (more than 5 cm) it is reasonable to monitor its size by periodic imaging. Surgical management should be reserved for those patients with hemangiomas that are causing symptoms or extrinsic compression of adjacent structures. Surgical management options of a hepatic hemangioma include resection, hepatic artery ligation, enucleation, and, rarely, liver transplantation. If a hemangioma is causing symptoms but surgical management is not feasible, the preferred non-surgical options then include hepatic artery embolization, radiotherapy, and treatment with interferon alpha-2a.

In women in whom hemangiomas have been identified it is not clear whether pregnancy should be avoided. This area remains controversial although it would be reasonable to advise a woman with a large hemangiomas to avoid exogenous hormone treatment.

Prevention

There is no way to prevent the development of hemangiomas. The complications of these lesions may be prevented by careful monitoring and definitive treatment when the lesions are causing symptoms or compression.

Hereditary hemorrhagic telangiectasia

Hereditary hemorrhagic telangiectasia is a familial disorder characterized by small vascular ectasias that may be located on the skin, mucous membranes, and in various organs throughout the body. Hereditary hemorrhagic telangiectasia is also called Rendu–Osler–Weber–Syndrome after the authors who individually described the clinical syndrome. The vascular ectasias of hereditary hemorrhagic telangiectasia may have protean locations with various complications depending on the organs involved. Classically, hereditary hemorrhagic telangiectasia is characterized by familial epistaxis in combination with telangiectasias. In patients with gastrointestinal tract involvement hereditary hemorrhagic telangiectasia may present with recurrent gastrointestinal bleeding. Involvement of the liver in hereditary hemorrhagic telangiectasia is rare but important to consider since the complications can be severe. When the liver contains arteriovenous malformations due to hereditary hemorrhagic telangiectasia, high cardiac output failure may result because of shunting of blood from the arteriole to the venous system within the liver. In addition hereditary hemorrhagic telangiectasia can lead to atypical cirrhosis.

Infantile hemangioendothelioma

Infantile hemagioendotheliomas are rare benign tumors composed of small, proliferating, capillary-like vascular channels. This tumor is not malignant but may cause hepatic failure or high-output cardiac failure if it becomes large enough.

Epithelioid hemangioendothelioma

Epithelioid hemagioendotheliomas are rare malignant tumors that are composed of epithelioid-appearing endothelial cells. These tumors may occur in soft tissue, bone, and rarely in the liver. These tumors were first described in 1982. Because of their rarity the natural history and malignant potential of these tumors has not been well characterized.

Angiosarcoma

Epidemiology

Angiosarcoma is a rare vascular tumor which may occur in the liver. It is composed of atypical endothelial cells that proliferate in the sinuisoids. This tumor is highly malignant. It occurs mainly in adults in the sixth to seventh decade. Men are affected more commonly than women with a male to female ratio of 4:1.

Risk factors for the development of angiosarcoma include exposure to thorium dioxide (Thortrast®), arsenic, and vinyl chloride.

Clinical picture

The most common presenting symptom is abdominal pain. Other features may include progressive liver failure, weight loss, nausea, and vomiting. Ascites may develop and may be blood stained. In approximately 15% of cases patients may present with hemoperitoneum after rupture of the tumor through the hepatic capsule wall.

Diagnosis

Laboratory studies may show rising bilirubin and markers of deteriorating liver function. Ultrasound may reveal a mass in the liver, but if the tumor is an infiltrating type it may not be discretely visualized. Hepatic angiography reveals a blush and puddling of contrast as the arteries have been displaced by the tumor tissue.

Liver biopsy

The hallmark is blood-filled cysts although there may be areas of solid growth. With progression of the tumor there is sinusoidal dilatation and disruption of normal hepatic architecture. The vascular spaces may enlarge to the point that the tumor takes on a cavernous appearance.

Prognosis

The prognosis of angiosarcomas of the liver is very poor. The tumors tend to grow rapidly and are highly malignant. Death usually occurs within 6 months of presentation.

Treatment

Angiosarcomas usually present at an advanced stage precluding curative surgery. Chemotherapy and radiation therapy have not been proven to have tremendous benefit.

Further reading

Bearman SI. Veno-occlusive disease of the liver. *Current Opinion in Oncology* 2000; 12: 103–109.

DeLeve LD, Shulman HM, McDonald GB. Toxic injury to hepatic sinusoids: sinuisoidal obstruction syndrome (veno-occlusive disease). *Semin Liver Dis* 2002; 22(1): 27–41.

Guttmacher AE, Marchuk DA, White RI. Hereditary hemorrhagic telangiectasia. *N Engl J Med* 1995; 333(14): 918–924.

Iqbal N, and Saleem A. Hepatic hemangioma: a review. *Texas Medicine* 1997; 93(5): 48–50.

Okuda K. Inferior vena cava thrombosis at its hepatic portion (obliterative hepatocavopathy). *Semin Liver Dis* 2002; 22(1): 15–26.

Sarin SK, Agarwal SR. Extrahepatic portal vein obstruction. *Semin Liver Dis* 2002; 22(1): 43–58.

Uchimura K, Nakamuta M, Osoegawa M *et al*. Hepatic epithelioid hemangioendothelioma. *J Clin Gastroenterol* 2001; 32(5): 431–434.

Valla D-C. Hepatic vein thrombosis (Budd–Chiari syndrome). *Semin Liver Dis* 2002; 22(1): 5–14.

Chapter 8

Fulminant Hepatic Failure

Abhasnee Sobhonslidsuk and K. Rajender Reddy

CHAPTER OUTLINE

Introduction

Fulminant hepatic failure is one of the more dramatic and lethal manifestations of acute liver injury. Its clinical features become evident as either an abrupt or an insidious onset of hepatic encephalopathy, after a variable interval between an apparently healthy state and the manifestations of liver failure. The diagnosis of acute liver failure is almost always made in a previously healthy person without known liver disease, although occasionally it can be made in asymptomatic patients with unrecognized chronic liver disease. Fulminant hepatic failure is an uncommon disease with an estimated 2000 reported cases annually in the US. Nonetheless, its mortality rate is exceedingly high, approaching 80% in individuals who do not receive rapid and appropriate therapeutic intervention. Over the years the survival of patients with fulminant hepatic failure has improved because of great advances in the early recognition of this presentation, an understanding of the poor prognostic indicators, more intensive clinical monitoring, and improved medical management. Liver transplantation has been the best and most definitive treatment for fulminant hepatic failure. However, the shortage of donor organs and lack of reliable criteria that can rapidly identify patients who require liver transplantation have been two major problems. New modalities of liver transplantation have been developed to overcome the difficulties of organ shortage. Biologic and artificial liver support devices, that support critically ill patients while waiting for a liver transplantation, have been under evaluation and appear promising. All of these efforts have led to a currently favorable outcome for individuals with fulminant hepatic failure.

Terminology and classification

The term fulminant hepatic failure was first introduced in 1970 by Trey and Davidson to describe a "potentially reversible condition, the consequence of severe liver injury, with an onset of encephalopathy within 8 weeks of the appearance of the first symptoms and in the absence of pre-existing liver disease." This term has been widely accepted with succeeding modifications. King's College Hospital in London proposed a category of late-onset hepatic failure in which encephalopathy occurs between 8 and 26 weeks after the onset of symptoms. More recently, a French group observed that the levels of coagulation factors produced by the liver, especially factors II and V, were important indicators of severe acute liver failure. The same group redefined fulminant hepatic failure by incorporating an interval between the onset of jaundice and the development of hepatic encephalopathy. They described fulminant hepatic failure as acute liver failure in which hepatic encephalopathy appeared within 2 weeks following the onset of jaundice, and subfulminant liver failure as acute liver failure in which hepatic encephalopathy manifested 2 weeks to 3 months after the onset of jaundice. The clinical features of

the latter are rather unique. Signs of portal hypertension, for example ascites, splenomegaly, and acute renal failure predominate in this group. Other complex definitions and classifications have been proposed to better define prognosis. The term hyperacute liver failure was used to describe a clinical presentation of encephalopathy occuring within 7 days of the onset of jaundice. An interval of 8 to 28 days from jaundice to encephalopathy has been another definition of acute liver failure. The term subacute liver failure was used to describe encephalopathy occuring within 5 to 12 weeks of the onset of jaundice. Acetaminophen, hepatitis A virus (HAV), and hepatitis B virus (HBV) commonly cause a clinical syndrome of hyperacute liver failure, in which the incidence of brain edema is very common, yet the chance of survival without transplantation among these patients is higher than that for acute or subacute liver failure (Table 8.1). Wilson's disease, autoimmune hepatitis, and reactivation of hepatitis B or superinfection with hepatitis D are exceptions where they at times manifest as a clinical syndrome of acute liver failure, although chronic parenchymatous disease of the liver with or without cirrhosis has been present for years. Interestingly enough, most western patients with acute liver failure usually develop hepatic encephalopathy within 12 weeks of the onset of jaundice, whereas eastern populations with acute liver failure usually present within 4 weeks of the onset of jaundice. The International Association for the Study of the Liver proposed that the definition of acute hepatic failure is when the interval between the onset of jaundice and encephalopathy was less than 4 weeks, and subacute hepatic failure is when encephalopathy appeared between 4 to 24 weeks after the onset of jaundice. No matter what classification is used to determine the prognosis of patients, an understanding of the pathophysiologic changes in fulminant hepatic failure is a prerequisite. The nomenclature of fulminant hepatic failure still demands more refinement in order to become a universally accepted terminology.

Etiology (Table 8.2)

Regardless of the initiating cause of fulminant hepatic failure, the typical pathological finding of a liver biopsy is of extensive coagulative necrosis of the liver with hepatocyte drop-out. The predominant area of liver injury depends on the etiologic agent. Drug-induced liver injury predominantly causes liver cell necrosis in zone 3 (centrizonal) of

Table 8.1 Subgroup classification of acute liver failure syndrome according to the interval of onset of jaundice and development of hepatic encephalopathy (Reproduced with permission from O'Grady *et al The Lancet* 1993; 342: 273–275)

	Hyperacute liver failure	Acute liver failure	Subacute liver failure
Duration of jaundice (days)	0–7 (0–1 week)	8–28 (> 1–4 weeks)	29–72 (5–12 weeks)
Commonest causes	acetaminophen, hepatitis A, hepatitis B	non-A, non-B hepatitis	non-A, non-B hepatitis
Cerebral edema (%)	common (69%)	common (56 %)	infrequent (14%)
Prothrombin time	prolonged	prolonged	least prolonged
Bilirubin	least raised	raised	raised
Survival rate (%)	36%	7%	14%

hepatic lobules. The incidence and etiology of fulminant hepatic failure has geographic variability. Nevertheless, globally, viral hepatitis is still the the most common cause of fulminant hepatic failure.

Viral hepatitis

Around 400 million people worldwide are HBV carriers. Globally, the most frequent cause of fulminant hepatic failure is HBV, especially in some regions of eastern and Mediterranean countries. In the US however, HBV infection is the cause of fulminant hepatic failure in only 10% of cases. In general, HBV-related fulminant hepatic failure has

Table 8.2 Common causes of fulminant hepatic failure

Group	Examples
Viral hepatitis	hepatitis A, B, C, D, E herpesvirus cytomegalovirus
Drug-induced hepatotoxicity	acetaminophen antituberculosis drugs troglitazone ecstasy
Herbal medicines	Jin bu huan comfrey
Toxins	*Amanita phalloides* carbontetrachloride trichloroethylene
Vascular causes	Budd–Chiari syndrome veno-occlusive disease ischemia or hypoxia heatstroke
Miscellaneous causes	malignant infiltration Wilson's disease autoimmune hepatitis (rare) acute fatty liver of pregnancy Reye's syndrome

been seen in 1% of adult cases who have acute hepatitis B. During acute hepatitis B infection, a robust immune response is needed to clear the infection. At times, the extensive immune-mediated lysis of infected hepatocytes causes severe liver injury, and hence leads to fulminant hepatic failure. The other condition that predisposes to fulminant hepatic failure through a similar mechanism is the abrupt withdrawal of steroids or chemotherapy. In such cases, HBV has the ability to reactivate and cause fulminant hepatic failure in patients where there may be an underlying low replicative state of HBV. Precore mutation of HBV, and hepatitis D virus (HDV), can also cause fulminant hepatic failure, although this is infrequent with HBV. The prevalence of HDV is high in the Mediterranean region, but in western countries it is largely confined to intravenous drug users. Hepatitis D virus is a virus that requires the concomitant presence of HBV infection. A large proportion of cases of HBV-related fulminant hepatic failure are found to have HBV and HDV co-infection. In addition, cases of fulminant hepatic failure associated with this co-infection tend to have a more severe course and a higher mortality rate than those with fulminant hepatic failure due to HBV infection alone.

Acute HAV infection leads to fulminant hepatic failure in less than 0.5% of cases. Previously, HAV accounted for 7% to 8% of fulminant hepatic failure cases in the US. Hepatitis A virus-related fulminant hepatic failure has the best outcome of the various viral hepatitis-related fulminant hepatic failures with spontaneous recovery and survival being higher than 60%. However, elderly patients and those with underlying chronic hepatitis C virus (HCV) infection tend to experience a severe clinical course of fulminant hepatic failure. The clinical course of HAV-related fulminant hepatic failure usually meets with the criteria of hyperacute liver failure.

Conflicting reports indicate that HCV may cause fulminant hepatic failure. In the US and Europe HCV-related fulminant hepatic failure in patients without underlying liver disease has rarely been reported to cause fulminant hepatic failure. In contrast, up to 50% of cases of non-A non-B fulminant hepatic failure, in Japan, have been found to have HCV RNA. Fulminant hepatic failure as a consequence of HCV is sometimes seen when there is a co-infection or superinfection of HCV along with other hepatotrophic virus.

Fulminant hepatic failure cases from hepatitis E virus (HEV) has rarely been reported in western countries. However, in countries such as India it is the most frequent cause of fulminant hepatic failure. Fulminant hepatic failure due to HEV is found rather specifically in pregnant women, and it requires medical attention and intensive care because of the extremely high mortality in these women. Other hepatotrophic viruses that are occasionally associated with fulminant hepatic failure in immunocompromised patients are cytomegalovirus, Epstein–Barr virus and herpesvirus types 1, 2, and 6. If the causative agent has been identified, urgent treatment with specific antiviral drugs is necessary to avoid liver transplantation.

In a substantial number of cases, even after a full serologic and virologic work-up, the causative factors cannot always be identified. These cases have been categorized as non-A, non-B hepatitis or cryptogenic hepatitis. Over time, the reported incidence of cryptogenic fulminant hepatic failure has decreased steadily because of our ability to diagnose the common viruses that cause fulminant hepatic failure more reliably and also because of a better recognition of the various drugs that cause fulminant hepatic failure. More recently, the reported contribution of the "unknown" causes to the overall cases of fulminant hepatic failure has ranged from 15% to 45%. Such cases usually have a subfulminant course with a mortality rate as high as 85%. Initial experiences indicated that some of the newly discovered viruses, GBV-C/HGV and TT viruses, cause fulminant hepatic failure but subsequent studies suggest that they may be innocent bystanders and not pathogenetically responsible.

Drug-induced hepatotoxicity

In the UK, 60% of fulminant hepatic failure cases occur as a consequence of acetaminophen overdose. In the US, however, acetaminophen overdose accounts for only 20% of the cases, though its incidence has increased considerably over the past decade. In 1998, a policy of smaller blister packaging of acetaminophen was implemented in the UK, and this has led to a reduction in the amount of drug taken in one single overdose. The prognosis of fulminant hepatic failure from acetaminophen is relatively better than from other causes, with a spontaneous recovery of more than 60%. Ingestion of acetaminophen of more than 150 mg/kg is likely to predictably cause acetaminophen hepatotototoxicity. The toxicity rarely occurs when the consumed dose is less than 12 g. In a healthy normal state, a small amount of acetaminophen is converted by cytochrome P450 2EII to a toxic intermediate metabolite N-acetyl-p-benzoquinoneimine. The toxic substance is then metabolized by intracellular glutathione and excreted as mercapturic-acid derivatives. Predisposing factors to acetaminophen toxicity are the conditions that increase the activity of P450 enzymes, such as the concomitant use of anticonvulsant therapy or alcohol abuse, and those that deplete gluthathione reserves, such as malnutrition. Hepatotoxicity in chronic alcoholics who take acetaminophen in a non-toxic dose has been well recognized and called a "therapeutic misadventure". N-acetylcysteine is an antidote of choice that is of proven benefit for the prevention of hepatotoxicity if it is given within 15 hours of acetominophen ingestion. It counteracts acetaminophen toxicity by replenishing gluthatione stores.

Other drugs often cause hepatotoxicity through an idiosyncratic mechanism. The unique feature of this type of hepatotoxicity is a rare and unpredictable event. Examples of this group are halothane, isoniazid, and antiretroviral drugs. Troglitazone, the first thiazolidinedione agent, for diabetes mellitus, was launched in the US in 1997. Three years later, the drug was withdrawn because at least 90 patients who took the drug subsequently developed acute liver failure. Moreover, 70 patients who took troglitazone for a certain period of time expired or underwent liver transplantation. One common cause of drug toxicity in patients younger than 25 years old is ingestion of ecstasy (3,4 methylenedioxy-metamphetamine) which may cause death, probably through the mechanisms of hypersensitivity and ischemia.

Herbal medicines

Nowadays, the use of herbal remedies is increasing and it has, to some extent, become fashionable in everyday life. Severe hepatotoxicity due to some herbs, such as Jin bu huan, chaparral, and comfrey has been reported.

Toxins

Mushroom poisoning, which often occurs following the ingestion of the mushroom *Amanita phalloides*, has a high mortality rate of between 10% and 40%. The principle toxin causing liver injury is alpha-amanitin, one of the amanatoxins. The minimum amount of toxin required to cause hepatotoxicity is approximately 50 grams which can be obtained from three middle-sized mushrooms. Clinical signs of fulminant hepatic failure usually appear several days after ingestion. Other toxins that can cause fulminant hepatic failure are the industrial chemical agents carbontetrachloride and trichloroethylene.

Vascular causes

Acute or subacute venous outflow obstruction, whether it affects the large hepatic veins (Budd–Chiari syndrome) or the centrilobular veins (veno-occlusive diseases), can cause fulminant hepatic failure. Veno-occlusive disease most often occurs after induction chemotherapy and bone-marrow transplantation. Ischemic liver necrosis usually results in mild liver injury and spontaneous recovery is frequently seen, except for the very rare case that needs liver transplantation.

Miscellaneous causes

Hematologic and non-hematologic infiltration may have a presenting feature of fulminant hepatic failure. Malignancy-related fulminant hepatic failure is one of the more catastrophic situations, with mortality reaching nearly 100%. Liver transplantation is contraindicated in these patients. In cases where a malignancy is suspected as causing fulminant hepatic failure, a liver biopsy, done transjugularly, is urgently indicated for an accurate diagnosis. Wilson's disease and autoimmune hepatitis share some common features; both diseases have underlying and unrecognized chronic liver disease but the onset of the diseases may simulate the features of fulminant hepatic failure. Awareness and recognition of these two uncommon diseases are necessary because acute liver failure associated with each disease is difficult to manage and usually ends up with liver transplantation. Two other uncommon causes of fulminant hepatic failure are acute fatty liver in pregnancy and Reye's syndrome. In acute fatty liver of pregnancy, the clinical manifestations of acute liver failure often appear in the third trimester, and may be associated with pre-eclampsia, hemolysis, and thrombocytopenia. Delivery of the baby is the definitive treatment. Acute, non-icteric liver failure in children or young adults occurring after taking aspirin, or following a viral infection should raise the clinical suspicion of Reye's syndrome. Liver histology in both diseases demonstrates microvesicular fatty infiltration with paucity of inflammatory cells. The pathogenesis of both these conditions is not known. Some women who suffer from acute fatty liver of pregnancy are found to have heterozygous deficiency of a mitochrondrial oxidation enzyme of fatty acids, long-chain 3-hydroxyl-acyl-CoA dehydrogenase. Impaired mitochondrial beta-oxidation and oxidative phosphorylation may be the basic mechanism of mitochondrial dysfunction in Reye's syndrome. The mechanism of mitochondrial dysfunction may explain the pathogenesis of both diseases.

Clinical manifestations

In the majority of cases the clinical syndrome of fulminant hepatic failure begins with the prodromal symptoms of malaise, anorexia, and low-grade fever, followed by the signs and symptoms of liver failure such as jaundice and encephalopathy. There are four clinical stages of acute hepatic encephalopathy. Patients with stage 1 display signs of slow thinking, slurred speech and sleep–wake disturbances. Patients with stage 2 are drowsy with asterixis. The consciousness of patients in stage III to IV worsens from semistupor to coma. Stages of hepatic encephalopathy can fluctuate, especially in patients with subfulminant hepatic failure. Cerebral edema and intracranial hypertension occur in 80% of cases who have grade III or IV hepatic encephalopathy. Clinical manifestations in such cases include profuse sweating, pupil dilatation, systemic hypertension and bradycardia, increased hyperventilation, increasing muscle tone and decerebrate posture, and apnea in the terminal stage, which infers the progression of brain herniation.

Complications and pathophysiology

In addition to hepatic encephalopathy, the clinical manifestations of fulminant hepatic failure include cerebral edema, sepsis, acute respiratory insufficiency, circulatory failure, and renal failure. Cytokines or mediators released by the failing liver, high levels of circulating endotoxins, and impaired metabolic functions of the liver precipitate disturbances of the systemic vascular circulation, diffuse organ dysfunction and, finally, multiple organ failure (Figure 8.1). Intensive medical support with a comprehension of the complex pathophysiology helps in better supporting patients who are awaiting liver transplantation.

Hepatic encephalopathy

The pathogenesis of hepatic encephalopathy in fulminant hepatic failure is multifactorial. Liver failure accompanied by porto-systemic shunting leads to an elevated blood concentration of potentially neurotoxic substances. Examples of circulating toxins involved in the pathogenesis of encephalopathy are ammonia, false neurotransmitters, endogenous benzodiazepines, and cytokines. Ammonia affects cerebral function by inducing a transient impairment of brain-energy metabolism and astrocyte swelling. The central noradrenergic system may also be associated in the pathogenesis of fulminant hepatic failure as supported by decreased levels of noradrenaline (norepinephrine) in the brain. The amelioration of encephalopathy in some cases, after the administration of the benzodiazepine receptor antagonist, flumazenil, suggests the potential role of endogenous benzodiazepines in the development of encephalopathy.

Brain edema

The most common causes of death in fulminant hepatic failure are brain edema and sepsis. Clinical features of brain edema become apparent in patients whose consciousness deteriorates to the level of grade III or IV hepatic encephalopathy. The pathogenesis of cerebral edema is unclear. Examination by electron microscope of brain biopsy derived from patients with fulminant hepatic failure has demonstrated evidence of both vasogenic and cytotoxic brain edema, but the changes suggestive of cytotoxic edema have been more evident. Several experimental models demonstrate a breakdown of the blood–brain barrier which is followed by an increased uptake of fluid and plasma resulting in vasogenic edema. However, the hypothesis of cytotoxic brain edema has been more widely studied and accepted than vasogenic edema.

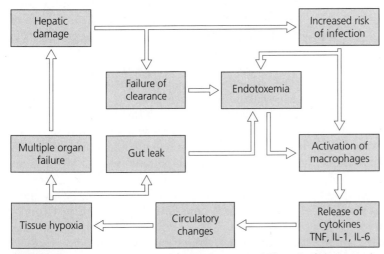

Figure 8.1 Pathogenesis of multiple organ failure in fulminant hepatic failure. Damaged liver releases toxic mediators that affect systemic organ functions, aggravating tissue oxygen extraction, and increasing the risk of infection (reproduced with permission from William R. Classification, etiology, and consideration of outcome in acute liver failure. (Reproduced with permission from *Semin Liver Dis* 1996; 16: 343–348).

Ammonia–glutamine hypothesis

The most appealing hypothesis for the pathogenesis of brain edema is one that involves ammonia and glutamine. The majority of circulating ammonia is synthesized from the hepatic–splanchnic region. When it enters the brain, the site of detoxification is in the astrocytes because the brain lacks a complete urea cycle. Astrocytes, cells with foot processes, are located between the cerebral blood vessels and neurons (Figure 8.2). Because of this ideal position, astrocytes function in maintaining a balance between energy consumption of neurons and glucose uptake from the capillaries, i.e. the metabolism–blood flow coupling. Ammonia elimination is through the change of glutamate to glutamine, which is catalyzed mainly by the enzyme glutamine synthetase. Inhibition of glutamine synthetase with methionine sulfoximine was shown to prevent the development of brain edema in an experimental study of rats. Glutamine acts as an osmolyte, promoting water diffusion into astrocytes. Astrocytes then swell, and this is the starting point of cytotoxic edema. The release of *myo*-inositol to re-establish normal astrocyte volume is a counter-balance mechanism for the increased intracellular osmolarity from the glutamine effect. Nevertheless, in fulminant hepatic failure, the rate of *myo*-inositol synthesis remains at the usual level and is unable to overcome the rapid liberation of glutamine. Not surprisingly, cerebral edema prevails in acute liver failure, especially in cases who have hyperacute clinical courses, and it rarely occurs in cases with chronic liver failure, suggesting a time-dependent process of brain edema. From one study, an arterial ammonia level higher than 230 µg/dL, measured within 24 hours after the development of grade III or IV hepatic encephalopathy, was associated with subsequent cerebral herniation from the development of brain edema (Figure 8.3).

Derangement of cerebral circulation

The pattern of change in cerebral blood flow in fulminant hepatic failure can be inconsistent. Studies in animal models of fulminant hepatic failure demonstrated that a fall in cerebral blood flow precedes the development of increased intracranial pressure. This suggests that cerebral hypoxia could be a cause of cerebral edema. In the normal situation, the cerebral blood flow is closely related to cerebral metabolism with a coupling system, which means that cerebral blood flow in fulminant hepatic failure should be lower because the cerebral metabolic rate for oxygen is uniformly reduced in this condition. The cerebral autoregulation keeps cerebral blood flow relatively constant by reactive dilatation or myotonic constriction of cerebral blood vessels. The finding of high cerebral blood flow is more frequently reported than that of low cerebral blood flow. So, in fulminant hepatic failure, the failure of cerebral autoregulation is very likely, and cerebral blood flow changes occur in parallel with systemic blood pressure (Figure 8.4). Cerebral edema and increased cerebral blood flow are

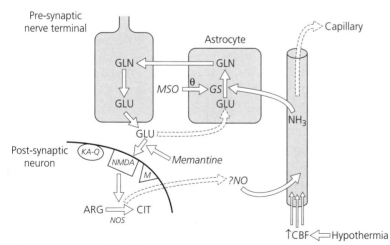

Figure 8.2 Model of ammonia-induced cerebral edema in fulminant hepatic failure and postulate sites of treatment. Effect of hypothermia, methionine sulfoximine (MSO) and memantine on cerebral blood flow (CBF), glutamine synthesis, and the NMDA receptor respectively. Nitric oxide (NO) may increase cerebral hyperemia directly (GLN: glutamine; GLU: glutamate; GS: glutamine synthetase) (reproduced with permission from Blei AT, Larsen FS. Pathophysiology of cerebral edema in fulminant hepatic failure. Reproduced with permission from *J Hepatol* 1999; 31: 771–776).

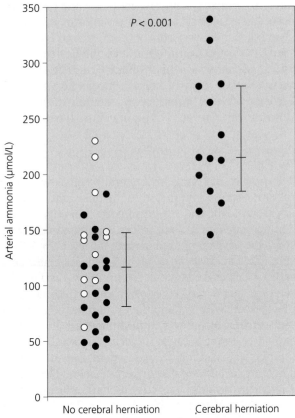

Figure 8.3 Arterial ammonia levels in patients with fulminant hepatic failure, with and without cerebral herniation. In the group with no cerebral herniation, there were 12 open circles, 7 of these underwent liver transplantation and 5 died from other reasons (reproduced with permission from Clemmesen JO, Larsen FS, Kondrup J, *et al.* Cerebral herniation in patients with acute liver failure is correlated with arterial ammonia concentration. *Hepatology* 1999; 29: 648–653).

two major factors causing increased intracranial pressure (ICP) due to the effect of cerebral volume expansion. The normal ICP in adults ranges from 0 to 10 mmHg. Cerebral perfusion pressure (CPP) is mathematically derived from mean arterial pressure minus the ICP. A CPP level below 50 mmHg or the elevation of ICP above 40 mmHg for longer than 2 hours has been suggested as an endpoint which would be a contraindication, although not an absolute contraindication, for liver transplantation because of a poor neurological outcome post-transplantation in such patients.

Cytokines from necrotic liver

Circulating cytokines that are released from a necrotic liver in fulminant hepatic failure are TNFα, IL-1β and

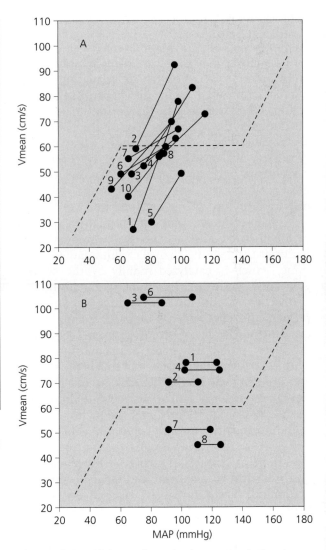

Figure 8.4 A) Loss of cerebral autoregulation in fulminant hepatic failure, and B) reversal after liver transplantation demonstrated by transcranial doppler (Vmean: mean flow velocity in the cerebral artery; MAP: mean arterial pressure) (reproduced with permission from Strauss G, Hansen BA, Kirkegaard P, *et al.* Liver function, cerebral blood flow autoregulation, and hepatic encephalopathy in fulminant hepatic failure. *Hepatology* 1997; 25: 837–839).

IL-6. These cytokines can affect multiple organs, including the brain. Cytokines may induce the synthesis of signal transduction, such as nitric oxide and prostacyclin, that further directly influence brain function. There are some reports that hepatectomy or total hepatic removal improved hemodynamic stability and helped control cerebral edema and intracranial hypertension, and this may be mediated via the removal of circulating cytokines.

Systemic hemodynamic changes

Several cytokines released from the necrotic liver activate vascular endothelium. Plugging of capillaries from migrating leukocytes and platelets compromises microcirculation. Reducing oxygen delivery to tissue occurs because blood is shunting away from the occluded capillary beds. Tissue hypoxia is an unavoidable phenomenon and aerobic metabolism is forcibly converted to anaerobic metabolism. Lactic acid is accumulated as time goes by, and it is accepted that lactic acidosis is a poor prognostic factor in fulminant hepatic failure. Tissue oxygen extraction is impaired in fulminant hepatic failure, so tissue oxygen consumption becomes dependent on oxygen delivery over a wider range of delivery (pathological supply-dependency) (Figure 8.5). Systemic vasodilatation from increased nitric oxide production induces hypotension, accentuating the degree of lactic acidosis, and probably decreasing cerebral blood flow. Patients with fulminant hepatic failure typically have hyperdynamic circulation with a low systemic vascular resistance and markedly increased cardiac output.

Infection and sepsis

Infection is a serious complication of fulminant hepatic failure in that approximately 25% of all

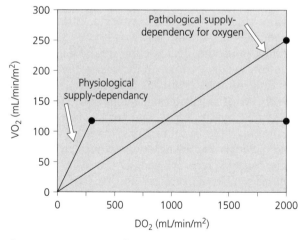

Figure 8.5 Due to the impairment of tissue oxygen extraction in fulminant hepatic failure, an increase in oxygen delivery (DO_2) results in a linear oxygen consumption (VO_2) (reproduced with permission from Ellis A, Wendon J. Circulatory, respiratory, cerebral, and renal derangements in acute liver failure: pathophysiology and management. *Semin Liver Dis* 1996; 16: 379–388).

deaths are caused by an infection. Furthermore, evidence of bacterial infection is found in 80% of patients with fulminant hepatic failure during its clinical course. Of all infections, gram-positive bacteria are responsible for 60% to 70% and gram-negative bacteria for 26% to 30% of infections. These observations sharply contrast with the studies conducted in developing countries, where infections due to gram-negative bacteria predominate in fulminant hepatic failure. The incidence of infection is higher in patients who have pre-existing hepatic encephalopathy, and infection itself can precipitate hepatic encephalopathy. An elevation of white blood cells and a high temperature are no longer useful as indicators of infection in fulminant hepatic failure because they are absent in 30% of cases. Fungal infection occurs in 30% of patients with fulminant hepatic failure, which is likely to be present concomitantly with bacterial infection often during the second week of hospitalization. Clinical features that lead to the suspicion of fungal infection are deterioration of coma after initial improvement, fever unresponsive to antibiotics, coexisting renal insufficiency and marked elevation of white blood count. Severe impairment of the immune system exists in these patients, and this is likely to be the reason for a higher incidence of infections. Reduced complement synthesis accentuates the defect of opsonization. Previous studies reported abnormal function of polymorphonuclear and Kupffer cells. An increase of inflammatory cytokines correlates with a high incidence of infection, systemic inflammatory response, and hepatic encephalopathy. Poor integrity of intestinal mucosa potentiates bacterial translocation and elevation of endotoxins. Patients with fulminant hepatic failure who have a prolonged stay in an intensive care unit have a high chance of superimposed infection because of the need for intravenous catheters for intensive monitoring, and for parenteral nutrition. Early administration of parenteral antimicrobial regimens alone, or combining with enteral antibiotics reduces the incidence of infection to 20% (Figure 8.6). Prevention of infection is necessary because the presence of sepsis precludes liver transplantation.

Hemostasis abnormalities

Coagulopathy, along with jaundice and hepatic encephalopthy, is an essential component of fulminant hepatic failure. Coagulation abnormalities are very common in fulminant hepatic failure because

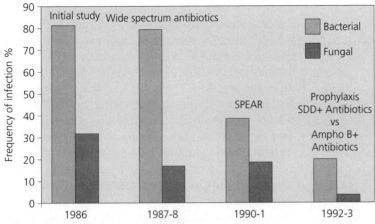

Figure 8.6 The benefit of antimicrobial prophylaxis in fulminant hepatic failure (reproduced with permission from Rolando N, Philpott-Howard J, William R. Bacterial and fungal infection in acute liver failure. *Semin Liver Dis* 1996; 16: 389–402).

the liver in this condition is incapable of synthesizing adequate coagulation factors, especially factors II, V, VII, IX, and X. The low levels of coagulation factors account for the prolonged prothrombin time and partial thromboplastin time. Levels of factors V and VII have been used as indicators of prognosis in fulminant hepatic failure. Low antithrombin III, frequently seen in fulminant hepatic failure, may interfere with the adjustment of heparin administration during hemodialysis. Cytokine release stimulates the fibrinolytic system and leads to disseminated intravascular coagulation DIC. Thrombocytopenia below 100 000 per mm³ is found in two thirds of patients. Abnormal morphology and functions of platelets is seen in some cases of fulminant hepatic failure.

Renal failure

Overall renal failure has been observed in 30% to 50% of fulminant hepatic failure cases but in acetaminophen-related fulminant hepatic failure, the number of cases complicating with acute renal failure approached 75%. Factors responsible for renal impairment in fulminant hepatic failure include microcirculatory impairment from the effects of circulating cytokines and endotoxins release. Reduced systemic vascular resistance and increased cardiac output aggravate hypotension and impair renal blood flow. Previous studies in cases with renal failure related to fulminant hepatic failure have demonstrated marked renal vasoconstriction with increasing plasma renin activity and reducing renal prostaglandin excretion, which represents an

imbalance between vasoactive mediators. Pre-renal azotemia and even acute tubular necrosis can occur in advanced cases. Hepatorenal syndrome can follow the clinical course of fulminant hepatic failure similar to that which occurs in end-stage liver disease.

Metabolic abnormalities

The inadequate gluconeogenesis from the massive loss of liver cell mass, the increasing energy expenditure due to marked systemic inflammatory response, the impairment of hepatic uptake of insulin, and the decrease of intake of nutrients result in hypoglycemia. An increasing breakdown of fat and muscle tissue as alternative sources of energy causes protein degradation. Hypophosphatemia, hypokalemia, and hypomagnesemia are commonly seen in fulminant hepatic failure. Metabolic acidosis and lactic acidosis from hypotension and tissue hypoxia are usually found in fulminant hepatic failure. Respiratory alkalosis is common in the early stages of hepatic encephalopathy. When consciousness deteriorates, the respiratory status progresses from hyperventilation to apnea. So, hypercapnia is frequent in patients who develop grade III and IV encephalopathy.

Assessment and prognosis

Because of the rapidly deteriorating course of the disease, patients who present with fulminant hepatic failure are in urgent need of early and accurate predictors that help to decide whether or not to list for liver transplantation. That ideal predictor has to identify patients who will not survive without liver transplantation before the development of a very advanced clinical condition. A third of patients with fulminant hepatic failure due to acetaminophen were initially suitable for liver transplantation but rapidly developed a contraindication. Among patients with hepatic encephalopathy grade I or II, spontaneous recovery can occur in 65% to 70% but when the clinical condition worsens to grade IV, recovery may occur in fewer than 20% of cases. The selection criteria for liver transplantation have not been standardized, but criteria that have been widely used in fulminant hepatic failure are the King's College Hospital criteria (Table 8.3) This criteria was developed from a retrospective study of 588 patients at King's College Hospital from 1973 to 1985. This study revealed that in acetaminophen-induced fulminant hepatic failure pH below 7.3, prothrombin time more than 100 seconds, creatinine above 300 μmol/L, and hepatic encephalopathy grade III or IV indicated a poor prognosis. In non-acetaminophen cases of fulminant hepatic failure etiologies of non-A, non-B hepatitis or drug toxicity, age less than 11 years and over 40 years, interval between jaundice and hepatic encephalopathy more than 7 days, bilirubin above 300 μmol/L, and prothrombin time over 50 seconds indicated a poor prognosis. Other groups from France proposed the Clichy criteria as a result of a prospective study of 90 fulminant hepatic failure cases related to acute viral hepatitis. They suggested that liver transplantation should be considered for comatose patients with a factor V level of less than 20% if their age is less than 30 years, or less than 30% if their age is over 30 years. The original reports of both groups showed high predictive accuracy, reaching 0.94 with the King's College Hospital criteria and 0.90 with the Clichy criteria, but subsequent studies that validated both criteria in other groups of fulminant hepatic failure revealed lower predictive accuracy. It is important to recognize that fulminant hepatic failure cases who do not fulfill either criteria cannot be excluded from consideration of liver transplantation, as some of the patients who do not meet the criteria may still not survive without a liver transplantation. Recent reports proposed the use of serum lactate after resuscitation (more than 3 mmol/L) in conjunction with the King's College Hospital criteria to improve the rapidity and accuracy of the prediction in acetaminophen-induced fulminant hepatic failure. Because the survival of fulminant hepatic failure cases depends on the extent of the liver injury and the rate of hepatocyte regeneration, many studies suggested using imaging studies, liver histology, and several markers of hepatic regeneration to improve the prognostic determination. In adults, spontaneous recovery rarely occurs when the liver volume has shrunk to less than 700 to 1000 milliliters. Transjugular liver biopsy, together with the King's College Hospital criteria, has been found to be useful for making diagnosis and predicting prognosis in some cases. In general, patients with 60% or less hepatocyte necrosis are likely to survive spontaneously, while liver transplantation is

Table 8.3 The King's College Hospital and the Clichy criteria for liver transplantation in fulminant hepatic failure

Clichy criteria	King's College Hospital Acetaminophen	Non-acetaminophen
grade III or IV encephalopathy with factor V less than 30% if patient's age is over 30 years	arterial PH < 7.3	prothrombin time > 100 s (or INR > 7.7)
or	*or*	*or*
factor V less than 20% if patient's age is younger than 30 years	all three of the following: 1. prothrombin time > 100 s (or INR > 7.7) 2. creatinine > 300 μmol/L (or > 3.4 mg/dL) 3. grade III or IV encephalopathy	any three of the following: 1. age <10 or > 40 years 2. etiologies: non-A, non-B or drug-induced hepatitis 3. jaundice > 7 days before encephalopathy 4. prothrombin time > 50 s (or INR > 3.85) 5. bilirubin > 300 μmol/L (or > 17.5 mg/dl)

mandatory for those with 90% or more cell necrosis. However, the idea of transjugular liver biopsy requires movement and repositioning of patients who are at risk of intracranial hypertension. This special type of procedure cannot be performed in many hospitals, and the issue of tissue sampling error is an issue with a transjugular liver biopsy. So, liver biopsy cannot be a recommended diagnostic tool in fulminant hepatic failure. A low level of plasma unbound Gc protein, an active scavenger, was reported to have high specificity in fulminant hepatic failure, but this test is beyond the technical capability of most laboratories. The levels of aminotransferases and alpha-fetoprotein have not been helpful in predicting prognosis.

Management of fulminant hepatic failure

General management

Patients presenting with acute or subacute onset of jaundice and mental changes must be hospitalized if the diagnosis of fulminant hepatic failure is suspected. Patients with jaundice and encephalopathy should be considered for admission to the intensive care unit. Investigation for a possible cause of fulminant hepatic failure should be reviewed from the history of the patient and relatives upon admission because of the urgent need for an antidote to some drugs and toxins such as N-acetylcysteine for acetaminophen overdose, and penicillin G and silibinin for mushroom poisoning. Assessment of the survival prognosis with either the King's College Hospital or the Clichy criteria must be done at the same time. Early listing for liver transplantation can be initiated for high-risk patients. Good medical management of complications at an early stage affects the likelihood of spontaneous survival or survival after liver transplantation.

Hemodynamic and metabolic management

Patients with fulminant hepatic failure usually present with hypotension and tachycardia. Management of fluid and electrolyte resuscitation requires the insertion of an arterial line, Swan–Ganz pulmonary artery pressure monitoring catheter, and foley catheter placement for the adjustment of fluid balance and for monitoring vital signs. Crytalloid-type fluid should be replaced by aiming at a pulmonary capillary wedge pressure of 12 to 14 mmHg because fluid overload can aggravate cerebral edema and pulmonary edema. Vasoconstritors, such as noradrenaline (norepinephrine), can be used for cases who do not respond to fluid replacement to keep a mean arterial pressure of 50 to 60 mmHg. However, adverse effects of noradrenaline (norepinephrine) in fulminant hepatic failure include a fall in tissue oxygen-extraction ratio and oxygen consumption, thus increasing tissue hypoxia. The addition of prostacyclin, a vasodilator agent, in some patients could increase oxygen consumption and oxygen extraction without reducing arterial blood pressure. Infusion of N-acetylcysteine may ameliorate the problem of hemodynamic changes in fulminant hepatic failure by enhancing the activity of the nitric oxide–soluble guanylate cyclase enzyme system. Nevertheless, reports of the benefit of infusions of N-acetylcysteine on systemic hemodynamics and oxygen kinetic in acetaminophen-induced fulminant hepatic failure are conflicting. The infusion form of N-acetylcysteine is not available in the US, so this precludes its for this purpose in the US. Hypoglycemia should be prevented by 5% to 10% dextrose, and following the blood glucose level every 2 to 3 hours. When the blood glucose level falls below 60 mg/dL, an infusion of 50% dextrose solution should be given promptly. Low potassium, phosphate, and magnesium should be corrected immediately. Supplement of calorie in fulminant hepatic failure cases needs to be in the order of 35 to 50 kcal/kg to compensate for a high catabolic state and enhanced energy expenditure. Enteral nutrition is preferable to the parenteral type for the purpose of maintaining the integrity of mucosa villi and preventing bacterial translocation from the gut.

Renal insufficiency

Early renal insufficiency can be prevented by low-dose dopamine although its efficacy has not been convincingly demonstated. When there are indications of dialysis, such as creatinine levels above 3.4 mg/dL, fluid overload, severe acidosis, and hyperkalemia, continuous hemodialysis or hemofiltration is a favorable method for the management of fulminant hepatic failure cases. The frequent hypotension episodes during intermittent hemodialysis result in a fall in CPP and thus aggravate cerebral edema.

Coagulopathy

Correction of coagulopathy using fresh frozen plasma is not recommended, unless there is symptomatic bleeding, because the one important parameter of recovery of liver synthetic function in fulminant hepatic failure, i.e. prothrombin time, becomes less useful, and also the large volume of plasma infusion may aggravate cerebral edema. Fresh frozen plasma is often given prior to an invasive procedure or when clinical bleeding is detected. Prophylactic treatment for upper gastrointestinal bleeding and stress ulcer is recommended with the use of a H$_2$ blocker, or sucralfate because of the high risk of bleeding from coagulopathy and stress conditions. Sucralfate may be preferred because it may prevent bacterial overgrowth and pneumonia that may be caused by ascending translocation of bacteria.

Infection

Most bacterial infections usually occur within 3 days of admission. Therefore, intensive daily culture of blood, urine, etc. is necessary. A prophylactic antibiotic, or early administration of an antibiotic when there is a clinically suspected infection is mandatory, nevertheless there is the risk of superinfection and the development of multiple resistant organisms. Selection of antibiotic regimens depends on the incidence, and type and etiology of infection at the hospital of admission. A parenteral antibiotic with or without gastrointestinal tract decontamination yields the same results. Antifungal medications should be given when patients have fever that does not respond to antibiotics, or if there is unexplained worsening of symptoms occurring after hospitalization of longer than 1 week.

Hepatic encephalopathy and brain edema

Most patients with an early grade of hepatic encephalopathy may not require respiratory support. When encephalopathy increases to grade III or IV, intubation should be carried out to protect the airway and provide oxygenation; however the possibility of increasing intracranial pressure during intubation should be recognized. Propofol and fentanyl are safe if patient sedation is necessary. Assisted ventilation should start when signs of hypoxia or hypercapnia occur. Accepted management of hepatic encephalopathy in fulminant hepatic failure is derived from similar experiences with clinical practice in chronic liver diseases. Control and prevention of all potential factors that could aggravate hepatic encephalopathy, such as high protein in the gastrointestinal tract, electrolyte imbalances, hypoxia, and sepsis are encouraged. Lactulose should be given when signs of encephalopathy appears, and an option of lactulose as retention enema form can be used in patients with grade III or IV encephalopathy. It is to be cautioned that the excessive administration of lactulose may cause fluid and electrolyte disturbances.

Clinical manifestations of intracranial hypertension commonly occur with an ICP above 30 mmHg, but the level of ICP is not correlated with specific neurologic signs. Computer tomography (CT) scans have not observed a correlation with increased ICP, and the use of transcranial doppler ultrasonography in measuring ICP is under investigation. The use of ICP monitoring in fulminant hepatic failure was first introduced in 1980. From a US survey of 91 transplantation centers in 1993, 59% had used ICP monitors. The epidural type is the most commonly used monitor (61%), with the lowest overall complication (4%). Intracranial pressure monitoring is helpful in directing therapy toward the control of ICP and prevention of brain herniation, for the selection of suitable patients for liver transplantation, for guiding the management of anesthetic agents during the operation and of medical care post-surgery, and for delisting the patients who have the potential for a poor outcome. Intracranial pressure monitoring is ideally continued 24 hours after transplantation. It is indicated in fulminant hepatic failure cases with hepatic encephalopathy grade III or IV. Correction of coagulopathy and thrombocytopenia before ICP placement is warranted, by aiming for a platelet count above 50 000 and international normalized ratio of less than 1.7. The goals of ICP monitoring are to maintain the ICP below 20 mmHg and CPP above 50 mmHg. The principles of supportive care in maintaining the CPP in fulminant hepatic failure are important. Patients need to stay in a quiet environment and repeated positioning or procedures that can aggravate ICP should be avoided. The elevation of the upper trunk to between 20° and 40° above the horizontal line is recommended for fulminant hepatic failure cases with grade III or IV encephalopathy, but further elevations create a significant increase in ICP. When ICP increases above

20 mmHg for longer than 5 minutes, 20% mannitol at a dose of 0.5 to 1 g/kg should be given as a bolus dose, and the dosage can be repeated as long as serum osmolality has not exceeded 320 mOsm/kg. Mannitol lowers ICP by reducing brain water and by changing the rheological characteristics of the blood. Improved survival has been observed in those who were administered mannitol. Mannitol expands plasma volume, so it is contraindicated in anuric patients unless the hypervolemic problem is managed with continuous hemofiltration. High-dose barbiturate is indicated when ICP elevation is resistant to mannitol. Pentobarbital is administered as a loading dose of 3 to 5 mg/kg (maximum 500 mg) over 15 minutes, followed by a continuous infusion at 0.5 to 2.0 mg/kg/h. The disadvantage of high-dose barbiturate administration is the risk of hemodynamic instability and the masking of brainstem function signs. The results of controlled hyperventilation in fulminant hepatic failure are unclear. A decrease in cerebral blood flow from hyperventilation in fulminant hepatic failure cases has been reported, which can possibly cause an adverse effect on cerebral edema. Steroids have not been shown to have any advantage in prophylaxis or treatment of cerebral edema in fulminant hepatic failure. Moderate hypothermia by reducing core temperature to 32 °C to 33 °C was effective in decreasing ICP, increasing CPP, and reducing arterial ammonia levels in seven fulminant hepatic failure cases with uncontrolled ICP. Hypothermia is an exciting innovation which warrants further proof in larger control studies before becoming a standard recommendation in fulminant hepatic failure.

Liver support devices

There is no more urgent medical condition than fulminant hepatic failure that needs abundant support because the function of the liver in the normal state encompasses several indispensable metabolic functions, including the biosynthesis of essential elements, transformation of macromolecules, biodegradation or detoxification of undesirable substances, and excretion of bile. When failure of the whole liver happens, it is difficult to find any support devices to replace all of its functions. The best method that can substitute the function of the failing liver is transplantation of the whole organ. However, it was estimated that only 41% of fulminant hepatic failure cases in the US received a liver transplant and 34% died while on the waiting list. Ideally, the hepatocytes of the injured liver have the ability to regenerate if the liver is freed of the detrimental cause, and enough time for its recovery is provided. Mortality from fulminant hepatic failure is multifactorial and is complicated by the systemic involvement of several toxins released from failing liver including ammonia, phenols, mercaptans, aromatic amino acids, fatty acids, cytokines, and nitric oxide moieties. Furthermore, hepatic regeneration is inhibited by some endogenous mediators, such as interferon-gamma, transforming growth factor (TGF-β), ammonia, and other toxins. The role of liver support devices is to help the liver in clearing such toxic substances, and in providing metabolic and synthetic functions until the liver recovers spontaneously or liver transplantation becomes available. Liver support devices can be classified into three types – non-biologic (artificial), biologic, and hybrid devices.

Non-biologic (artificial) support devices

Hemodialysis

The idea of using hemodialysis in fulminant hepatic failure stemmed from the good results of hemodialysis treatment in renal failure. Hemodialysis removes small molecules including ammonia and the false neurotransmitters that are believed to be the major causes of hepatic encephalopathy. Neurologic improvement has been seen in 40% to 58% of patients in uncontrolled studies with no change in patient survival. In 1993 a more complex system was developed by modifying the hemodialysis method; it is called the Molecular Adsorbent Recirculating System (MARS) and is used in cases of fulminant hepatic failure. Protein-bound and water-soluble toxins from blood are transferred into a dialysate compartment via an albumin-impregnated membrane. The dialysate is perfused through an anion-exchange absorbent charcoal and with secondary dialysis, to reconstitute itself. Studies without a control group revealed improvement in encephalopathy and brain edema, and a reduction in ammonia and other toxic substances. The positive results of MARS need to be confirmed in larger control trials.

Hemofiltration

The important substances causing multiple organ failure in fulminant hepatic failure are not only the small molecules, but also middle-sized molecules such as inflammatory cytokines. Continuous venous–venous hemofiltration is the more favorable method for the management of fulminant hepatic failure rather than hemodialysis, because hemofiltration is able to remove middle- and large-sized molecules more efficiently, and it can avoid the problem of brain edema from significant fluid shifts during the procedure. Hemofiltration has not demonstrated benefit in a controlled study and its adverse effect is of severe thrombocytopenia, thus discouraging its role in the therapy of fulminant hepatic failure.

Hemoperfusion

Perfusion of blood through adsorbent systems can remove many large toxins. Charcoal hemoperfusion was evaluated extensively in the 1970s and 1980s. Problems reported in patients treated with hemoperfusion are the loss of leukocytes and platelets, and hypotension. The efficacy of prostacyclin in preventing platelet loss was reported. Early studies of charcoal hemoperfusion showed encouraging results of better survival but subsequent controlled trials failed to demonstrate this positive outcome.

Plasma exchange and plasmapheresis

An increase in survival was reported following the use of plasmapheresis in a small number of patients. High-volume plasmapheresis was developed for use in fulminant hepatic failure. An improved effect on oxygen extraction parameters systemically and in the brain has been reported in one study using high-volume plasmapheresis. It may be beneficial as a bridge to liver transplantation.

At the time of writing, results of artificial support devices are all inconclusive, and the results of multicenter trials are still pending. More complex and better systems to replace the functions of the liver while awaiting transplantation or spontaneous recovery are under development.

Biologic support devices

Extracorporeal liver perfusion

The attempt to search for the highly effective treatment for fulminant hepatic failure led to the concept of using the whole liver as an extracorporeal perfusion system in 1965. Blood from patients is perfused through an extracorporeal liver by using the liver from cows, dogs, baboons, and harvested human liver that is unfit for liver transplantation. Uncontrolled studies with a small number of patients showed neurologic improvement, reduction of toxic substances, and complete recovery in a few cases. Controlled trials have not yet been carried out. An important problem of extracorporeal liver perfusion is biocompatibility. Pre-existing antibodies activate complement in the endothelial cell of the extracoporeal liver and the formation of immune complex, creating vascular thrombosis and malfunction of the liver. Moreover, there is some concern for a transmission of zoonosis from xenograft to human although there have never been reports in clinical studies.

Hepatocyte transplantation

The better outcome following transplantation of hepatocytes in animal models gave rise to an evaluation of this approach in humans as a bridge to liver transplantation. Administration of the hepatocytes obtained from liver graft unacceptable for use in liver transplantation is technically accomplished by infusion of the cells into the splenic artery, portal vein, or peritoneum under immunosuppression. Successful engraftment of the transplanted hepatocytes has been observed, in a few case series, to result in improvements in encephalopathy, brain edema, and biochemical markers of fulminant hepatic failure. Hepatocyte transplantation is not without risks. Pulmonary emboli from the migration of the hepatocytes to the lungs were reported in a patient who had hepatocyte transplantation through portal vein infusion. The quantity of hepatocytes obligated for basic liver function and an interval of cell engraftment are not yet known. Although the development of hepatocyte transplantation is in its infancy, its actual application as a bridge to liver transplantation is not impossible. The development of viable hepatocyte cell culture in proper condition, and reducing cell immunogenecity can solve some of the difficulties.

Hybrid devices

The concept of hybrid devices originated from combining the features of both artificial and biologic support systems in the 1970s. A hybrid device or a bioreactor consists of fully competent hepatocytes, an extracorporeal perfusion or delivery system to bring blood (or plasma) from patients to hepatocytes, and a semipermeable membrane separating hepatocytes from blood and allowing adequate exchange. Two hybrid systems that have been developed and evaluated in phase I and II clinical trials are the ELAD (extracorporeal liver assisted device) and the BAL (bioartificial liver) (Table 8.4).

The currently developed bioreactors are composed of multiple hollow-fiber capillaries passing through a sealed housing, and hepatocytes which are contained in the extracapillary space. In the ELAD system, blood is perfused through the intracapillary space of the hepatocyte-containing hollow cartridge (Figure 8.7). Its design carries the risk of consumptive coagulopathy and requires prophylaxis with heparin. In the BAL system, separated plasma is first perfused through a charcoal column for filtration of cytotoxins before it enters the bioreactor (Figure 8.8).

The ideal hepatocytes in artificial biologic systems should be human in origin, of non-malignant phenotype, readily available, rapidly grown in cell culture, stable in a well-differentiated status for a long period, and finally should maintain the full range of hepatocyte functions. The limitations of hepatocyte development are the shortage of availability of such cells and the rapid loss of differentiated function in tissue culture. The attempts to solve the difficulties are to use hepatocytes from other species, or hepatocytes in differentiated cell lines. The ELAD system uses the cells grown from a C3A hepatoblastoma cell line, in the extracapillary space of a cartridge. The long-term safety of using the C3A cell line has been a concern because of the reports of cell-line leakage into the patient's systemic circulation. Primary porcine hepatocytes have been utilized in the BAL system because they have similar physiologic functions to those of human hepatocytes. Nevertheless, there have been

Table 8.4 Comparison between the bioartificial liver and the extracorporeal liver assist device

	Bioartificial liver	Extracorporeal liver assist device
Perfusate	plasma	blood
Cell type	porcine	hepatoblastoma-derived C3A cells
Anticoagulant	citrate	heparin
Bioreactor	hollow-fiber	hollow-fiber
Perfusion	intermittent	continuous
Cell site	outer surface of the fiber	outer surface of the fiber
Cell mass (% normal human cell mass)	2%	20%
Additional features	charcoal sorbent column plasma separator	no charcoal column

From Maddrey, WC. Bioartificial Liver in the treatment of hepatic failure. Liver Transplantation 2000; 6: S27–S30.

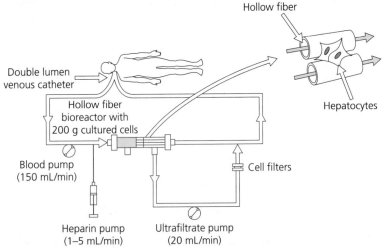

Figure 8.7 Diagram of an extracorporeal liver assist device using whole-blood perfusion and a bioreactor containing a C3A hepatoblastoma cell line) (reproduced with permission from Palmes D, Qayumi AK. Liver bridging techniques in the treatment of acute liver failure. *J Invest Surg* 2000; 13: 299–311 published by Taylor & Francis Ltd; http://www. tandf.co.uk/journals/titles/08941939.html).

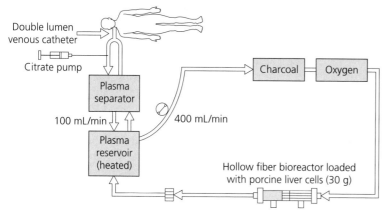

Double lumen
venous catheter

Citrate pump

Plasma
separator

100 mL/min

Plasma
reservoir
(heated)

Charcoal — Oxygen

400 mL/min

Hollow fiber bioreactor loaded
with porcine liver cells (30 g)

Figure 8.8 Diagram of a bioartificial liver in which plasma is perfused first through a charcoal column and then through the bioreactor containing porcine liver cells (reproduced with permission from Palmes D, Qayumi AK. Liver bridging techniques in the treatment of acute liver failure. *J Invest Surg* 2000; 13: 299–311 published by Taylor & Francis Ltd; http://www. tandf.co.uk/journals/titles/08941939.html).

some debates about the risk of zoonosis and pre-existing human antibodies directed against porcine tissue.

A pilot controlled trial of the ELAD was conducted in 1996. Although there was no clinical benefit in survival, improvement of encephalopathy and galactose elimination time were demonstrated. The beneficial effect of the BAL as a bridge for liver transplantation and on neurological parameters has also been reported. Recently, a preliminary result of the first large-scale controlled trial conducted in the US and Europe using the BAL revealed a promising survival advantage.

Liver transplantation

The definitive treatment for fulminant hepatic failure is liver transplantation. In the US, approximately 7% of all liver transplantations were carried out for fulminant hepatic failure and 41% of fulminant hepatic failure cases underwent orthotopic liver transplantation. Up to 50% died while awaiting orthotopic liver transplantation. Over time, survival after orthotopic liver transplantation has improved significantly. One-year and five-year patient survival, over time, has improved from 68% to 92% and 61% to 80% respectively. The factors responsible for low patient and graft survival in the past were the urgent use of reduced-size, steatotic, and ABO-incompatible grafts and the critical condition of patients. All of these factors account for the lower survival of fulminant hepatic failure patients after transplantation, compared to patients transplanted for other causes. There is a trend

toward a poorer survival after transplantation in patients with a higher grade of encephalopathy. According to grade of coma, survival rate of patients who underwent orthotopic liver transplantation in grade 1 to 2 coma was 71%, in grade 3 coma was 80%, and in grade 4 coma was 48%. Some centers have done a hepatectomy in cases of fulminant hepatic failure to remove the necrotic liver while awaiting orthotopic liver transplantation, but this approach had a limiting window period of 24 to 36 hours, and this two-step operation cannot generally be encouraged in practice. Brain edema and sepsis are the most common causes of death occurring during transplantation and in the first 3 months postoperatively. The key factors that create an excellent survival rate are the rapid assessment of prognosis by using the clinical criteria of the King's College Hospital or the Clichy group or other available criteria, the enforcement of ICP monitoring, the aggressive and intensive treatment of complications, an early listing for orthotopic liver transplantation, and a careful delisting patients who are deemed unlikely to survive after orthotopic liver transplantation. The contraindications of orthotopic liver transplantation in fulminant hepatic failure are active ongoing sepsis, uncontrolled hemodynamic instability, adult respiratory distress syndrome, the development of fixed dilated pupils for more than 1 hour, a prolonged elevation of ICP greater than 35 mmHg or a CPP of less than 40 mmHg for longer than 1 to 2 hours, and the presence of malignancy. Early referral of patients prior to the development of grade III encephalopathy to a specialized center will increase the opportunity for survival by providing enough time for transplant centers to find liver organs. However, the shortage

Living donor liver transplantation

In the US, over the past several years, the number of patients listed for orthotopic liver transplantation has increased more than 15-fold but the number of available liver organs has increased only 3-fold. The median waiting time for orthotopic liver transplantation has lengthened from 34 days to 496 days. This long waiting time and the increasing demand led to the urgent development of living donor liver transplantation. This technique in Asian countries, especially in Japan, has advanced more rapidly than cadaveric liver transplantation because of the traditional and religious beliefs against the latter. From the United Network of Organ Sharing data, living donor liver transplantation accounted for 1% of all liver transplantation carried out in the US during 1990 to 1996. Living donor liver transplantation is performed by removing the whole native liver of the recipient, and by replacing it orthotopically with either the right or left lobe graft from a living donor. Living donor liver transplantation with the right lobe liver has gained more popularity in western countries because of the problem of small-for-size living donor grafts of adult patients. Irrespective of type of liver graft, it is recommended that mean graft volume:standard volume ratio and mean graft volume:body weight ratio are not less than 40% or 0.8 respectively. Living donor liver transplantation is not without a donor risk. The mortality rate of donors reported thus far ranges from 0% to 0.8% although the actual number may be higher than the reported number. Ideally, therefore, candidate patients considered for living donor liver transplantation should be those carrying an urgent need of transplantation and having an expectation of favorable outcomes, such as patients with fulminant hepatic failure. Owing to the cautious selection of patients and donors, the 1-year and 5-year survival rates of patients with fulminant hepatic failure who underwent living donor liver transplantation have been around 90%.

Auxiliary liver transplantation

The concept of auxiliary liver transplantation for fulminant hepatic failure is to transplant a liver graft sufficient to support patients with a failing liver in anticipation that the native liver will recover and immunosuppression will be withdrawn. A follow-up study of the fulminant hepatic failure cases who had been supported with auxiliary liver transplantation revealed a complete regeneration of native liver in 68%, incomplete regeneration in 14%, and severe fibrosis or cirrhosis in 18% of cases. Favorable predictors of complete regeneration of the native liver are patient's age younger than 40 years, viral hepatitis (HAV and HBV) and acetaminophen-related causes, and an interval between the onset of jaundice and the development of hepatic encephalopathy of less than 7 days. Auxiliary liver transplantation does not seem to be beneficial for cases with subfulminant liver failure or either acute or chronic liver diseases, because of the difficulty of hepatocytes to regenerate. Auxiliary partial orthotopic liver transplantation is performed by right or left lobe hepatectomy of the native liver and replacing it with a liver graft orthotopically (Figure 8.9). In heterotopic auxiliary liver transplantation, a liver graft is placed lower than the position of the native liver without requiring hepatectomy of the native liver (Figure 8.10). One study reported that 65% of patients surviving 1 year after auxiliary liver transplantation were free of immunosuppresion within

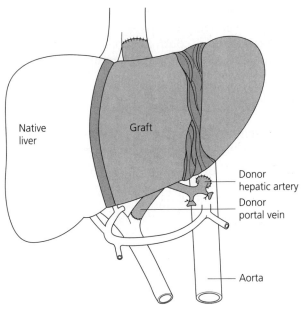

Figure 8.9 An auxiliary partial orthotopic liver transplantation is performed by replacing the resected part of the recipient liver with an auxiliary graft (gray color) to the recipient's site (reproduced with permission from Palmes D, Qayumi AK. Liver bridging techniques in the treatment of acute liver failure. *J Invest Surg* 2000; 13: 299–311 published by Taylor & Francis Ltd; http://www.tandf.co.uk/journals/titles/08941939.html).

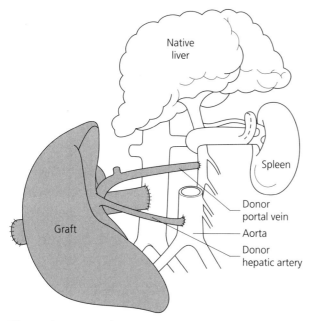

Figure 8.10 In a heterotopic auxiliary liver transplantation the auxiliary graft (gray color) is positioned in the abdominal cavity below the native liver (reproduced with permission from Palmes D, Qayumi AK. Liver bridging techniques in the treatment of acute liver failure. *J Invest Surg* 2000; 13: 299–311 published by Taylor & Francis Ltd; http://www.tandf.co.uk/journals/titles/08941939.html).

1 year after transplantation. Auxiliary partial orthotopic liver transplantation offers advantages over orthotopic liver transplantation in fulminant hepatic failure in that it provides a chance of life free from immunosuppression with an equal survival rate. Patients survival after heterotopic auxiliary liver transplantation is inferior to that of either auxiliary partial orthotopic liver transplantation or orthotopic liver transplantation. Graft compression and venous obstruction from the insufficient space of abdomen, and a toxic liver syndrome from the remaining native liver are the major problems of heterotopic auxiliary liver transplantation. The longer operative time for hepatectomy is also a concern of auxiliary partial orthotopic liver transplantation.

Conclusion

A great deal of endeavor from the past to the present has made a revolution to the knowledge of fulminant hepatic failure. Many serious complications have been recognized and managed intensively from the onset of the illness. Undoubtedly, overall

survival rate and positive outcomes of the disease at the present time are exceedingly higher than those of the past decade. Despite the improvements, there still remain a number of patients who die while awaiting liver transplantation. Liver support devices currently are not capable of substituting all the functions of the liver. Several questions regarding liver support devices, such as the appropriate end point of clinical trials, remain. Results of previous small studies are awaiting confirmation by large, multicenter, control trials.

Further reading

Bernuau J, Rueff B, Benhamou J-P. Fulminant and subfulminant liver failure: definitions and causes. *Semin Liver Dis* 1986; 6: 97–106.

Canalese J, Gimson AES, Davis C, *et al.* Controlled trial of dexamethasone and mannitol for the cerebral edema of fulminant hepatic failure. *Gut* 1982; 23: 625–629.

Ferenci P, Lockwood A, Mullen K, *et al.* Hepatic encephalopathy – definition, nomenclature, diagnosis and qualification: final report of the working party at the 11th World Congress of Gastroenterology, Vienna, 1998. *Hepatology* 2002; 35: 716–721.

Gimson AES, O'Grady J, Ede RJ, *et al.* Late-onset hepatic failure: clinical, serological and histological features. *Hepatology* 1986; 6: 288–294.

Hoofnagle JH, Carithers RL, Shapiro C, *et al.* Fulminant hepatic failure: summary of a workshop. *Hepatology* 1995; 21: 240–252.

Lee WM. Acute liver failure. *N Engl J Med* 1993; 329: 1862–1872.

O'Grady JG, Alexander GJM, Hayllar KM, *et al.* Early indicators of prognosis in fulminant hepatic failure. *Gastroenterology* 1989; 97: 439–445.

O'Grady JG, Schalm SW, Williams R. Acute liver failure: redefining the syndromes. *Lancet* 1993; 342: 273–275.

Schiot FV, Atillasoy E, Shakil AO, *et al.* Etiology and outcome for 295 patients with acute liver failure in the US. *Liver Transpl Surg* 1999; 5: 29–34.

Seef LB, Cuccherini BA, Zimmerman HJ, *et al.* Acetaminophen hepatotoxicity in alcoholics: a therapeutic misadventure. *Ann Intern Med* 1986; 104: 399–404.

Shakil AO, Kramer D, Mazariegos GV, *et al.* Acute liver failure: clinical features, outcome analysis and applicability of prognostic criteria. *Liver Transpl Surg* 2000; 6: 163–169.

Stange J, Mitzner SR, Risler T, *et al.* Molecular Adsorbent Recycling System (MARS): clinical results of a new membrane-based blood purification system for bioartificial liver support. *Artif Organs* 1998; 23: 319–330.

Stevens AC, Busuttil R, Han S, *et al.* An interim analysis of a phase II/III prospective randomized, multicenter, controlled trial of the Hepatassist bioartificial liver support system for the treatment of fulminant hepatic failure. *Hepatology* 2001; 34: 299A.

Trey C, Davidson LS. The management of fulminant hepatic failure. In Popper H, Schaffner F (eds) *Progress in Liver Disease*. New York, Grune and Stratton, 1970, p. 282.

Trotter JF, Wachs M, Everson GT, *et al*. Adult to adult transplantation of the right hepatic lobe from a living donor. *N Engl J Med* 2002; 346: 1074–1082.

Chapter 9

Benign Solid and Cystic Tumors of the Liver

Arie Regev and K. Rajender Reddy

Benign solid tumors

Introduction

Benign tumors of the liver are detected with increasing frequency because of the frequent use of imaging studies of the abdomen. Technical advances in imaging modalities have led to the identification of smaller lesions. Patients with benign hepatic tumors may be symptomatic or asymptomatic, and the relationship between symptoms and the hepatic lesion may be difficult to corroborate. In most cases patients have no pre-existing liver disease. Benign tumors and tumor-like masses of the liver may represent a diagnostic dilemma for the clinician. Benign hepatic tumors may be difficult to differentiate from malignant ones by laboratory investigations and imaging studies. Moreover, some of the benign tumors may have malignant potential. Histopathological evaluation remains essential in the clinical management of most tumors or masses in the liver; possible exceptions include focal nodular hyperplasia, hemangioma, and focal fatty change that may be unequivocally diagnosed by imaging studies. Unfortunately, in many benign lesions (e.g. hemangioma and hepatic adenoma) liver biopsy carries a high risk of bleeding and is therefore contraindicated. A fundamental knowledge of the various lesions and their characteristic features should help in the differential diagnosis.

Benign tumors of the liver may arise from hepatocytes, bile-duct epithelium, the supporting mesenchymal tissue, or a combination of two or more of these tissues (Box 9.1).

The most common benign tumors are hepatic adenoma, hemangioma, and focal nodular hyperplasia, however, many other lesions may present as a mass in the liver.

Hepatocellular adenoma

Epidemiology

Hepatocellular adenoma (hepatic or liver-cell adenoma) is a solid tumor, seen mainly in women of child-bearing age. It was considered to be rare until the mid-1960s. Since the 1970s there has been a dramatic increase in the number of reported cases, probably related to the introduction of oral contraceptives in the 1960s. The association between hepatocellular adenoma and oral contraceptives is well established. In addition, adenomas occur in association with diabetes mellitus, glycogen storage diseases, and pregnancy. There are also reported cases in men and children without known predisposing factors. Adenomas are present more commonly in women using estrogen at higher doses and for a longer duration. The greatest risk occurs in women after the age of 30 years, who took oral contraceptives for more than 5 years. Women who use oral contraceptives for more than 9 years have been estimated to have 25 times the average risk of developing hepatic adenoma. However, in 10% of cases the exposure may be as short as 6 to 12 months. Adenomas have been shown to regress with cessation of oral contraceptive therapy, and to increase in size during pregnancy. Rarely, hepatic adenoma has been associated with long-term administration of an androgenic anabolic steroid. In women who have never used oral contraceptives, the annual incidence is 1 to 1.3 per million. The incidence increases to 3 to 4 per 100 000 in long-term users of oral contraceptives. The incidence has decreased in the last decade, compared to the 1970s and 1980s, probably as a result of lower concentrations of estrogens in oral contraceptives.

Multiple hepatic adenomas occur in association with glycogen storage disease types I and III. They usually occur before the third decade of life. Their frequency averages 50% in glycogen storage disease type I, and 25% in type III. A rare condition in which ten or more adenomas are encountered is called liver adenomatosis. This may occur in both men and women and may not be associated with the use of oral contraceptives.

Clinical manifestations and natural history

Many of these tumors are noted incidentally by physical examination or ultrasonography. About one fourth present with abdominal symptoms, most commonly pain or discomfort in the epigastrium or right upper quadrant. Abdominal symptoms occur more frequently during menstruation or shortly thereafter. Acute or severe abdominal pain may be due to hemorrhage into the tumor, or, less frequently, rupture into the peritoneum, or tumor necrosis. Rupture and bleeding may lead to hypotension and shock. These complications seem to be more common during pregnancy or within 6 weeks post-partum. Patients with hepatic adenoma are also at increased risk of transformation into carcinoma within the tumor. The frequency of this uncommon complication is not well established. Other signs and symptoms may include abdominal mass in 25% to 35% and hepatomegaly. Laboratory studies are usually normal. Alkaline phosphatase and gamma-glutamyl transpeptidase may occasionally be elevated, mainly in patients with bleeding or rupture. Serum levels of alphafetoprotein are not elevated. Liver adenomatosis (10 or more adeno-

---

Box 9.1 Benign solid tumors of the liver

Epithelial tumors
   hepatocellular adenoma
   bile duct adenoma
   biliary cystadenoma

Mesenchymal tumors
   cavernous hemangioma
   infantile hemangioendothelioma
   fibroma
   angiomyolipoma
   lipoma
   lymphangioma
   benign mesenchymoma

Mixed tumors
   teratoma

Tumor-like lesions
   focal nodular hyperplasia
   nodular regenerative hyperplasia
   mesenchymal hamartoma
   microhamartoma (von Meyenburg complex)
   inflammatory pseudotumor
   focal fatty change
   pseudolipoma
   macroregenerative nodule

---

mas) is more likely to be associated with elevated serum levels of alkaline phosphatase and gamma-glutamyl transpeptidase.

Pathology

Hepatic adenoma usually appears as a well-circumscribed light-brown to yellow tumor that may or may not be encapsulated. It arises in an otherwise normal liver and is usually subcapsular. Adenomas are usually solitary tumors although occasionally two or more lesions may be present. They range from 1 to 30 cm in size, the majority being 8 to 15 cm in diameter. Foci of hemorrhage or necrosis are frequently observed. Microscopically adenoma may mimic normal liver tissue. It is composed of cells closely resembling normal hepatocytes, which are arranged in plates separated by sinusoids. Consequently, a liver biopsy not only carries an increased risk of bleeding, but also may lack pathognomonic characteristics and is commonly non-diagnostic. Nevertheless, adenoma cells may have a slightly atypical appearance and are usually larger than normal liver cells. The sinusoids are frequently dilated. There are few or no bile ducts, portal tracts, or central veins within the adenoma. In addition Kupffer cells may be either markedly reduced in number or absent. There is no fibrosis, although bile stasis may be present in bile canaliculi. Since adenomas have no portal tracts, they are perfused solely by peripheral arterial feeders. The tendency to bleed may arise from the hypervascular nature of the adenoma, which contains dilated sinusoids with thin walls, and poor connective tissue support under arterial pressure.

Imaging studies (Table 9.1)

Ultrasonography On ultrasonography hepatic adenoma appears as a well-demarcated mass with variable internal echogenicity. Doppler may show venous signals within the lesion. This appearance is not diagnostic and further studies are required.

Computed tomography scan Computed tomography does not provide a diagnostic picture either. Adenoma appears as either a hypo- or isodense mass that enhances in an irregular pattern upon injection of contrast material. (Figure 9.1A) The absence of a central scar helps in differentiating adenoma from focal nodular hyperplasia. Nevertheless, in cases where a prior bleeding has occurred, the center may remain hypodense after contrast injection, and may be indistinguishable from a central scar. In the presence of multiple lesions the diagnosis of hepatic adenomas

should be considered a diagnosis of exclusion, since metastatic disease, or multifocal hepatocellular carcinoma are more common causes.

Magnetice resonance imaging Magnetic resonance imaging shows a low-to-slightly hyperintense signal on T1-weighted images, with a well-defined low-intensity capsule (Figure 9.1B). On T2 the lesion enhances heterogeneously, and may show low-signal intensity in the center of the lesion in the presence of central necrosis (Figure 9.1C).

Hepatic arteriography Hepatic arteriography may add important information for diagnosis. Hepatic adenoma is frequently associated with enlargement of the hepatic artery. About half of the hepatic adenomas are hypovascular, with draping of hepatic arteries around the lesion. The remainder is hypervascular. Blood vessels are frequently seen entering the lesion from the periphery in a parallel pattern (spoke-wheel appearance). Arteriovenous shunting and portal venous invasion suggest hepatocellular carcinoma rather than adenoma.

99mTechnetium colloid scan These scans were frequently used in early studies. They often demonstrated decreased uptake of the colloid, especially in lesions larger than 4 cm. This has been attributed to decreased numbers of Kupffer cells in these lesions, however it is an inconsistent finding, and is not reliable in differentiating an adenoma from a focal nodular hyperplasia.

Management

Because of the high risk of bleeding, liver biopsy is best avoided when the diagnosis of hepatic adenoma is suspected. Even when a biopsy is performed, the diagnosis remains uncertain in a significant number of patients (approximately 25%). In light of the risks of bleeding, rupture, and malignant transformation, the recommended approach for hepatic adenoma is segmental or lobar resection whenever possible. When rupture has occurred, emergency resection should be performed if possible. If resection cannot be performed, embolization of the hepatic artery feeding the tumor, should be considered. Many authors recommend avoiding pregnancy in patients with unresected adenoma, because of the reported increase in size as well as increased risk of hemorrhage and rupture. Mortality from elective resection of hepatic adenoma is less than 1%, however it may increase to 5% or 8% for

Table 9.1 Imaging features of cavernous hemangioma, hepatocellular adenoma, and focal nodular hyperplasia

	Hemangioma	Adenoma	Focal nodular hyperplasia
Ultrasonography	Hyperechoic lesion. Well-defined borders.	Usually non-diagnostic.	Variable echogenicity. Occasionally shows central scar.
Doppler	No internal flow.	Venous signals within the lesion (non-diagnostic).	Arterial flow within the lesion.
Contrast-enhanced spiral CT scan	Hypodense lesion pre-contrast.	Hypo- or isodense lesion pre-contrast.	Hypo or isodense pre-contrast. Homogenous arterial enhancement.
	Centripetal enhancement.	Irregular enhancement with peripheral arterial enhancement post-contrast.	Hypodense central scar.
	Retained contrast on delayed venous phase.	May turn isodense post-contrast.	
Magnetic resonance imaging unenhanced	Well-circumscribed homogenous lesion.	Low to slightly hyperintense area on T1.	Low signal on T1. Slightly hyperintense on T2.
	Low signal on T1. Very high signal on T2.	Well-defined low intensity capsule. Heterogeneous enhancement on T2.	Central scar hyperintense on T2.
Gadolinium-enhanced MRI	Progressive centripetal enhancement. Similar to CT.	Enhancement as in CT. Hypodense central scar.	Homogenous arterial enhancement. Contrast accumulates in central area on delayed T1.
Scitigraphy with 50%–^{99m}Tc-labeled red red blood cells	Increased uptake in the lesion during venous phase. Retention on delayed images.	Hypo-concentration of the colloid (focal defect) in most patients.	Equal or increased uptake in 70% of the patients.
Angiography	Venous lakes with well-defined circular shape. Displaced arterial branches. Delayed venous phase.	Hypervascular lesion-50%. Hypovascular lesion-50%. Peripheral vascular supply.	Dilated hepatic artery. Highly vascular lesion, with a central vascular supply. Spoke-wheel pattern in one third of patients.

emergency resection in bleeding or ruptured lesion.

The increased frequency of bleeding and the increased malignant potential has prompted consideration of liver transplantation in patients with glycogen storage disease type-1 and multiple adenomas. This has been successfully performed in several patients, achieving not only the removal of the malignant potential, but also the elimination of the metabolic defect responsible for type 1A glycogen storage disease.

Hemangioma

Epidemiology

Hemangioma is the most common benign tumor of the liver. The reported prevalence at autopsy ranges from 0.4% to 7.4%. Most often they are found incidentally and have no major clinical implications. Hemangiomas are more prevalent in women, and in the right hepatic lobe. The sex ratio is between 4:1 and 6:1. They may present at all ages, but are most common between the third and fifth decades, and are rare in young children. There is some controversy regarding the term cavernous hemangioma. While some authors use it as a general name for hemangiomas, others use it to describe a stage of development of the lesion.

Clinical manifestations and natural history

In most cases hemangiomas are small and asymptomatic. Infrequently they may grow to a large size and may press or displace adjacent structures. Hemangiomas larger than 4 cm in diameter are referred to as giant hemangiomas. Large hemangiomas are uncommon, however they are more

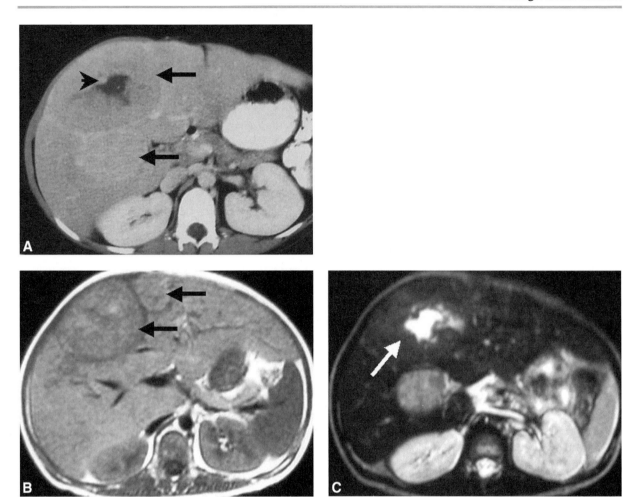

Figure 9.1 Hepatocellular adenoma. (A) Abdominal CT scan shows two well-circumscribed mass lesions in the liver (arrows). The anterior lesion shows central necrosis (arrowhead). (B) Abdominal MRI, T1-weighted image of the same patient shows two lesions with slightly decreased intensity and well-defined low-intensity capsule (arrows), which are suggestive of hepatocellular adenoma. (C) T2-weighted image shows central high-signal intensity (arrow), which is consistent with central necrosis. (Courtesy of J. Casillas, MD, Department of Radiology, University of Miami, Miami, FL. USA)

likely to cause symptoms. The most common complaints are of abdominal pain or discomfort, but early satiety, nausea, and vomiting may also occur. Pain may be due to infarction or necrosis, pressure on adjacent structures, or distention of the liver capsule. However, the relationship between the symptoms and the hemangioma may be difficult to ascertain, and in many cases other causes are discovered.

Physical examination is usually unremarkable unless a palpable mass is encountered.

Rarely a bruit may be heard over the hemangioma. Hepatic biochemical tests are usually normal, and are therefore of little help in the diagnosis of a hemangioma. On rare occasions serum aminotransferases may be mildly elevated. Hemangiomas have been reported to grow rapidly during preg-

nancy and following the use of estrogens, however, the effect of pregnancy and estrogens on growth is inconsistent. There are rare reports of a spontaneous rupture of hepatic hemangiomas. Very rarely, patients with giant hemangiomas may develop consumption coagulopathy within the hemangioma and may present with evidence of disseminated intravascular coagulation, the so-called Kasabach–Merritt syndrome.

Imaging studies (Table 9.1)

Radiography Plane abdominal radiographs may rarely show calcification.

Ultrasonography The ultrasonographic appearance of a hemangioma is usually of an echogenic, homogenous lesion with well-defined borders (Figure 9.2A). Posterior acoustic enhancement is a common feature. Doppler usually does not detect flow within the hemangioma because of the slow blood flow.

Dynamic, contrast-enhanced computed tomography scan

This shows a hypodense lesion on the pre-contrast scan (Figure 9.2B), and diffusion of the contrast from the periphery to the center of the lesion on serial scans, until opacification is homogenous (see Figure 9.2D). Opacification is usually completed in 3 minutes, and the lesion remains isodense or hyperdense on delayed scans up to 60 minutes after injection. Foci of globular enhancement, representing venous lakes are seen in the majority of large hemangiomas. The center of the lesion may remain hypodense with increasing frequency as the size increases. A non-homogenous filling may be seen caused by previous bleeding or thrombus formation within the hemangioma. Triphasic CT has a sensitivity and specificity of more than 85% for lesions greater than 2 cm in size.

Magnetic resonance imaging

Magnetic resonance imaging shows a high degree of specificity in the diagnosis of hemangioma, and is of special value in the diagnosis of small lesions. Sensitivity is greater than 90%. Hemangiomas appear as well-circumscribed, homogenous lesions, with low signal intensity on T1-weighted images and high signal intensity on T2. Intravenous contrast enhancement with gadolinium shows a centripetal opacification similar to contrast-enhanced CT. Magnetic resonance imaging is most useful for lesions smaller than 2 cm in size, or in patients with contraindications to the use of iodine-based intravenous contrast material.

99mTechnetium pertechnetate-labled red blood cells pool study

99mTechnetium pertechnetate-labled red blood cell (99mTc-RBC) scans show initial hypoperfusion during the arterial flow phase, followed by gradual increase in the isotope in the lesion, with retention of the isotope in the lesion in delayed images (Figure 9.2C, 9.3A–D). A 99mTc-RBC scan has a low sensitivity for lesions smaller than 2 cm. Sensitivity for lesions larger than 2 cm ranges from 69% to 82%, with specificity close to 100%.

Single photon emission computed tomography

Single photon emission CT (SPECT) with 99mTc-RBC shows persistent isotope activity within the lesion. This modality has sensitivity and specificity close to those of MRI (90% to 95% in lesions

greater than 2 cm). It is best used to clarify lesions doubtful on CT.

Angiography Angiography is rarely needed for the diagnosis of a hemangioma. It is used only when other modalities have failed to yield a definitive diagnosis. Hemangiomas are typically shown to displace large hepatic arterial branches to one side. The hepatic arteries are not enlarged and taper normally to small vessels before filling the vascular spaces. The vascular space usually has a well-defined circular shape because of a central fibrosis, and it usually shows a prolonged opacification.

Pathology

Hemangiomas appear on gross examination as spongy, purple, compressible lesions (Figure 9.4A). Microscopically they are composed of endothelial-lined vascular walls of varying thickness (Figure 9.4B). Intraluminal thrombi may be present. Fibrous septa and calcifications represent resolution of remote thrombosis. Biopsy is usually not necessary for diagnosis and may result in significant bleeding.

Management

Normally hemangiomas require no treatment. The rare reports of rupture should not be considered as an indication for resection. Indications for surgery include

1. a large symptomatic lesion
2. complications such as bleeding
3. uncertainty about the lesions true nature, especially when hepatocellular carcinoma cannot be excluded.

Resection or enucleation of the lesion may be performed safely, by an experienced surgical team, with mortality rate near 0%. Other modalities of therapy, such as hepatic artery ligation or embolization and radiation therapy, although reported, are not likely to yield good long-term results.

Focal nodular hyperplasia

Epidemiology

Focal nodular hyperplasia (FNH) is the second most common benign solid tumor of the liver. Its

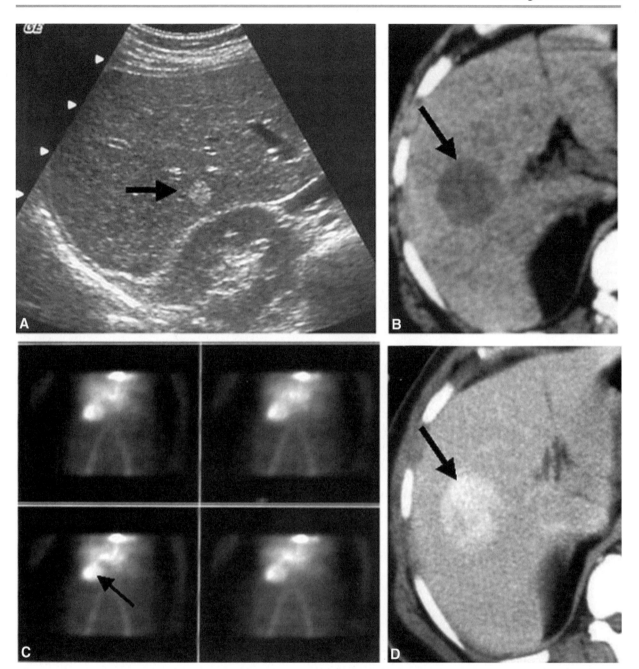

Figure 9.2 Hemangioma. (A) Ultrasonography, a transverse view of the right hepatic lobe shows a well-circumscribed echogenic mass measuring 2 × 2 cm, which is consistent with a hemangioma (arrow). (B) Abdominal CT scan, pre-contrast injection, shows a well-circumscribed mass with low attenuation in the right hepatic lobe (arrow). (C) Tagged erythrocyte (^{99m}Tc-RBC) study in a patient with a single large hemangioma in the right hepatic lobe. The scan shows gradual increase in the isotope within the lesion, with retention of the isotope in the lesion in delayed images. (D) Abdominal CT scan, the hemangioma demonstrated in 2B is shown in a delayed image (5 min), following the administration of intravenous contrast. The lesion shows a persistent enhancement in a globular pattern, typical of a hemangioma. (Courtesy of J. Casillas, MD, Department of Radiology, University of Miami, Miami, FL.)

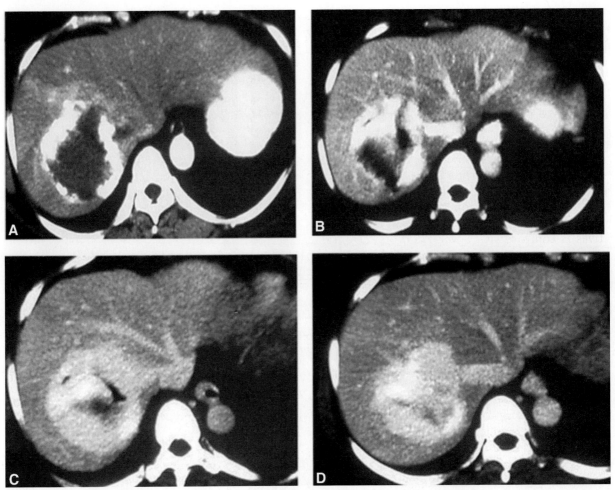

Figure 9.3 Hemangioma. Dynamic, contrast-enhanced CT scan demonstrates globular enhancement from the periphery to the center of the lesion at consecutive stages of intravenous contrast injection. (A) 40 sec (B) 60 sec (C) 90 sec (D) 120 sec. (Courtesy of J. Casillas, MD, Department of Radiology, University of Miami, Miami, FL.)

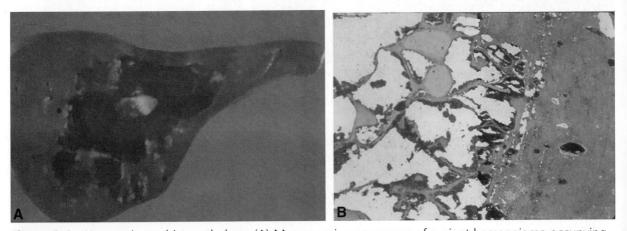

Figure 9.4 Hemangioma, histopathology. (A) Macroscopic appearance of a giant hemangioma occupying a large part of the right and left hepatic lobes. (B) Histologic examination exhibits numerous dilated vascular channels with thickened, acellular fibrous septa. (Courtesy of P.A. Bejarano, MD, Department of Pathology, University of Miami, Miami, FL.)

prevalence at autopsy is between 0.3% and 0.6%. FNH has been reported to occur most frequently in young women, although it may occur in both genders, and the sex difference is less striking than that for hepatic adenoma. The peak incidence is between the third and fifth decades of life, although it is seen at any age. FNH is thought to originate in a vascular malformation that leads to local hyperplastic response of hepatic parenchyma. It is sometimes associated with other vascular malformations such as hepatic hemangiomas and neoplasms of the brain. Generally, it is more common than hepatic adenoma, and its association with the use of oral contraceptives is controversial. Several authors have found an association between FNH and both hepatic hemangioma and adenoma. This occurs more commonly among users of oral contraceptives.

Clinical manifestations and natural history

FNH is usually asymptomatic (50% to 90% of the cases). About three quarters of the lesions are discovered incidentally on a routine ultrasonography or during abdominal surgery. The lesion may present as a non-tender mass in the right upper abdomen. However, rarely patients may present with abdominal pain resulting from hemorrhage, rupture, or necrosis in the lesion. These complications have been said to occur more frequently in patients taking oral contraceptives, although this association is still controversial. Physical examination is normal in four fifths of the patients. The remainder may present with hepatomegaly, abdominal mass, or tenderness. Hepatic biochemical tests are usually normal, and are of little value in the diagnosis of FNH. Malignant transformation has not been described in FNH, and the prognosis of an unresected lesion is excellent. The majority of FNH lesions will not increase in size after diagnosis, and will probably remain asymptomatic. Rupture causing hemoperitoneum and shock is exceedingly rare.

Imaging studies (Table 9.1)

Imaging and histologic features usually make it possible to distinguish between FNH and hepatic adenoma, although in an occasional case this may be extremely difficult. Detection of a central scar is characteristic.

Ultrasonography This commonly identifies a nodular mass, with variable echogenicity, but it is usually non-diagnostic. It may occasionally demonstrate the central scar and Doppler may show arterial flow inside the lesion. A hypoechoic rim may be demonstrated and should raise the possibility of malignancy.

Computed tomography Computed tomography scans may show a hypodense or isodense lesion that enhances homogenously during the arterial phase of contrast injection, and returns to its pre-contrast density within 1 minute (Figure 9.5A,B). Central scar is demonstrated in 60% of patients. In contrast to a hemangioma no venous pooling is seen during late images.

Magnetic resonance imaging Magnetic resonance imaging usually shows an isointense homogenous lesion on T1-weighted images, and an isointense to slightly hyperintense mass on T2-weighted images. The central scar is demonstrated in 78% of the cases. Injection of gadolinium shows early enhancement of the lesion and may increase the intensity of the central scar, showing delayed intensity of the scar in T1-weighted images (Figure 9.5D). Gadolinium injection helps to distinguish focal nodular hyperplasia from malignant vascular tumors.

^{99m}Technetium sulfur colloid liver scans These scans demonstrate equal or enhanced uptake in the lesion compared to the rest of the hepatic parenchyma in 50% to 70% of patients (Figure 9.5C). This is in contrast to hepatic adenoma, which usually shows hypoconcentration of the colloid (defect), and shows increased uptake in less than 7%. This has been attributed to the high numbers of Kupffer cells within the focal nodular hyperplasia, compared to lower numbers or decreased function in hepatocellular adenoma. It may assist in distinguishing focal nodular hyperplasia from hepatocellular adenoma, however, the reliability of this modality is poor in lesions less than 4 cm in size.

Single photon emission computed tomography Single photon emission CT may enhance the sensitivity compared to planar scintigraphy, but also shows low reliability in lesions smaller than 2 cm in size.

Angiography Although it is seldom required for the diagnosis of focal nodular hyperplasia, angiography demonstrates a dilated hepatic artery with one or more highly vascular lesions. The vessels

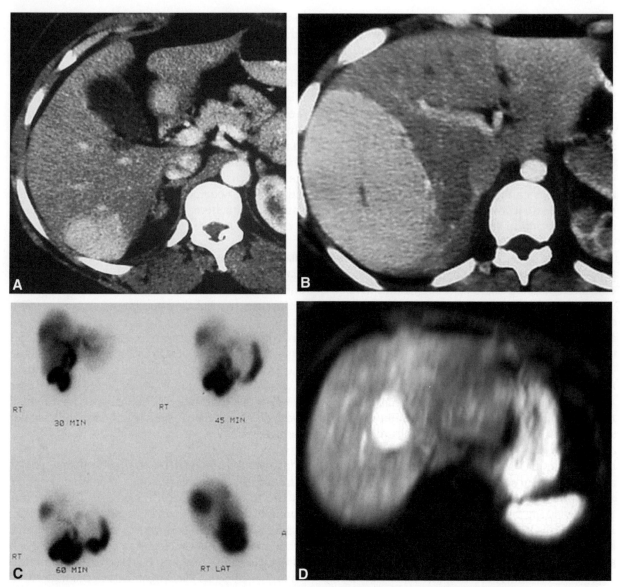

Figure 9.5 Focal nodular hyperplasia (FNH). (A) Contrast-enhanced CT scan shows a lesion in segment 6, which enhances homogenously during the arterial phase of contrast injection. (B) Arterial phase of a contrast-enhanced CT scan shows an enhanced lesion in segments 5 and 6, with a non-enhancing central scar. (C) 99mTc sulfur colloid liver scan demonstrates a focal lesion with enhanced uptake in the right hepatic lobe. (D) MRI, arterial phase after the injection of gadolinium, demonstrates homogenous enhanced lesion in the right lobe of the liver. (Courtesy of J. Casillas, MD, Department of Radiology, University of Miami, Miami, FL.)

within the lesion are very torturous, and septation of the tumor mass may be visible in about half of the cases during the capillary phase. A "spoke wheel" pattern with central arterial supply and radiating vessels is seen in about one third of the cases. Nevertheless, angiographic findings frequently do not distinguish between focal nodular hyperplasia and hepatocellular adenoma, especially in lesions smaller than 3 centimeters in size.

Pathology

Macroscopically, focal nodular hyperplasia is a firm sharply demarcated nodular lesion, which is devoid of a capsule. It is frequently single, although multiple lesions have been described. It is usually found in peripheral areas of the liver and may occasionally be pedunculated. Its color is light brown to yellow, and average size is less than 5 cm, rarely exceeding 10 cm in diameter. Typically, it has a dense central scar with radiating fibrous septa, which divide the lesion into lobule-like structures (Figure 9.6A). These nodules may be small resembling cirrhotic nodules, or they may be very large. Occasionally foci of hemorrhage or necrosis may be encountered. A single artery supplies the lesion and is not accompanied by a portal vein or a bile duct. Microscopically, focal nodular hyperplasia closely resembles cirrhosis (Figure 9.6B). The septa typically contain numerous bile ductules, blood vessels, and inflammatory cells. The hepatocytes, between the septa, are indistinguishable from those of a normal liver. They are arranged in cords forming sinusoids, however they lack portal tracts and central veins. Kupffer cells are present.

Differential diagnosis

The differential diagnosis of focal nodular hyperplasia includes benign lesions such as hepatocellular adenoma and giant hemangioma, and malignant tumor such as hepatocellular carcinoma, fibrolamellar carcinoma, intrahepatic cholangiocarcinoma, and metastases.

Although lacking the characteristic central scar, many of these lesions may bleed internally or may show a central necrosis. This may create a similar appearance to the central scar of focal nodular hyperplasia on CT, but may usually be differentiated on MRI; central hemorrhage or necrosis show a low signal on T2 as opposed to a high signal in focal nodular hyperplasia. Hepatocellular adenoma is usually larger than focal nodular hyperplasia and lacks the characteristic central scar. Giant hemangioma shows a characteristic centripetal enhancement on contrast injection. Similar to adenoma, prior bleeding or fibrosis may be difficult to differentiate from the central scar of focal nodular hyperplasia on CT scan, but is identified on MRI. In contrast with focal nodular hyperplasia, hepatocellular carcinoma usually appears in patients with pre-existing liver disease. It may show vascular invasion and metastatic spread. In fibrolamellar carcinoma a calcified central scar may be seen in up to 55% of cases. Intrahepatic cholangiocarcinoma is less vascular than focal nodular hyperplasia although it also may have a central scar. It may also show local invasion, which is not a feature of focal nodular hyperplasia. Hepatic metastases may be hypervascular, but usually lack a central scar. Most are hypodense, showing a ring enhancement on the vascular phase of enhanced CT scan.

Management

Since the frequency of complication is very low, the recommended treatment in asymptomatic patients is observation. It is recommended to repeat abdominal imaging 3 months, 6 months and 1 year after the diagnosis. If the lesion is highly suggestive of focal nodular hyperplasia, and does not change over a period of 1 year, no further observation is indicated. If the lesion is enlarging on consecutive imaging studies, resection should be considered. There are several reports of a decrease in size of focal nodular hyperplasia following the discontinuation of oral contraceptives. Patients should probably be advised to discontinue oral contraceptive therapy. Although there is no convincing data on the risk of pregnancy in patients with focal nodular

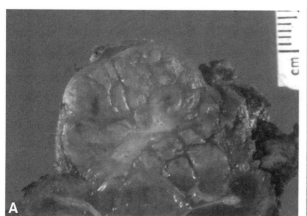
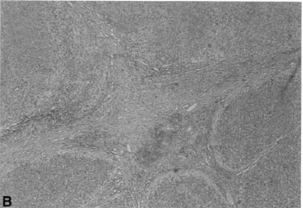

Figure 9.6 Focal nodular hyperplasia (FNH). (A) Cut surface of a resected specimen of focal nodular hyperplasia. Note central scar and cirrhosis-like appearance. (B) Low-power view of a focal nodular hyperplasia shows a central fibrous scar with fibrous septa forming nodule-like structures. (Courtesy of P.A. Bejarano, MD, Department of Pathology, University of Miami, Miami, FL.)

hyperplasia, several authorities recommend that the patient avoids pregnancy, or undergoes resection of the lesion if pregnancy is contemplated. Large or pedunculated lesions have rarely been reported to undergo torsion or necrosis, and may require local resection. Resection is also recommended for severely symptomatic lesions, however, other possible causes for symptoms should be ruled out and the association between the lesion and the symptoms needs to be clearly ascertained prior to surgery.

Other benign tumors

Bile duct adenoma

Bile duct adenoma is a rare hepatic tumor which is usually diagnosed incidentally at laparotomy or autopsy. It is found more commonly after the fifth decade of life, and is virtually never symptomatic. Size is usually less than 1 cm. Bile duct adenomas are almost always solitary and are found predominantly in the right hepatic lobe, frequently in a subcapsular position. Microscopically, they are characterized by a local proliferation of normal-appearing small bile ducts and fibrous stroma containing numerous lymphocytes.

Its main significance is in the differential diagnosis from metastatic carcinoma, cholangiocarcinoma, or other focal hepatic lesions.

Angiomyolipoma

Angiomyolipoma is a rare liver tumor composed of fat tissue, epithelioid cells, smooth muscle cells and thick-walled vascular channels. Clusters of hematopoietic cells may be present. It is diagnosed most commonly in women in the fourth to seventh decade. Unlike angiomyolipoma of the kidney, that of the liver is less common and is rarely associated with tuberous sclerosis. Size ranges from 0.8 to 36 cm, and symptoms are usually associated with the larger lesions. On ultrasonography these are homogeneous, highly echogenic, well-circumscribed lesions. Computed tomography scan shows a hypodense lesion with density measurement characteristic of fat tissue. Nevertheless, in most reported cases this tumor is initially misdiagnosed as hepatocellular adenoma, hepatocellular carcinoma, liposarcoma, or focal nodular hyperplasia. For symptomatic or suspicious lesions resection is the treatment of choice.

Infantile hemangioendothelioma

Although infrequently encountered, infantile hemangioendothelioma is the most common benign hepatic tumor in children accounting for more than 50% of cases.

This tumor presents almost always in the first 6 months of life and is twice as common in girls. It is associated with a high incidence of congestive heart failure resulting from massive arteriovenous shunting, which may lead to a high mortality rate (up to 70%) among the affected children. Spontaneous regression occurs frequently.

Pseudolipoma

Pseudolipoma of the liver is a rare lesion composed of mature adipose tissue, it is found outside the liver but within the Glisson's capsule. The speculated origin is from epiploicae appendices or omental fat. Fat necrosis and calcification may occur.

Tumor-like lesions

Inflammatory pseudotumor

This is a rare hepatic lesion of uncertain origin. Similar lesions have been reported in almost every organ in the body. It affects all ages, men more often than women, with a ratio of 8:1. Inflammatory pseudotumor typically presents with fever, pain, and weight loss associated with a liver mass. Hepatic biochemical tests are elevated and jaundice may occur. Reported size ranges from 1 to 35 cm. The pathogenesis is unclear. Macroscopically the lesion is devoid of a capsule and has no distinct borders. Microscopically it is composed of spindled cells mixed with mononuclear inflammatory cells, predominantly plasma cells, in a fibrous stroma. It has been reported to infiltrate intrahepatic veins and bile ducts, and may initially be misdiagnosed as a liver abscess, Hodgkin's disease, or sarcoma. Cultures from the lesion are invariably negative. The natural history is variable. The lesion may regress and disappear spontaneously, or may persist and cause severe symptoms. Resection should be considered only in those instances in which the mass effect of the lesion is producing symptoms, or in those cases in which a firm histologic diagnosis cannot be made preoperatively. Liver transplantation may be required for unresectable lesions.

Macroregenerative nodules

Macroregenerative nodules occur in the setting of chronic liver disease with advanced fibrosis or cirrhosis. This is in contrast with all other tumor-like lesions, which usually occur in patients with no pre-existing liver disease. They are found in cirrhotic livers associated with any underlying liver disease, and are currently considered a premalignant condition. Recently the term dysplastic nodules has been proposed by the International Working Party on terminology of nodular hepatocellular lesions. Similar lesions have been described in massive or submassive necrosis due to acute liver injury.

On gross examination, macroregenerative nodules appear distinct from the surrounding cirrhotic parenchyma because of a difference in color and a tendency to protrude from the liver's surface. Central necrosis or hemorrhage within the nodule suggest hepatocellular carcinoma. The hepatocytes within a macroregenerative nodule may show both low-grade and high-grade dysplastic features, but they do not meet the criteria of hepatocellular carcinoma. On T1-weighted MRI images this lesion appears isointense, or slightly hyperintense, compared with the normal hepatic parenchyma. On T2-weighted images this lesion is hypodense. These features assist in differentiating between macroregenerative nodule and hepatocellular carcinoma, which would have a variable signal on T1 but will become hyperintense on T2, and will enhance during the arterial phase of gadolinium injection. Patients in whom these lesions are recognized should be followed closely by repeat imaging studies and serum levels of alfa-fetoprotein.

Focal fatty change

Focal fatty change in the liver may manifest as a focal lesion or as diffuse infiltration. It is usually a large lesion which may be single or multiple, however, it may vary in size, and may or may not be associated with diffuse fatty infiltration. Focal fatty change may be associated with obesity, diabetes mellitus, hypercholesterolemia, corticosteroid therapy malnutrition, total parenteral nutrition, and alcoholism. Hepatic biochemical tests may be normal or mildly elevated, although they are nonspecific. Imaging studies, such as ultrasonography, CT scan, and MRI, may usually delineate this lesion and differentiate it from other processes. Ultrasonography shows a hyperechoic lesion with ill-defined borders. Computed tomography scan shows a hypodense, sharply demarcated area, with no mass effect on hepatic and portal veins. Helical contrast-enhanced CT scan typically demonstrates normal vessels coursing through the hypodense lesion. Magnetic resonance imaging shows increased intensity in T1, which is a typical finding for fatty infiltration and may appear only rarely in other conditions such as malignant melanoma and iron overload. When the diagnosis is uncertain a liver biopsy should be performed which is usually diagnostic.

Biliary microhamartoma (von Meyenburg complex)

This is a frequent incidental finding at surgery and autopsy. It usually measures a few millimeters, but may be as large as 0.5 cm in diameter. It may appear as a solitary lesion or it may be multiple. It is asymptomatic and is associated with normal hepatic biochemical tests. Histologically it appears as an abnormal proliferation of ductules or small bile ducts of various sizes, which are surrounded by fibrous stroma. Von Meyenburg complex is a frequent finding (more than 90%) in patients with adult polycystic kidney disease. It is also associated with solitary hepatic cysts.

Clinical approach to a solid liver lesion

There is a wide spectrum of conditions that needs to be considered when a focal solid lesion is noted in the liver. Detailed history, physical examination, hepatic biochemical tests, and imaging studies are all of major importance in making the diagnosis. Based on the results of these studies the clinician needs to decide whether the lesion is benign or malignant, whether a biopsy is needed to confirm the diagnosis, and if surgical treatment is required. The specific approach may vary with the presentation of the lesion, the demographic details of the patients, and the medical history. For example the diagnostic approach in a solid tumor found in a young, previously healthy woman, should focus on the differential diagnosis of hemangioma, focal nodular hyperplasia, and adenoma. Focal nodular hyperplasia and hemangioma typically have characteristic features on imaging studies, and are diagnosed with a high degree of accuracy with no histological examination. In contrast in a middle-aged man with a recent history of colon cancer the most likely diagnosis will be a metastatic lesion, whereas in a patient with pre-existing cirrhosis or chronic hepatitis B or C, the likely diagnosis would be hepatocellular carcinoma or a macroregenerative nodule. These tumors have a characteristic appearance on CT scan and MRI. High serum levels of alfa-fetoprotein may confirm the diagnosis of hepatocellular carcinoma (a level of more than 400 IU/mL is considered diagnostic). The diagnostic approach should therefore include a detailed history and physical examination to assess whether underlying liver disease or a comorbid illness is present. In addition, hepatic biochemical tests, tumor markers, serological markers for viral hepatitis, and contrast-enhanced dynamic CT scan should be obtained. Ultrasonography is a useful screening test, however in most instances it is not sufficient for a final diagnosis. Triphasic contrast-enhanced CT scan is usually necessary for an accurate diagnosis. It also assists in detecting additional small hepatic masses and evaluating for other intra-abdominal lesions. When hemangioma is suspected, delayed venous phase images should be requested. In the absence of a history or clinical evidence suggestive of malignancy or pre-existing liver disease, a solid liver lesion is most likely benign. The most common solid benign hepatic lesions are hemangioma (approximately 4%), focal nodular hyperplasia (0.4%), and adenoma (less than 0.004%). In questionable lesions contrast-enhanced MRI may add important information. Either MRI or ^{99m}Tc-RBC SPECT may be used to confirm the diagnosis of hemangioma in questionable cases. Calcifications detected in a solid lesion suggest the diagnosis of fibrolamellar carcinoma, and a hemorrhage within the lesion is more suggestive of adenoma. When the likely diagnosis is focal nodular hyperplasia in an asymptomatic patient, this patient may be followed by ultrasonography or CT scans every 3 months for 1 year. The therapeutic approach may vary based on the history and physical examination. For example a severely symptomatic lesion is likely to require surgery, regardless of the findings of imaging studies or histology. When the likely diagnosis is adenoma, surgical therapy is usually recommended. Resection is also recommended when imaging studies cannot establish the diagnosis of focal nodular hyperplasia or hemangioma. Occasionally, a diagnostic laparoscopy in a specialized medical center may help in establishing the diagnosis and avoiding surgery. Angiography may also add important information and should be considered prior to surgery. Liver biopsy is usually not recommended, and is better avoided when adenoma is suspected, because of the risk of bleeding and low diagnostic yield. In malignant lesions there is the additional risk of seeding, which may lead to dissemination of the tumor.

Cystic lesions of the liver

Introduction

Cystic lesions of the liver consist of a heterogeneous group of disorders which differ in etiology, prevalence, and clinical manifestations (Box 9.2). Liver cysts may be single or multiple. They may vary in size and location, and are usually found in patients with no pre-existing liver disease. There is still a considerable controversy regarding the definition and classification of cystic lesions of the liver. Most liver cysts are found incidentally on imaging studies and tend to have a benign course. However, a minority may cause symptoms and rarely may be associated with serious morbidity and mortality.

The distinction between the different cystic lesions of the liver can be difficult, but is extremely important as these lesions may have different clinical significance. Larger cysts are more likely to cause complications such as spontaneous hemorrhage, rupture into the peritoneal cavity, compression of biliary ducts, and rupture into the biliary tree. Specific types of cysts may have unique complications such as malignant transformation in cystadenoma, or anaphylactic shock because of a hydatid cyst. Some of these

---

Box 9.2 Classification of hepatic cysts

Simple (solitary) cyst

Ciliated foregut cyst

Polycystic disease

Parasitic
  hydatid (echinococcal)

Neoplastic
  Primary
  cystadenoma, cystadenocarcinoma, squamous cell carcinoma
  Secondary
  carcinoma of ovary, pancreas, colon, kidney, neuroendocrine

Duct related
  Caroli's disease
  bile duct duplication

False cysts
  traumatic liver cyst
  intrahepatic infarction
  intrahepatic biloma

complications may occasionally mandate surgical intervention.

Simple cyst

Epidemiology

Simple cysts of the liver are cystic formations containing clear fluid that do not communicate with the intrahepatic biliary tree. They are found in approximately 1% of necropsied adults, and may be diagnosed at any age. Their size ranges from a few millimeters to massive lesions of 30 cm or more, occupying large volumes of the upper abdomen, however the vast majority are under 4 cm in diameter. Simple cysts are usually solitary, but occasionally multiple cysts may be found. Only a small minority cause symptoms. Simple cysts tend to occur more commonly in the right lobe, and are more prevalent in women. The female-to-male ratio is approximately 1.5:1 among those with asymptomatic simple cysts, while it is 9:1 in those with symptomatic or complicated simple cysts. Huge cysts are found almost exclusively in women over 50 years old.

Clinical manifestations and natural history

Most simple cysts of the liver are asymptomatic and are detected incidentally by abdominal ultrasonography or CT scan.

Symptoms usually occur with larger cysts or with complications. Symptomatic patients may present with abdominal discomfort, pain, or nausea. A very large cyst may present with increased abdominal girth, which may be accompanied by a palpable abdominal mass. Complications are rarely encountered in patients with simple cysts. They include spontaneous hemorrhage, bacterial infection, torsion of pedunculated cyst, or biliary obstruction because of extrinsic pressure. Laboratory findings are typically normal.

Imaging studies

Ultrasonography This is the most useful method for the diagnosis of a simple cyst. A simple cyst appears as an anechoic, unilocular, fluid-filled space with imperceptible walls, and with posterior acoustic enhancement. Clinical features combined with the sonographic findings are usually sufficient to distinguish simple cysts from other lesions that can appear cystic such as a liver abscess, necrotic malignant tumor, hemangioma, and hamartoma.

Computed tomography On a CT scan a simple cyst appears as a well-demarcated water-attenuation lesion that does not enhance following the administration of intravenous contrast (Figure 9.7A). Uncomplicated simple cysts are virtually never septated. However, hemorrhage into a simple cyst can lead to confusion in the sonographic and tomographic differentiation from a cystadenoma or cystadenocarcinoma (Figure 9.7B). In one report, hemorrhage was associated with the appearance of septa in 2 of 57 patients (3.5%) with large simple cysts (4 cm or more). Hemorrhage is much less frequent in smaller cysts.

Magnetic resonance imaging Magnetic resonance imaging demonstrates a well-defined water-attenuation lesion that does not enhance following the administration of intravenous gadolinium. On T1-weighted images the cyst shows a low signal, whereas a very high signal is shown on T2-weighted images (Figure 9.7C).

Pathology

Macroscopically, a simple cyst appears as a unilocular fluid-filled formation, which is well separated from the surrounding liver tissue. The external surface is smooth and usually translucent. Large cysts may produce atrophy of the adjacent hepatic tissue, and a huge cyst may result in complete atrophy of a hepatic lobe with compensatory hypertrophy of the other lobe. Histological examination is seldom needed for establishing the diagnosis. However, when histology is available the following criteria can be used for a definitive diagnosis

- an outer layer of a thin dense fibrous tissue
- an inner epithelial lining consisting of a single layer of cuboidal or columnar epithelium, this layer is found in most but not in all simple cysts
- lack of mesenchymal stroma or cellular atypia.

Differential diagnosis

The differential diagnosis of a simple cyst includes a variety of hepatic lesions that can have a cystic appearance such as hepatobiliary cystadenoma, cystadenocarcinoma, hydatid cyst, hepatic abscess, necrotic malignant tumor, hemangioma, and hamartoma. Rarely hepatic metastasis from a neu-

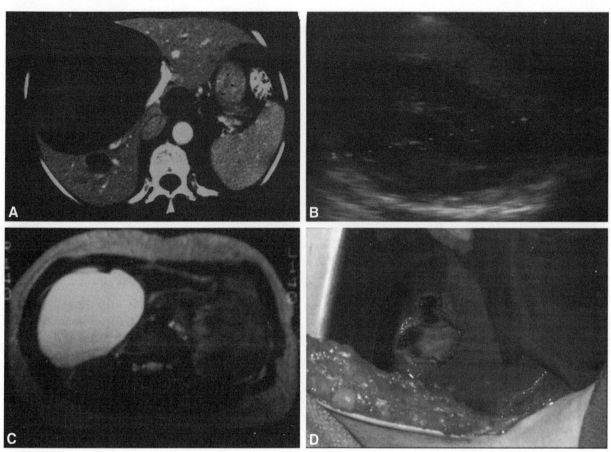

Figure 9.7 Simple cyst. (A) Abdominal CT scan shows a well-defined water attenuation lesion in the left hepatic lobe. (B) Post-bleeding into the cyst cavity. Abdominal ultrasound demonstrates an unilocular space, with internal echoes. (C) T2-weighted MRI image, demonstrating a typical high signal. (D) Wide unroofing in the right hepatic lobe (reproduced with permission from the American College of Surgeons, Regev A, Reddy KR, Berho M, *et al*. Large cystic lesions of the liver in adults: a 15-year experience in a tertiary center. *J Am Coll Surg* 2001; 193: 36).

roendocrine tumor may present as an asymptomatic sharply defined necrotic area. Certain clinical manifestations and radiologic findings may point against the diagnosis of a simple cyst and requires further work-up to rule out another diagnosis (Table 9.2). The distinction can usually be made based on the clinical setting and radiographic findings. Aspiration is usually not required for diagnosing cysts that have a typical sonographic appearance. When it is performed, the aspirated fluid is always sterile and cytologically negative. It may vary from a clear straw color to brown. Hydatid disease should be ruled out before aspiration is performed.

Treatment

The majority of simple cysts do not require treatment. However, it is recommended to monitor large cysts (4 cm or more in diameter) periodically with ultrasonography to ensure that they have remained stable. Further monitoring is usually unnecessary if the cyst remains unchanged for 2 years. The presence of symptoms related to the cyst or increasing size should raise concern that the lesion could be a cystadenoma or a cystadenocarcinoma. Such patients may require surgical intervention. The causal relationship between abdominal pain or discomfort and a simple cyst must be admitted with caution, and accepted only if the cyst is large and other possible causes of the symptoms have been excluded. Percutaneous aspiration has been advocated as a diagnostic test for relief of symptoms, however, this test is not without risk and has not been widely accepted.

Several therapeutic approaches have been described for symptomatic, large, simple cysts including needle aspiration with or without injection of sclerosing solution, internal drainage with

Table 9.2 Clinical manifestation and imaging findings pointing against the diagnosis of a simple cyst

Manifestation/imaging finding	Differential diagnosis
Progressive symptoms	cystadenoma, cystadenocarcinoma, metastasis
Abnormal hepatic biochemical tests	cystadenocarcinoma, metastasis
Rapid growth on periodical follow-up	cystadenoma, cystadenocarcinoma, metastasis
Calcifications or daughter cysts	echinococcal cyst
Thick or irregular cyst wall	cystadenoma, cystadenocarcinoma, metastasis, echinococcal cyst
Non-homogenous cyst content	cystadenoma, cystadenocarcinoma, echinococcal cyst, bleeding into a simple cyst
Septations or multilocular cyst space	cystadenoma, cystadenocarcinoma, echinococcal cyst, bleeding into a simple cyst

cystojejunostomy, wide unroofing, and varying degrees of liver resection. In most series, needle aspiration was associated with a high failure rate and rapid recurrence. On the other hand, wide unroofing or cyst resection (Figure 9.7D) has been associated with a relatively low incidence of cyst recurrence or complications. The laparoscopic approach has proven to be safe, achieving a wide unroofing without the need for a debilitating incision. Several centers have reported recurrence rates ranging from 0% to 14.3% and morbidity rates of 0% to 25% after laparoscopic unroofing of solitary simple cysts. These results support the notion that surgical therapy is the only definitive treatment for symptomatic simple cysts, and that laparoscopic unroofing should be the procedure of choice for accessible cysts. Reported complications of laparoscopic unroofing include wound infection, chest infection, bile leak, subphrenic hematoma, and prolonged post-operative drainage through an abdominal drain (> 3 days). Laparoscopic unroofing may not be possible in patients with a superior or posterior location of the cyst.

Hepatobiliary cystadenoma

Epidemiology

Hepatobiliary cystadenoma is a rare cystic tumor that occurs within the liver parenchyma or, less frequently, in the extrahepatic bile ducts. The published experience with this lesion is limited to single case reports and small series. Cystadenomas occur in adulthood, more often in women. They occurred more often in the right lobe than in the left in one report, while two other series reported frequent involvement of the left lobe. These tumors

grew to a large size and required surgical intervention in most reports.

Clinical manifestations

The most commonly reported presenting symptoms were a sensation of an upper abdominal mass, abdominal discomfort or pain, and anorexia. These symptoms may be present for several years prior to diagnosis. However, many patients were asymptomatic and the lesions were found incidentally on abdominal imaging studies.

Diagnosis and imaging studies

The appearance of cystadenoma on ultrasonography can usually differentiate it from a simple cyst (Figure 9.8A). Septations are seen in a cystadenoma whereas an uncomplicated simple cyst should not have septations. On a CT scan a cystadenoma appears as a low attenuated mass, which may be uni- or multilocular, or may have septations (Figure 9.8B). The cyst wall is usually thickened and/or irregular.

Pathology

Histologic examination is required for definitive diagnosis, although the lesion may be suspected on imaging studies. A cystadenoma is usually a multilocular cystic lesion with a smooth external surface, and a thin wall with smooth internal lining. The cyst frequently contains blood or chocolate-colored material. Microscopically, cystadenomas are lined by biliary type, mucus-secreting, cuboidal, or columnar epithelium, supported by dense cellular (mesenchymal) fibrous stroma resembling ovarian tissue (Figure 9.8 C,D). The lining is surrounded by a loose and less cellular layer of collagen. It has been suggested that hepatobiliary cystadenoma

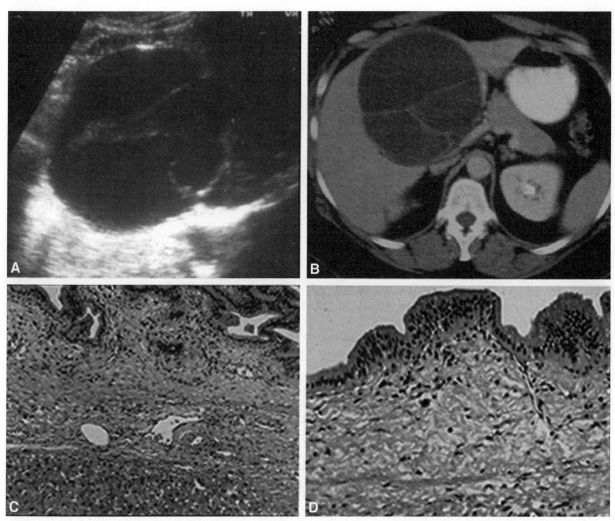

Figure 9.8 Hepatobiliary cystadenoma in a 62-year-old woman. (A) Ultrasound shows a large cystic lesion with septations and slightly irregular wall. (B) CT scan demonstrates the same cyst occupying most of the left hepatic lobe. (C) Histologic appearance, low-power magnification showing the wall of the cyst composed of a layer of loose vascular, spindle cell stroma lined by tall columnar epithelium. Note polypoid projections (hematoxylin and eosin, original magnification × 400) *(see plate section for color)*. (D) Closer view demonstrates the layer of simple columnar epithelium with focal areas of pseudostratification. No cellular atypia or pleomorphism is noted (hematoxylin and eosin, original magnification × 2000), (reproduced with permission from the American College of Surgeons, Regev A, Reddy KR, Berho M, *et al*. Large cystic lesions of the liver in adults: a 15-year experience in a tertiary center. *J Am Coll Surg* 2001; 193: 36).

may be composed of two distinct groups that differ in the presence or absence of a mesenchymal stroma surrounding the epithelial lining of the cyst.

Treatment

The preferred treatment for cystadenomas is resection, which should be performed whenever possible since malignant transformation of the cyst lining has been described in as many as 15% of patients. Removal of the cyst can be accomplished by enucleating it from the surrounding liver. Partial exci-

sion is invariably associated with recurrence and with worse prognosis compared to complete resection. Aspiration is also associated with rapid recurrence of fluid and symptoms.

Cystadenocarcinoma

Epidemiology

Cystadenocarcinomas probably arise from malignant transformation of a cystadenoma. This tumor is significantly less common than cystadenoma. It is usually found in the elderly although it has been reported in patients in their thirties.

Diagnosis and imaging studies

The distinction between a cystadenoma and cystadenocarcinoma can be difficult to make based upon clinical, radiologic, and histological evidence. Cystadenocarcinomas are usually multilocular and resemble cystadenomas in their ultrasonographic and tomographic appearance (Figure 9.9A). If metastatic spread has occurred metastatic lesions may be identified within the liver or in distant sites.

Pathology

If the tumor has not spread the gross features of cystadenocarcinoma are similar to those of cystadenoma. The external surface is smooth similar to cystadenoma. However, in contrast to cystadenoma, which has a thin wall with smooth lining, cystadenocarcinoma has a thicker wall that may show large tissue masses protruding from the internal cyst lining (Figure 9.9B). Malignant changes are typically found in the inner epithelial lining (Figure

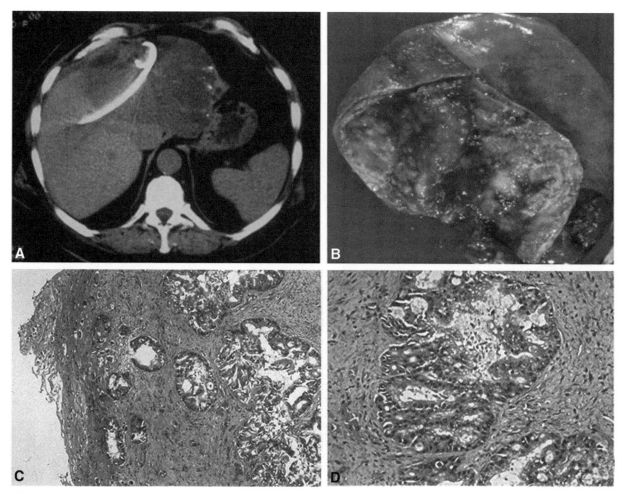

Figure 9.9 Cystadenocarcinoma. (A) CT scan, during a percutaneous aspiration. Note irregular thick cyst wall with nonhomogenous content. (B) Gross pathological examination, revealing a thick wall with multiple papillary projections *(see plate section for color)*. (C) Histologic examination: Scanning magnification showing complex glandular structures embedded in the stroma of the wall (hematoxylin and eosin, original magnification: × 400). (D) Higher power demonstrates glands with a cribriform growth pattern and nuclei displaying mild atypia (hematoxylin and eosin, original magnification: × 2000) *(see plate section for color)*, (reproduced with permission from the American College of Surgeons, Regev A, Reddy KR, Berho M, *et al.* Large cystic lesions of the liver in adults: a 15-year experience in a tertiary center. *J Am Coll Surg* 2001; 193: 36).

9.9 C,D). Cystadenocarcinomas have occasionally been identified preoperatively by aspiration and examination of the contents of the cyst, but this procedure carries the risk of peritoneal seeding of the tumor.

Treatment

In contrast to a cystadenoma, if cystadenocarcinoma is suspected treatment should consist of a formal liver resection. Enucleation is not recommended as it probably carries an increased risk of recurrence. The lesion is potentially curable by complete excision. The effect of non-surgical therapy (e.g. radiation or chemotherapy) is unknown. Although this tumor can invade adjacent tissues and metastasize, its prog-

nosis has generally been better than that associated with cholangiocarcinoma.

Echinococcal cyst

Epidemiology

Echinococcal (hydatid) cysts of the liver are caused by the larval form of *Echinococcus granulosus*, which is usually acquired from infected dogs. These are fluid-filled structures limited by a parasite-derived membrane which contains germinal epithelium. Hydatid cysts of the liver are uncommonly encountered in the US.

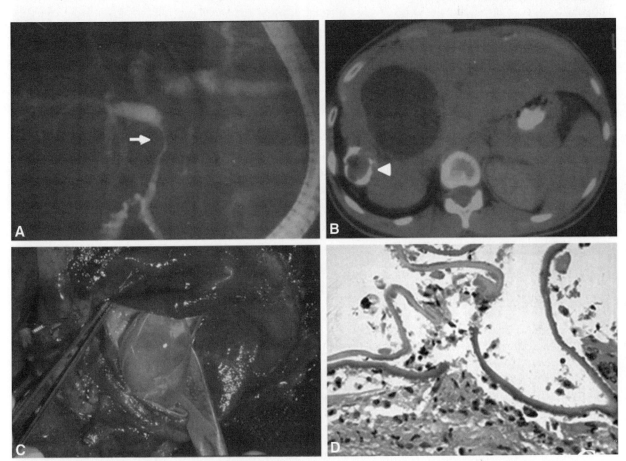

Figure 9.10 Echinococcal cyst. (A) ERCP demonstrating external compression of the hepatic duct by the cyst. (B) CT scan shows a complex septated cyst and a heavily calcified daughter cyst in the right hepatic lobe (arrowhead), in a 38-year-old man. (C) Post-resection *(see plate section for color)*. (D) Histologic appearance of a degenerated cyst containing fragments of the germinal membrane (hematoxylin and eosin, original magnification × 2000) *(see plate section for color)*, (reproduced with permission from the American College of Surgeons, Regev A, Reddy KR, Berho M, *et al*. Large cystic lesions of the liver in adults: a 15-year experience in a tertiary center. *J Am Coll Surg* 2001; 193: 36).

Clinical manifestations and natural history

Patients are often asymptomatic. Hydatid cysts usually evolve over a long period of time before they become large enough to produce symptoms. Many may remain asymptomatic even into advanced age. When symptoms do occur, they are usually caused by the mass effect of an enlarging cyst or complications such as intraperitoneal leakage, infection, or biliary obstruction (Figure 9.10A). The cyst can rupture into the biliary tree and produce biliary colic, obstructive jaundice, cholangitis, or pancreatitis. Communication with the biliary tree is found in at least 25% of the patients. Pressure or mass effects on the bile ducts, portal and hepatic veins, or on the inferior vena cava can result in cholestasis, portal hypertension, venous obstruction, or Budd–Chiari syndrome. Liver cysts can also rupture into the peritoneum causing peritonitis, or transdiaphragmatically into the bronchial tree causing pulmonary hydatidosis or a bronchopleural fistula. Minor leakage of cyst content into the peritoneal cavity may produce a mild acute allergic reaction usually manifested with urticaria and abdominal discomfort. In the case of major rupture there are often acute peritoneal signs and associated acute anaphylaxis that may be fatal. Secondary bacterial infection of the cysts can result in liver abscesses.

Diagnosis

Echinococcal cyst most often presents as a hepatic mass with typical appearance on abdominal imaging, coupled with confirmatory serologic testing by indirect hemagglutination or ELISA. These tests have a sensitivity of 85% to 100% and specificity of 88% to 96% for echinococcal infection. Routine bloodwork may show abnormal hepatic biochemical tests in some patients and eosinophilia in most of them. Examination of the stool is unhelpful since fecal eggs are not present in the human host. Skin testing (Casoni's test) has largely been abandoned because of its low specificity and potential danger of severe local allergic reaction.

Imaging studies

Ultrasonography, computed tomography, magnetic resonance imaging These studies typically demonstrate a multilocular cystic lesion with daughter cysts and/or calcification of the cyst walls (Figure 9.10B). In complicated disease they may also show communication of the cyst with the biliary system or external leakage of cyst material.

Pathology

Histological examination of an echinococcal cyst usually shows the parasite-derived laminated membrane (see Figure 9.10D), and may reveal scolices in the cyst lumen. However, histopathology is not essential for the diagnosis in most cases.

Treatment

Asymptomatic cysts that have a completely calcified wall and negative or low indirect hemagglutination test may contain no active scolices. These cysts have a very low likelihood of complications and should probably be treated conservatively. In the rest of the cases the treatment of choice consists of either surgery or percutaneous drainage. Medical therapy with mebendazole or albendazole is reportedly not effective in most cases of hydatid disease, however, it has been advocated as a preoperative measure. A variety of surgical procedures have been described. The therapeutic approaches used in most centers in North America consist of surgical evacuation, resection or excision of the cysts with prior irrigation by hypertonic saline as a scolicidal agent (Figure 9.10C). Other scolicidal agents have been tried for this purpose, including formalin, hydrogen peroxide, silver nitrate, and absolute alcohol, however, most of them have been associated with significant morbidity and mortality. Recently it has been suggested that percutaneous drainage combined with albendazole therapy, may be an effective and safe alternative to surgery for the treatment of uncomplicated hydatid cysts of the liver, although this approach has not been widely accepted in North America.

Polycystic liver disease

Epidemiology

Polycystic liver disease is thought to be caused by failure of intralobular bile ducts to involute during fetal development. These intralobular ducts become distorted and eventually degenerate into cysts. Polycystic liver disease is considered by many authorities to be a part of a clinical spectrum which includes congenital hepatic fibrosis, microhamartoma (von Meyenburg complex), choledochal cyst, and Caroli's disease. Although it arises in early fetal life, polycystic liver disease is usually diagnosed in the forth to fifth decade, with the development of symptoms. It is frequently associated with autosomal dominant polycystic kidney disease, which is the most common hereditary disorder of the kidney, occurring in 1:1 500 to 1:5 000 of the general population. Fifty per cent of patients with autosomal dominant polycystic kidney disease have liver cysts, and this frequency increases to 75% over the age of 60. There are reported cases of patients with multiple liver cysts and no apparent renal disease. It is not clear whether these patients represent a distinct group, or whether they have autosomal dominant polycystic kidney disease in which renal involvement is inconspicuous or has been overlooked. The number and size of liver cysts are greater in females than in males, and increase with the age of the patient. In addition to cysts, some of the other conditions in this spectrum of diseases may coexist in patients with autosomal dominant polycystic kidney disease. These include cystic dilatation of the ductal system, von Meyenburg complex, and ductal plate malformation. In addition, these patients have increased frequency of asymptomatic intracranial aneurysms, as well as cysts in other organs such as the pancreas, spleen, and uterus.

Clinical manifestations and natural history

Symptoms usually develop in the fourth to fifth decade of life. The patient may complain of abdominal discomfort, distention, nausea, and vomiting. Rupture or bleeding into a cyst may be associated with severe abdominal pain and occasionally fever. Contrary to a previously held notion, polycystic liver disease may be associated with significant morbidity and mortality. About 10% of the deaths in patients with autosomal dominant polycystic kidney disease result from complications of the liver disease. Hepatic complications include infection of a cyst, bleeding into a cyst, rupture, portal hypertension, obstruction of the biliary system, and, rarely, cholangiocarcinoma. In uncomplicated cases results of hepatic biochemical tests are usually normal or mildly abnormal. Obstruction of biliary ducts by large cysts may result in obstructive jaundice.

Ascites may occur in patients with portal hypertension, however in most cases synthetic liver function tests are normal.

Imaging studies

Ultrasonography This demonstrates multiple fluid-filled cystic lesions which usually show no internal echoes. The sonographic features are similar to those of simple cysts. Internal echoes may be detected in complicated cysts, i.e. post-bleeding or infection.

Computed tomography Computed tomography scans show multiple well-defined low-attenuation lesions which do not enhance following the administration of intravenous contrast (Figure 9.11A).

Magnetic resonance imaging On MRI these cysts show low signal on T1-weighted images and high signal on T2-weighted images, that do not enhance following intravenous injection of gadolinium (Figure 9.11 B–D).

Pathology

The liver may be normal in size or greatly enlarged, and its outer surface may be deformed. Cysts may vary in size from several millimeters to more than 10 cm. They may be diffused or restricted to one lobe, usually the left. The cysts are macroscopically and microscopically similar to simple cysts of the liver. They are unilocular, thin walled, and lined by a single-layered columnar or cuboidal biliary epithelium. They are surrounded by a fibrous tissue capsule, and usually contain clear or brown serous fluid. Although the cysts are lined by biliary-type epithelium they do not contain bile and typically do not communicate with the biliary tree. The only exception to this rule is in cases where a cyst ruptures into an adjacent bile duct. The adjacent liver tissue appears normal, but may contain multiple biliary microhamartomas (von Meyenburg complexes).

Treatment

Asymptomatic liver cysts require no treatment. In patients with large cysts causing abdominal pain or discomfort there is no satisfactory treatment. Extensive fenestration, with or without hepatic resection, may result in a dramatic improvement, however liver cysts and symptoms may recur a few months after surgery in many patients. The appearance of symptoms, or changes in hepatic biochemical tests, should alert the physician to the development of complications. Antibiotic treatment may not suffice in cases of an infected cyst and surgical drainage is often required. Obstructive jaundice due to extrinsic compression of the biliary tree has been treated by unroofing of the larger cysts, although the rate of recurrence is high.

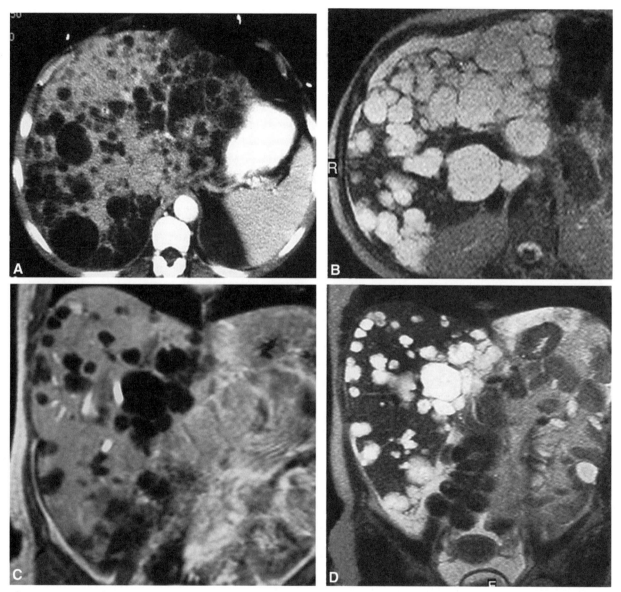

Figure 9.11 Polycystic liver disease. (A) Contrast-enhanced CT scan, arterial phase, exhibits hepatomegaly and multiple, well-defined, low-attenuation lesions, which do not enhance following the administration of intravenous contrast. (B) T2-weighted MRI image demonstrates multiple well-defined high signal lesions. (C) Enhanced MRI (coronal image) demonstrates multiple lesions of low signal intensity that do not enhance following intravenous injection of gadolinium. (D) T2-weighted MRI (coronal image) shows multiple lesions of high signal intensity. (Courtesy of J. Casillas, MD, Department of Radiology, University of Miami, Miami, FL.)

Patients with portal hypertension may benefit from portocaval shunting, however combined renal and liver transplantation may be necessary in patients with advanced liver and kidney disease. Since asymptomatic intracranial aneurysms appear to be more frequent in people with autosomal dominant polycystic kidney disease than in the general population, high-resolution brain CT scan has been recommended as a routine screening test for these patients.

Caroli's disease and Caroli's syndrome

Epidemiology and pathogenesis

Caroli's disease is a rare congenital abnormality characterized by saccular dilatations of segmental intrahepatic bile ducts, without other hepatic abnormalities. The dilated ducts form cysts of various sizes which are connected by normal portions of bile duct. The inheritance of this disease is uncertain. It probably belongs to a family of abnormalities that include ductal plate malformation, congenital hepatic fibrosis, and polycystic liver disease, however, there is still a considerable controversy regarding the classification of these diseases. The term Caroli's syndrome is applied to the coexistence of Caroli's disease and congenital hepatic fibrosis. This occurs in about half of the patients and is usually transmitted as an autosomal recessive trait. Many authors classify Caroli's disease and Caroli's syndrome within the spectrum of congenital biliary dilatation (or choledochal cyst) as type IVa. In contrast to polycystic liver disease, in Caroli's disease the dilated ducts communicate with the biliary tree, and are therefore more prone to infections and intrahepatic stone formation. Similar to polycystic liver disease, Caroli's disease may also be associated with a kidney disease, however in this case the renal disease is usually infantile medullary spongiosis, which is characterized by dilatation of the collecting ducts. Caroli's disease may present at any age, but is usually diagnosed in childhood or early adult life. About 75% of affected patients are male.

Clinical manifestations and natural history

Caroli's disease, although usually present at birth, remains asymptomatic for the first 5 to 20 years of the patient's life, and occasionally much longer. Asymptomatic disease may remain unrecognized throughout the patient's life or may be diagnosed incidentally on an imaging study. Hepatic biochemical tests are usually normal. Occasionally, there is a mild to moderate increase in AlkP and GGT. Symptomatic patients may present with abdominal pain, hepatomegaly, and fever, which are usually manifestations of gram-negative sepsis due to cholangitis. However, cholangitis tends to present without abdominal pain and jaundice, in contrast to bacterial cholangitis complicating bile-duct stones. As a consequence, the first episodes of fever may not be attributed to bacterial cholangitis. Jaundice, which is initially mild or absent, may increase during the course of cholangitis. Patients may develop intrahepatic biliary stones that may cause obstruction and contribute to the development of cholangitis and abscess formation.

Patients with Caroli's disease usually do not have manifestations of liver failure or portal hypertension. In patients with Caroli's syndrome associated with congenital hepatic fibrosis, manifestations of portal hypertension are usually present.

Cholangiocarcinoma has been described in approximately 7% of patients with Caroli's disease.

Imaging studies

Ultrasonography This shows multiple intrahepatic biliary cysts.

Contrast-enhanced computed tomography scan This technique demonstrates the dilated intrahepatic bile ducts with adjacent enhanced radicles of the portal vein (Figure 9.12A). The contrast-enhanced portal vein within the dilated intrahepatic bile duct has been named the central dot sign.

Cholangiography Either endoscopic (ERCP) or percutaneous cholangiography is a diagnostic test for Caroli's disease (Figure 9.12B). It demonstrates bulbous dilatations of the intrahepatic bile ducts with normal ducts between them, and a normal common bile duct. These invasive procedures can induce bacterial cholangitis, and must be performed only for therapeutic purposes or if diagnosis cannot be ascertained by non-invasive imaging studies.

Magnetic resonance cholangiopancreatography Magnetic resonance cholangiopancreatography (MRCP) may be used as a non-invasive alternative to ERCP and percutaneous cholangiography. Although it is probably less accurate than cholangiography in most medical centers, this test may be diagnostic in many patients with Caroli's disease and should be used prior to the use of invasive tests.

Diffuse involvement of the common bile duct and intrahepatic ducts showing strictures and dilatations is suggestive of primary sclerosing cholangitis as opposed to Caroli's disease. Cholangiocarcinoma may be demonstrated in a CT scan, MRCP, or cholangiography.

Treatment

Cholangitis should be treated promptly with intravenous antibiotics. Endoscopic or surgical drainage of the biliary system may be required for removal of an obstructing stone. Prolonged treatment with ursodeoxycholic acid has been successful for intrahepatic stones in patient with Caroli's disease. In cases where there is unilateral or segmental involvement, surgical resection may be effective. Even with preventive antibiotic treatment, the patient may suffer from recurrent infections by resistant bacterial strains, which may be difficult to control. Diffuse disease with recurrent episodes of cholangitis may require a liver transplantation, although the biliary infection is usually a contraindication. Without a surgical intervention or liver transplantation the long-term prognosis is poor.

Other cystic lesions of the liver

A variety of other cystic lesions of the liver with variable clinical significance have been described.

Traumatic cyst

Traumatic cyst (or post-traumatic cyst) is an extremely rare finding. It occurs as a result of intrahepatic hemorrhage. The resulting blood collection is liquefied and resorbed creating a cavity that frequently communicates with bile ducts. The blood collection is replaced by bile creating a bile-containing cyst. These cysts are more prevalent in the right lobe of the liver and may vary considerably in size. Most reported patients were young. Traumatic cysts are usually diagnosed some time after a blunt abdominal trauma. They typically present with abdominal pain, distention, and anorexia. A history of a significant abdominal trauma is usually obtained. Perforation and secondary infection are rare complications. Most of these cysts contain bile, and their wall is composed of fibrous tissue with variable amounts of inflammation. The treatment of choice is wide unroofing or partial excision with marsupialization to the abdominal wall. Simple percutaneous or surgical aspiration is an inadequate treatment in most cases.

Ciliated hepatic foregut cyst

A ciliated foregut cyst is a rare, benign, solitary cyst consisting of ciliated pseudostratified columnar epithelium, subepithelial connective tissue, a smooth muscle layer, and an outer fibrous capsule. Unlike simple solitary cysts, they occur more frequently in men and are found most commonly in the left lobe. There are about 60 reported cases of ciliated foregut cyst, the size of which ranges from 0.4 to 9.0 cm. There are no cases reported of malignant transformation in ciliated hepatic foregut cyst, and the clinical importance of its diagnosis lies in the distinction between this entity and other, potentially malignant hepatic lesions.

Primary squamous cell carcinoma

There are several reports of primary squamous cell carcinoma arising in hepatic cysts lined predominantly by stratified squamous epithelium. These lesions appear to have a poor prognosis, although the information in the literature is sparse.

Liver metastases

Rarely, certain liver metastases may appear as cystic lesions, usually because of the occurrence of

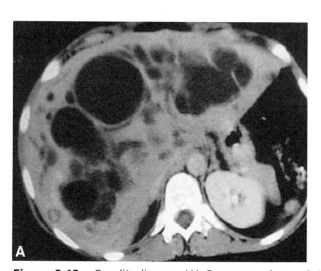
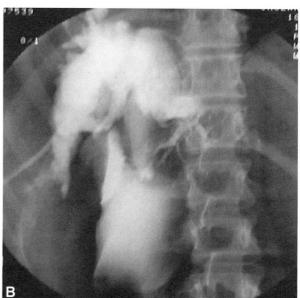

Figure 9.12 Caroli's disease. (A) Contrast-enhanced CT scan demonstrates multiple cystic and tubular structures consistent with dilated intrahepatic bile ducts. (B) Percutaneous transhepatic cholangiography (PTC) shows bulbous dilatation of the intrahepatic bile ducts. (Courtesy of J. Casillas, MD, Department of Radiology, University of Miami, Miami, FL.)

central necrosis. These include metastases from ovarian carcinoma, pancreas, colon, kidney, and neuroendocrine tumors.

Summary and recommendations

Cystic lesions of the liver may pose a diagnostic and therapeutic dilemma.

Simple cyst is by far the most common lesion encountered. Clinical features combined with typical sonographic findings are usually sufficient to distinguish simple cysts from other cystic lesions (Table 9.1). Needle aspiration is usually not indicated for diagnosis. Nevertheless, certain clinical manifestations and radiologic findings may point against the diagnosis of a simple cyst and require further work-up to rule out another diagnosis such as cystadenoma, cystadenocarcinoma, or hydatid cyst (Box 9.2).

In large asymptomatic, non-complicated, simple cysts, it is recommended to monitor by periodical ultrasonography for the first 2 to 3 years following diagnosis. Significant growth, progressive symptoms, or any suspicion of neoplastic cyst mandate surgical intervention. In symptomatic patients, the possibility of coexisting pathology must be excluded. When symptoms are the only indication for surgery, selection of patients with truly symptomatic cysts is crucial before considering any intervention. The procedure of choice for simple cysts is laparoscopic wide unroofing which is often curative. Percutaneous aspiration is ineffective and should be avoided. Prior to surgery it is recommended to rule out echinococcal disease by serologic testing. On opening the cyst roof, close inspection of the interior for neoplastic components is extremely important. Any suspicion regarding underlying malignancy (e.g. solid or thickened cyst wall, nodules, etc.) mandates a biopsy for frozen-section histopathology. Enucleation may be sufficient for cystadenoma, whereas formal hepatic resection is indicated in cases of cystadenocarcinoma.

Further reading

Benhamou JP, Menu Y. Non-parasitic cystic diseases of the liver and intrahepatic biliary tree. In: Blumgart, LH (ed.) *Surgery of the Liver and Biliary Tract* 2nd edn, vol. II. Churchill Livingstone, New York, 1994: p. 1197.

Brunt EM. Benign tumors of the liver. *Clin Liver Dis* 2001; 5: 1.

Martin IJ, McKinley AJ, Currie EJ, *et al*. Tailoring the management of nonparasitic liver cysts. *Ann Surg* 1998; 228: 167.

Molina EG, Schiff ER. Benign solid lesions of the liver. In: Schiff, ER, Sorrell, MF, Maddrey, WC (eds) *Schiff's Diseases of the Liver* 8th edn, vol. II, Lippincott-Raven, Philadephia, 1999: p. 1245.

Nisenbaum HL, Rowling SE. Ultrasound of focal hepatic lesions. *Semin Roentgenol* 1995; 30: 324.

Reddy KR, Kligerman S, Levi J, *et al*. Benign and solid tumors of the liver: relationship to sex, age, size of tumors, and outcome. *Am Surg* 2001; 67: 173.

Reddy KR, Schiff ER. Approach to a liver mass. *Semin Liver Dis* 1993; 13: 423.

Regev A, Reddy KR, Berho M, *et al*. Large cystic lesions of the liver in adults: a 15-year experience in a tertiary center. *J Am Coll Surg* 2001; 193: 36.

Sherlock S. Cystic disease of the liver. In: Schiff, ER, Sorrell, MF, Maddrey, WC (eds) *Schiff's Diseases of the Liver* 8th edn, vol. II, Lippincott-Raven, Philadephia, 1999: p. 1083.

Taylor BR, Langer B. Current surgical management of hepatic cyst disease. *Adv Surg* 1997; 31: 127.

Chapter 10

Hepatocellular Carcinoma

Steven B. Porter and K. Rajender Reddy

CHAPTER OUTLINE

Introduction

Hepatocellular carcinoma is the most common primary malignancy of the liver, resulting in as many as 1 million deaths annually worldwide. In some parts of the world, hepatocellular carcinoma is the most common cause of death from cancer. The reported survival rates for untreated and symptomatic hepatocellular carcinoma vary from 0% at 4 months to 1% at 2 years.

Among all cancers, hepatocellular carcinoma is the fifth most common in the world with over 500 000 new cases per year, accounting for more than 5% of all cancers. It remains the most common cause of death in patients with cirrhosis. Although hepatocellular carcinoma is less common in most parts of the developed western world, its incidence is increasing substantially. There has been an 80% increase in the incidence of hepatocellular carcinoma in the US alone over the past 20 to 30 years with approximately 15 000 new cases each year. This has been attributed to the hepatitis C and hepatitis B virus-related hepatocellular carcinoma primarily in immigrants.

Because of the usual development of hepatocellular carcinoma in patients with chronic liver disease, it is often diagnosed and managed by gastroenterologists and hepatologists. In this chapter we will discuss the epidemiology, risk factors, clinical presentation, diagnosis, prognosis, and treatment of hepatocellular carcinoma from a hepatologist's perspective. The magnitude of the hepatocellular carcinoma problem is growing in the US and remains a significant problem in parts of Africa and the Far East. Treatment regimens are improving as biochemical and technological advances in the practice of hepatology allow for more insight into the molecular basis of hepatocellular carcinoma. However, without the eradication of both hepatitis B and hepatitis C viruses, hepatocellular carcinoma will remain a significant cause of morbidity and mortality.

Epidemiology

The highest incidence of hepatocellular carcinoma is found in sub-Saharan Africa and the Far East. In these regions, the death rate ranges from 23 to 150 per 100 000 per year. Hepatocellular carcinoma is relatively uncommon in North America, northern Europe, and Australia. In these areas the death rate is less than 5 per 100 000 per year. In regions with a high incidence of hepatocellular carcinoma, the neoplasms are found more frequently in the young adult population, while in areas of low risk it generally occurs in older individuals.

Hepatocellular carcinoma is found more frequently in males than females in a ratio of 3 to 1. Because of the prevalence of perinatally transmitted hepatitis B virus infection in sub-Saharan Africa and the Far East, hepatocellular carcinoma related to hepatitis B virus infection is more often seen in a younger population. In contrast, in the developed world where this malignancy is related to hepatitis C virus infection, the age of presentation is relatively older because of the later acquisition in life of hepatitis C virus infection and its associated slow progression of disease. In the US and Europe the tumor prevalence has been found to be low until the fifth decade and thereafter it increases briskly peaking in the seventh decade (Figure 10.1). In addition, in areas where hepatitis B virus infection

is endemic, there may be an oncogenic role for aflatoxin and, further, hepatocellular carcinoma may develop more frequently in a non-cirrhotic liver. In contrast, hepatocellular carcinoma related to hepatitis C virus in the developed world is seen primarily in patients with cirrhosis and, to a lesser extent, in patients with bridging fibrosis.

Risk factors

The chief risk factor for hepatocellular carcinoma is cirrhosis, regardless of its etiology. The annual risk of developing hepatocellular carcinoma in patients with cirrhosis ranges from 1% to 6%. Moreover, 20% to 50% of patients presenting with symptomatic hepatocellular carcinoma have previously undiagnosed cirrhosis. The other main risk factors for hepatocellular carcinoma are infection with hepatitis C virus and hepatitis B virus, coinfection with both (which results in a greater risk than either virus alone), and concomitant alcohol use in the background of viral hepatitis. Relatively infrequent causes for hepatocellular carcinoma include use of oral contraceptives, genetic hemochromatosis, autoimmune chronic hepatitis, and primary biliary cirrhosis. Recently, non-alcoholic fatty liver disease and cirrhosis has emerged as a condition that has a high risk for development of hepatocellular carcinoma.

The annual incidence of hepatocellular carcinoma in hepatitis B virus cirrhotics exceeds 2% while the annual incidence in non-cirrhotic chronic hepatitis B virus is 0.5%. The annual incidence for the development of hepatocellular carcinoma in hepatitis C virus cirrhosis has been reported to range between 1% and 4% per year.

Clinical presentation

In the symptomatic patient the classic clinical features of hepatocellular carcinoma are right upper quadrant pain, a palpable mass or enlarged liver, and weight loss (Figure 10.2). There should be a high index of suspicion for hepatocellular carcinoma when worsening hepatic function is observed in a patient with previously diagnosed cirrhosis. Dyspnea and jaundice are both late symptoms. Rare presentation includes acute abdominal catastrophe from the rupture of a liver tumor and resultant intra-abdominal bleeding. Although hyperbilirubinemia may be present, the degree of abnormality of the hepatic biochemical profile does not correlate with the size of the tumor. Various

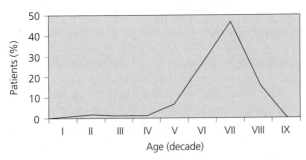

Figure 10.1 Age distribution trends in 461 Italian patients with hepatocellular carcinoma. (Reproduced from Trevisani *et al* Clinical and pathologic features of hepatocellular carcinoma in young and older Italian patients. *Cancer* 1996; 77: 2223–2232. © American Cancer Society. Reprinted with permission of Wiley-Liss, Inc., a subsidiary of John Wiley & Sons. Inc.)

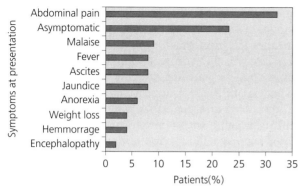

Figure 10.2 Symptoms at the initial presentation of hepatocellular carcinoma in a series of 461 Italian patients. (Reproduced from Trevisani *et al* Clinical and pathologic features of hepatocellular carcinoma in young and older Italian patients. *Cancer* 1996; 77: 2223–2232. © American Cancer Society. Reprinted with permission of Wiley-Liss, Inc., a subsidiary of John Wiley & Sons. Inc.)

paraneoplastic manifestations have been described with hepatocellular carcinoma, erythrocytosis due to excessive production of erythropoeitin is an occasional feature and hypoglycemia either due to liver failure or high insulin levels is found in about one third of patients with hepatocellular carcinoma. Other uncommon manifestations include gynecomastia and hyperthyroidism.

However, in many patients, hepatocellular carcinoma is diagnosed in an asymptomatic patient because of rigid screening procedures. Such diagnoses are likely to lead to the best outcomes.

Diagnosis

Tumor markers

There are three major serological markers of hepatocellular carcinoma: alpha-fetoprotein (AFP), the L3 subfraction of AFP (AFP-L3), and PIVKA-II (also known as des-γ-carboxy prothrombin). These three makers, when coupled with imaging techniques (see Radiology), serve the following functions

1. early diagnosis of hepatocellular carcinoma in patients at risk and differential diagnosis of space-occupying lesions in the liver
2. therapeutic outcome of hepatocellular carcinoma as well as early detection of relapse
3. assessment of the biology of the malignancy and prognosis of hepatocellular carcinoma (AFP and PIVKA-II do not correlate and, therefore, they are

used as complementary investigations and are not mutually exclusive).

Alpha-fetoprotein

Alpha-fetoprotein is a glycosylated protein with a molecular size of approximatley 70 000 Daltons, it contains an asparagine-binding, double-chain complex sugar. Alpha-fetoprotein is produced in the fetal yolk sac and intestine and remains present at high concentrations in fetal life. Apart from hepatocellular carcinoma, elevated levels of AFP can be found in pregnant women, in patients with germ-cell tumors, cirrhosis, and acute and chronic hepatitis. The measurement of serum AFP may be helpful in the diagnosis and management of hepatocellular carcinoma although the sensitivity and specificity are quite variable. In healthy individuals, AFP exists in sera at concentrations around 10 ng/mL. Alpha-fetoprotein is elevated above 20 ng/mL, twice the upper limit of normal, in more than 70% of patients with hepatocellular carcinoma. However, AFP elevations from 10 to 500 ng/mL and even occasionally to 1000 ng/mL may be seen in patients with a high degree of necroinflammatory activity, such as with chronic viral hepatitis, who do not have hepatocellular carcinoma.

The sensitivity, specificity, and positive predictive value of AFP in three well-performed screening studies for hepatocellular carcinoma ranged from 39% to 64%, 76% to 91%, and 9% to 32% respectively. Alpha-fetoprotein is further useful in monitoring response to treatment and detecting recurrence after treatment of hepatocellular carcinoma, if the AFP was elevated before treatment. If AFP levels increase abruptly or are gradually elevated within low ranges, unaccompanied by signs of inflammation such as elevated alanine aminotransferase and/or aspartate aminotransferase, they can signal the development of hepatocellular carcinoma. The proportion of patients with hepatocellular carcinoma who are seronegative for abnormal AFP has been increasing gradually during the past 20 years. Also, AFP has been found to be insensitive in the diagnosis of hepatocellular carcinoma in African Americans. The role of AFP alone is shifting from that of a diagnostic tool to one of confirmation of hepatocellular carcinoma.

Alpha-fetoprotein

A subfractionation of AFP, designated AFP-L3, has been observed to be a more sensitive and specific serologic marker for hepatocellular carcinoma. In addition, it has prognostic significance. Alpha-fetoprotein-L3 is the *Lens culinaris* agglutinin-reactive fraction of AFP, is a fucosylated variation of AFP, and is measured by using a lectin-affinity assay. The cutoff value for normal AFP-L3 has been set at 10% of total AFP. Values exceeding 10% are strongly indicative of hepatocellular carcinoma even when the total AFP value is increased only slightly. Alpha-fetoprotein-L3 over 10% of total AFP signals the development of hepatocellular carcinoma in the foreseeable future so these patients need to be put on stringent surveillance with frequent follow-up. An elevated AFP-L3 has been observed to be associated with certain pathologic features of poorly differentiated hepatocellular carcinoma in tumors less than 2 centimeters in diameter and also with multifocality. Further, AFP-L3 values in small hepatocellular carcinomas are significantly higher for hypervascular rather than for iso- or hypovascular tumors and also are closely associated with intrahepatic metastases.

Following treatment of hepatocellular carcinoma, AFP in serum decreases much earlier than AFP-L3. If AFP-L3 stays elevated despite AFP reaching a trough level, residual hepatocellular carcinoma should be suspected. Residual malignancy should be a concern if AFP-L3 does not decrease to less than 10% following treatment and a relapse should be suspected if it re-elevates after having reached the normal range. Finally, AFP-L3 has a prognostic significance in that survival in patients with hepatocellular carcinoma is longer in those with normal AFP-L3. This marker, however, is investigational in the US and is not available for routine use.

Prothrombin induced by vitamin K absence or antagonist-II

Prothrombin induced by vitamin K absence or antagonist-II (PIVKA-II) in serum is another marker of hepatocellular carcinoma. Prothrombin is the major vitamin K-dependent blood coagulation protein synthesized in the liver, and its presence in serum has correlated with hepatocellular carcinoma. In the presence of vitamin K, γ-carboxylation of prothrombin takes place in the liver. Without vitamin K, or in the presence of vitamin K antagonists such as warfarin, the prothrombin remains uncarboxylated prior to release into the bloodstream and, thus, PIVKA-II is also known as des-γ-carboxy prothrombin.

The marker PIVKA-II behaves independently of AFP. The upper limit of normal is set at 40 mAU/mL (AU = arbitrary units) based on the sensitivity of second-generation immunoassays. These tests report a sensitivity estimated at 48% with specificity of 96%. As with AFP, PIVKA-II can be elevated in non-hepatocellular carcinoma situations. These include obstructive jaundice and intrahepatic cholestasis that lead to long-standing deficiency of vitamin K, as well as the presence of drugs such as warfarin or other antibiotics.

Levels of PIVKA-II increase in parallel to the size of the tumor and abnormal values are more prevalent in patients with poorly or moderately differentiated hepatocellular carcinoma as compared to well-differentiated malignancy. In patients with chronic hepatitis or cirrhosis, if PIVKA-II levels reach the 30 to 40 mAU/mL level, there is a high probability that either hepatocellular carcinoma has escaped detection by imaging techniques or it will develop in the foreseeable future.

The half-life of PIVKA-II is 40 to 70 hours, which is much shorter than the 5-day half-life of AFP. Hence PIVKA-II can reflect the therapeutic efficacy on hepatocellular carcinoma much more rapidly than AFP. Following treatment, the two markers behave differently. The mutual complementary nature of the serologic tests allows for better surveillance since small hepatocellular carcinomas tend to raise one marker but not both in concert (Figure 10.3).

Radiology

Recent improvements in imaging modalities have led to the diagnosis of hepatocellular carcinoma in the earlier stages. Previously imaging studies were mainly of two types: radioisotope scans and angiography. Radioisotope scans lacked sensitivity and specificity, especially in the case of tumors less than 2 centimeters in size, while angiography has since faded from the forefront and is now only used in the administration of therapies such as chemoembolization. Angiography without a tumor-retaining contrast such as lipiodol has poor ability to discern tumors smaller than 2 centimeters.

Ultrasound is able to locate small tumors, although the technique is limited by the experience of the radiologists performing the examination, obesity of the patient, and the overlying amount of gas in the bowel. The focus is primarily on different echogenicity from the surrounding liver tissue: small tumors may be hypoechoic and become hyperechoic as they grow larger. Ultrasound is almost exclusively used as a screening tool, while CT is more commonly used for diagnosis. Computed tomography if often used as a confirmatory tool to rule out false positive ultrasound examinations, and magnetic resonance imaging (MRI). However, ultrasound is still able to depict vascular

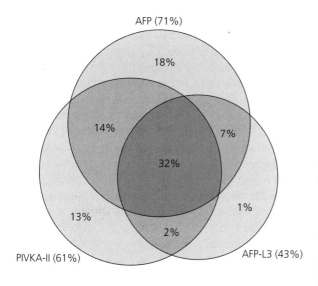

AFP (71%)

18%

14%   7%

32%

13%   1%

2%

PIVKA-II (61%)   AFP-L3 (43%)

(n = 189, No markers: 13%)

Figure 10.3 Reproduced from Fujiyama *et al.*
Tumor markers in early diagnosis, follow-up and
management of patients with hepatocellular
carcinoma. Fujiyama *et al.* Tumor markers in early
diagnosis, follow-up and mangement of patients
with hepatocellular carcinoma. *Oncology* 2002; 62
(suppl 1): 57–63. © S. Karger AG, Basel.

involvement. Currently, new contrast agents (e.g.
intra-arterial carbon dioxide) are being looked at to
aid in ultrasound.

The vast improvements in CT technology over
the past two decades include the introduction of
spiral scanners that allow for very rapid imaging
after infusion of intravenous contrast agents. With
the development of increasingly better scanning
protocols, CT has come to displace ultrasound as a
primary method of diagnosing hepatocellular carcinoma. Since hepatocellular carcinoma derives its
blood supply predominantly from the hepatic
artery, hepatocellular carcinomas enhance early on
during the infusion of contrast in the arterial phase.
The surrounding parenchyma, on the other hand,
enhances during the portal venous phase. Triphasic
CT scan describes three discrete time zones in the
imaging study: before contrast, arterial phase, and
portal venous phase, and is the preferred method of
CT imaging for hepatocellular carcinoma. While
CT scanning has much improved, there are still
many tumors that it is unable to identify.

Magnetic resonance imaging is the preferred imaging modality used at some institutions. Typically
hepatocellular carcinoma appears hypointense on T1-
and hyperintense on T2-weighted images, but there
exists considerable variability. In addition MRI may
not identify tumors less than 2 centimeters in size.

Histology

While histologic examination of liver tissue is an important element in the diagnosis of hepatocellular carcinoma, the routine use of needle biopsy of hepatocellular
carcinoma is controversial. The inherent risk, albeit low
at 1%, is of needle-track seeding of hepatocellular carcinoma and this is particularly undesirable if liver transplantation is a serious consideration. It is for this reason
that many institutions are reluctant to perform a liver
biopsy in suspected hepatocellular carcinoma. A more
relevant risk is that of bleeding from the biopsy site after
the procedure because of the hypervascularity of the
tumor. However, if therapeutic interventions, such as
ablative therapies that have associated risks are
planned, it is worth considering needle biopsy for confirmation of hepatocellular carcinoma.

In the case of a massive tumor or extensive
spread throughout the liver, a blind needle biopsy is
sufficient, especially if the mass can be palpated.
Outside of that setting, needle biopsies are generally guided by either ultrasound or CT. If necessary,
laparoscopic or open surgical biopsies can be performed if no radiographic means can locate the cancer. The tissue sample can be evaluated
histologically, cytologically, or by both methods. Histologically, hepatocellular carcinoma at times may
be indistinguishable from benign hepatic masses
such as macroregenerative nodules, adenoma, or
focal nodular hyperplasia.

Several histologic classifications for hepatocellular
carcinoma have been proposed and validated. Hepatocellular carcinoma is classified into well-differentiated, moderately differentiated, poorly differentiated,
and undifferentiated types. Such grading has prognostic significance. There is a World Health Organization Histologic Classification that is accepted
worldwide and is based on the following histologic
patterns: trabecular, pseudoglandular, compact, scir-
rhous, and fibrolamellar carcinoma. Another well-
recognized histologic classification is the
Edmondson–Steiner Classification which grades this
malignancy based on histologic differentiation from
grade 1 to grade 4.

Surveillance

The earlier that the hepatocellular carcinoma lesion
is detected, the more effective is the therapy that
can be given. The goal of surveillance protocols is to
detect hepatocellular carcinomas less than 2 centimeters in size. The time that it takes for an unde-

tectable lesion to grow to 2 centimeters is about 4 to 12 months and, as such, the suggested interval for surveillance is set at 6 months. Patients with a particularly high risk do not warrant more intensive surveillance since higher risk does not correlate with faster growth. The overall reported annual detection rate of hepatocellular carcinoma in surveillance studies, which included patients with chronic hepatitis in addition to cirrhosis, is 0.8% to 4.1%. The standard for 6-month surveillance is serological markers and ultrasound.

Since it is very difficult to distinguish between stage III fibrosis and cirrhosis, the 6-month protocol may be started when cirrhosis is suspected since it is not justified to perform repeated liver biopsies just to initiate surveillance. Biochemical diagnostic tools for cirrhosis are not yet established.

Recall

Currently there are no well-defined recall policies regarding hepatocellular carcinoma. In cases where a hypo- or hyperechoic nodule smaller than 1 centimeter is observed in ultrasound evaluation, it is reasonable from a clinical perspective to repeat ultrasound every 3 months until the lesion grows larger than 1 centimeter, at which time additional diagnostic modalities can be pursued. It is important to recognize, however, that some of the cancers may be of a slow-growing nature and therefore the absence of a change within a year in the size of an observed lesion should not be misconstrued as the lesion being benign. If a lesion exceeds 1 centimeter in size on ultrasound imaging, it is recommended that further investigations such as CT or MRI be performed (Figure 10.4).

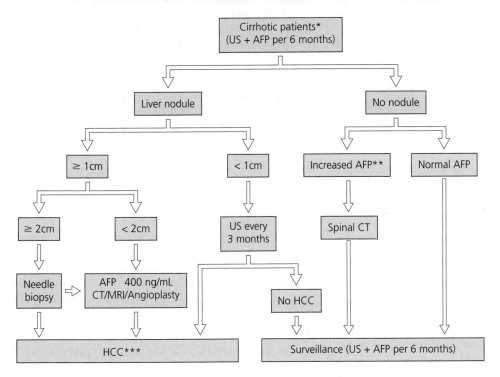

* Available for curative treatments if diagnosed with HCC
** AFP levels to be defined
*** pathological confirmation or non-invasive criteria
Non-invasive criteria (restricted to cirrhotic patients)
1. Radiological criteria: two coincident imaging techniques[1],
focal lesion >2cm with arterial hypervascularization.
2. Combined criteria: one imaging technique associated with AFP,
focal lesion > 400ng/mL.
[1] Four techniques considered: US, spiral CT, MRI and angiography.

HCC	=	hepatocellular carcinoma
US	=	ultrasound
AFP	=	alpha-fetoprotein
CT	=	computerized tomography
MRI	=	magnetic resonance imaging

Figure 10.4 Reproduced from Bruix J, Sherman M, Llovet JM, *et al.* Clinical management of hepatocellular carcinoma: conclusions of the Barcelona 2000 EASL conference. *Journal of Hepatology* 2001; 35:421–430

Hepatocellular carcinoma can now be confidently diagnosed following two imaging techniques showing a nodule greater than 2 centimeters with arterial hypervascularization or a single positive imaging technique associated with AFP greater than 400 ng/mL. With other serologic studies that may serve complementary to AFP, the target level of AFP for the diagnosis of hepatocellular carcinoma can perhaps be lowered, although this has to be further investigated. In patients with a negative ultrasound and an AFP over 20 ng/mL during follow-up after an initial normal baseline AFP, a triphasic CT scan is recommended. At the very least, this scan will provide a baseline image to be used for comparison in the event of new findings.

Prognosis

The five staging systems or prognostic classifications currently used for hepatocellular carcinoma are

- the Okuda stage
- the Tumor Node Metastases (TNM) classification
- the Cancer of the Liver Italian Program (CLIP) system
- the Barcelona Clinic Liver Cancer (BCLC) classification
- the Groupe d'Etude et de Traitement du Carcinome Hépatocellulaire (GETCH) classification.

Okuda staging system

The Okuda staging system is commonly referred to as the most simple and widely used system in practice. It consists of three stages (I, II, and III) and is based on tumor size, the presence of ascites, serum albumin, and serum bilirubin. When created this staging system was based on a retrospective analysis of 850 patients with hepatocellular carcinoma in Japan between 1975 and 1983 (see Table 10.1). In the earlier years, the Okuda stage was widely used because of its simple calculability. It takes into consideration both tumor size and liver functional status, and is very useful in classifying those with advanced or end-stage disease (Okuda stage III patients). However, the differentiation of disease severity between stage I and stage II patients is not precise. Therefore, this staging system is deficient at stratifying stage I and stage II patients for effective treatment regimens, in part because it was created in an era when treatment options, including liver transplantation, were sparse. It should also be noted that the relative tumor size is poorly reproducible by the various imaging modalities even with their respective advancements.

Tumor node metastases classification

The TNM classification created by the International Union Against Cancer looks at single or multiple tumors, characterizes their size (relative to 5 centimeters) and their vascular invasiveness, and considers the involvement of regional lymph nodes (the hilar, hepatic, periportal, and those along the abdominal inferior vena cava above the renal veins), and distant metastases. The tumor consideration is the most stratified (Table 10.2).

The downside of the TNM classification is that it does not incorporate parameters of hepatic function and, thus, is unhelpful in guiding us regarding surgical and non-surgical treatment. Also, this staging method requires a biopsy of hepatic lymph

Table 10.1 The Okuda staging system

Criteria	Points	
	0	1
Tumor size	< 50% of total liver volume	> 50% of total liver volume
Ascites	No	Yes
Albumin	> 3 mg/dL	< 3 mg/dL
Bilirubin	< 3 mg/dL	> 3 mg/dL

Stage I patients have a total score of 0.
Stage II patients have a total score of 1–2.
Stage III patients have a total score of 3–4.
Source: Okuda K, Ohtsuki T, Obata H, et al. Natural history of hepatocellular carcinoma and prognosis in relation to treatment: study of 850 patients. Cancer 1985; 56: 918–928. © 1985 American Cancer Society. Reproduced with permission of Wiley-Liss, Inc., a subsidiary of John Wiley & Sons, Inc.

Table 10.2 The TNM classification

	Tumor	Node	Metastases
Stage I	T1	N0	M0
Stage II	T2	N0	M0
Stage IIIA	T3	N0	M0
Stage IIIB	T4	N0	M0
Stage IIIC	Any T	N1	M0
Stage IV	Any T	Any N	M1

T1: solitary tumor without vascular invasion.
T2: solitary tumor with vascular invasion or multiple tumors, none more than 6 cm in greatest dimension.
T3: multiple tumors more than 5 cm or tumor involving a major branch of the portal or hepatic vein(s).
T4: tumor(s) with direct invasion of adjacent organs other than the gallbladder or with perforation of visceral peritoneum.
N0: there is no regional lymph node metastasis.
N1: the regional lymph nodes are involved.
M0:
M1:
Source: Sobin LH, Wittekind CH (eds). International Union Against Cancer (UICC). TNM Classification of Malignant Tumours 6th edn. New York: Wiley-Liss, 2002, pp. 81–83.

nodes which carries a risk of complication in the patient with portal hypertension.

Cancer of the Liver Italian Program system

The CLIP system (Table 10.3) was created to improve the stratification of the Okuda staging method. This system incorporates hepatic function as determined by Child–Pugh class, tumor morphology, portal vein thrombosis, and AFP. In a retrospective study of 435 patients with hepatocellular carcinoma (almost 100% with underlying cirrhosis

and 80% with histologic or cytologic confirmation of hepatocellular carcinoma) at sixteen Italian institutions between 1990 and 1992, the Italian group found four independent predictive factors of survival in multivariate analysis.

The inclusion of tumor type, portal vein thrombosis, and AFP level provides additional indices of tumor burden over that of the Okuda staging system. The CLIP system has a higher number of categories and a greater discriminant ability than the Okuda system. The scoring ranges from 0 (Child–Pugh Class A, normal AFP, no portal vein thrombosis, and a solitary tumor with extension less than 50% of the total liver volume) to 6 (Child–Pugh Class C, high AFP, portal vein thrombosis, and a solitary massive tumor or cancer spread to more than 50% of the total liver volume).

While the CLIP system has more stratification of patients than the Okuda staging system, it will have to update the scoring to adjust to the move to the MELD score as preferred over the Child–Pugh stage. Also, new cellular and molecular markers such as p73, p53, interleukin-2 receptor, and intercellular adhesion molecule 1 may or may not be added to the independent factors on survival in the future.

The Barcelona Clinic Liver Cancer classification

The BCLC staging system was created under the shifting paradigm of management of hepatocellular carcinoma since the advent of improved imaging studies and regular screening in the last decade (Figure 10.5). Now, approximately 25% of hepatocellular carcinoma patients may benefit from radical therapies (resection, orthotopic liver transplant, or percutaneous ethanol injection) while only 25% of

Table 10.3 The CLIP scoring system

Criteria	Points		
	0	1	2
Child–Pugh stage	A	B	C
Tumor morphology	Uninodular and extension ≤ 50%[1]	Multinodular and extension ≤ 50%[1]	Massive or extension > 50%[1]
Portal vein thrombosis	No	Yes	
AFP	< 400 ng/dL	> 400 ng/dL	

[1] *percentage of total liver volume.*
Source: The Cancer of the Liver Italian Program Investigators. A new prognostic system for hepatocellular carcinoma: a retrospective study of 435 patients. Hepatology 1998; 28: 751–755.

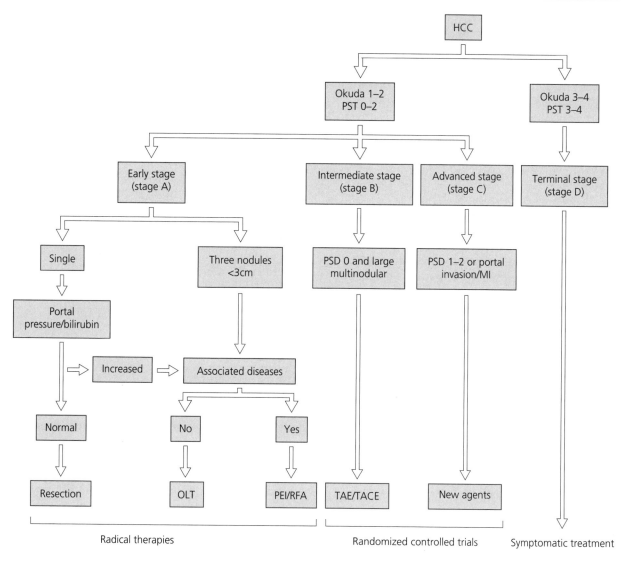

Figure 10.5 The Barcelona Clinic Liver Cancer staging classification of hepatocellular carcinoma.

current hepatocellular carcinoma patients have what is now considered to be end-stage disease.

The BCLC model matches strata with treatment options. Focusing on two preoperative factors

1. clinically relevant portal hypertension – defined as the presence of either esohageal varices, splenomegaly with a platelet count less than 100 000/mm³, or a hepatic vein pressure gradient of 10 mmHg or more
2. bilirubin levels differentiated at the 1 mg/dL level

allowed the workers to stratify three different groups of surgical candidates: the group without either of the above predictors had a 5-year survival rate of 74%, whereas the group with both adverse predictors had a 5-year survival rate of 25%.

Four stages of hepatocellular carcinoma were identified.

1. Stage A1 through A4 describes early stage hepatocellular carcinoma from a single tumor and the absence of relevant portal hypertension and normal bilirubin (A1) to a single tumor

with both relevant portal hypertension and increased bilirubin (A3) to three tumors smaller than 3 centimeters regardless of liver function (A4).

2. Intermediate hepatocellular carcinoma (Stage B) includes asymptomatic patients with multinodular tumors without vascular invasion or extrahepatic spread.

3. Advanced hepatocellular carcinoma (Stage C) includes symptomatic tumors (performance status test = 1–2, constitutional syndrome) or with an invasive tumoral pattern reflected by the presence of vascular invasion or extrahepatic spread.

4. End-stage hepatocellular carcinoma (Stage D) characterized by a performance status test = 3–4, Okuda stage III, with patients displaying severe cancer-related symptoms reflected by a deteriorated performance status or tumors in the setting of very advanced liver functional impairment.

The Groupe d'Etude et de Traitement du Carcinome Hépatocellulaire classification

The Groupe d'Etude et de Traitement du Carcinome Hépatocellulaire studied 506 patients (with 418 deaths) in a training sample and 255 patients (with 200 deaths) in a test sample to validate a new prognostic system (see Table 10.4). The scoring system relies on five variables that correlated with survival in a Cox regression analysis in the training sample

- Karnofsky index < 80% (relative risk of death 2.15)
- bilirubin ≥ 50 μmol/L (relative risk of death 2.08)
- AFP ≥ 35 μg/L (relative risk of death 1.68)
- alkaline phosphatase ≥ twice the upper limit of normal (relative risk of death 1.61)
- portal obstruction (relative risk of death 1.33).

Three strata were defined as follows

- Group A with a total score of 0
- Group B with a total score of 1 to 5
- Group C with a total score of 6 or more.

In the training sample, 16% of patients were classified in group A, 47% in group B, and 37% in group C. Observed 1- and 2-year survival rates were 71.6% and 51.1% for Group A, 33.8% and 16.8% for Group B, and 7.4% and 3.1% for Group C. The mean predicted survival at 1 and 2 years was 64% and 47% for Group A, 36% and 19% for Group B, and 7.4% and 3.1% for Group C.

Overall, the CLIP and BCLC classifications are given the most weight in the recent literature. The CLIP system has been shown to have discriminatory ability and predictive power over the Okuda stage and TNM system. The strength of the BCLC system lies in its ability to stratify patients for treatment. However, all of the prognostic models thus far are not precise enough because of their dependence on variables that are not central to the fundamental biochemical or molecular causes of liver disease. Until further information on the molecular basis of hepatocellular carcinoma is elucidated, these systems will fall short of true prognostic ability. However, with the recent creation of the BCLC, CLIP, and GETCH systems, at the very least, multicenter and regional interest is on the rise to find the correct system to track the most common primary malignancy of the liver.

Table 10.4 The Groupe d'Etude et de Traitement du Carcinome Hépatocellulaire classification

Points	0	1	2	3
Karnofsky index (%)	≥ 80			< 80
Serum bilirubin (μmol/L)	< 50			≥ 50
Serum alkaline phosphatase (ULN)	< 2		≥ 2	
Serum AFP (μg/L)	< 35		≥ 35	
Portal obstruction (ultrasound)	no	yes		

Source: Chevret S, Trinchet JC, Mathieu D, et al. Groupe d'Etude et de Traitement du Carcinome Hépatocellulaire. A new prognostic classification for predicting survival in patients with hepatocellular carcinoma. J Hepatol 1999; 31: 133–141.

Treatment

The optimal method to demonstrate the benefit of any treatment for hepatocellular carcinoma in a randomized controlled trial would have to involve a no treatment control arm. Because of the ethical implications of that type of study, it will never be performed. Thus far, palliative approaches have been studied in the advanced and terminal strata of patients who would not benefit from surgical methods (hepatic resection or orthotopic liver transplant), ablative methods, or chemoembolization and chemotherapy. Therefore, there is a bias toward palliative therapies that offer limited benefit given the selection of poor candidates for such therapy. Each center is likely to perform whatever therapy best suits the patient given the local abilities of the center itself. However, in patients with early hepatocellular carcinoma in decompensated liver disease, orthotopic liver transplant is the preferred treatment protocol.

Surgical methods

Resection

Hepatic resection is second only to orthotopic liver transplant in its ability to effectively eliminate hepatocellular carcinoma, and is an approved method of treatment in resectable livers. To be a successful candidate for resection, patients must have a single, non-diffuse tumor and preferably be asymptomatic without hepatic decompensation. However, resection does not eliminate remaining portions of the liver at risk for malignant transformation, nor does it improve hepatic function. In non-cirrhotics who have technically resectable cancers and no evidence of vascular invasion or spread outside the liver, or other decompensation, resection is undoubtedly the treatment of choice. Unfortunately, non-cirrhotic asymptomatic hepatocellular carcinomas represent less than 5% of all hepatocellular carcinomas found in western patients. In a cirrhotic patient, the accepted guidelines for resection are that it be a solitary lesion in the left lobe or it be amenable to a segmental resection if in the right lobe. Further, it should be considered in patients with well-compensated liver disease and without portal vein thrombosis and metastatic disease.

On average, a 5-year survival rate of approximately 50% has been observed in resected patients when the following criteria were met

- the tumor is solitary and less than 5 centimeters in diameter
- there is no evidence of vascular invasion or extrahepatic spread, and
- there is no evidence of either cirrhosis or well-compensated Child–Pugh class A cirrhosis including no evidence of portal hypertension.

However, recurrence of tumor exceeds 50% even when the strict criteria are enforced. An increased risk of recurrence can be predicted by pathologic characteristics such as vascular invasion, satellites, and the degree of poor differentiation.

The use of intraoperative ultrasound is necessary to detect additional tumor nests as well as to guide anatomical resection to eliminate unrecognized local spread. Indocyanine green retention rate has been used to assess hepatic synthetic function and thus identify the best candidates for surgery. Established portal pressure hypertension and hyperbilirubinemia have also predicted poor outcomes after surgical resection. The balance of resection versus orthotopic liver transplant may shift pending further data on the outcomes of living donor liver transplantation.

Orthotopic liver transplantation

Orthotopic liver transplantation is theoretically the best treatment for hepatocellular carcinoma.

It results in the widest possible resection margins for the cancer, it removes the risk for *de novo* tumors by replacing the diseased organ with a graft, and it restores hepatic function. But with the limited availability of donors and increasing wait times once listed, orthotopic liver transplantation has become a less effective way of dealing with the increasing incidence of hepatocellular carcinoma. Living donor liver transplantation, a procedure with increasing acceptability, may help to alleviate some of these problems but currently there are limited data on the outcome.

Orthotopic liver transplant results in an approximately 15% 1-year mortality rate overall for adults and thus may not be appropriate for early cancers that have a better prognosis if left untreated or treated with non-surgical modalities. Contraindications for orthotopic liver transplantation include

- extrahepatic spread
- a single tumor greater than 5 centimeters in diameter
- the presence of more than three tumors, or
- at least three lesions present with one of them greater than 3 centimeters in diameter.

Helical CT or MRI can often help to detect extrahepatic spread.

Tumor recurrence is strongly correlated to tumor size, number of nodules, and presence of vascular invasion. While 3-year survival rates varied from 21% to 47% and with recurrence rates as high as 29% to 54% in advanced tumors, 3-year survival in patients with ideal criteria has been close to 80% which is comparable to survival in patients who undergo orthotopic liver transplant for end-stage liver disease without hepatocellular carcinoma. However, those figures come from an era when the waiting time was less than 6 months. More recent data from the United Network for Organ Sharing suggest an average wait time of approximately 18 months because of a relatively fixed number of donor organs with a rising transplant candidate pool. As median wait time increases, it is likely that the transplant candidate with hepatocellular carcinoma may be delisted because of an increase in tumor burden, the development of metastatic disease, or they may die while waiting for a transplant. The adoption of the MELD score for liver allocation in the ultrasound may ameliorate this issue somewhat, since it favors patients with hepatocellular carcinoma when compared to the Child–Pugh classification.

Living donor liver transplantation eliminates waiting time and thus theoretically is preferred when there is a waiting time longer than 6 months. In 2000, according to the United Network for Organ Sharing, 6.5% of all transplants were living donor liver transplantation. This number may eventually increase to 20% if application criteria remain stable. A Markov model of living donor liver transplantation versus cadaveric transplantation showed substantial gains in life expectancy and cost effectiveness when the waiting list for orthotopic liver transplant exceeded 7 months. However, full outcomes analysis are still forthcoming and will prove extremely important in the implementation of living donor liver transplantation in the future.

There is, as yet, no evidence that the choice of primary immunosuppression or withdrawal from steroids has any effect on survival after orthotopic liver transplant for hepatocellular carcinoma or recurrence of cancer.

Non-surgical therapy

Ablation

There are two main ablative methods at the time of writing – percutaneous ethanol injection and radiofrequency ablation.

Percutaneous ethanol injection is performed under CT or ultrasound guidance and involves 8 to 10 mL of alcohol injected per session. Injection begins at the distal end of the tumor and the needle is advanced proximally while the patient is under conscious sedation. Serious complications are rare and the most common complaints of the procedure are pain and a feeling of intoxication immediately after the injection. Percutaneous ethanol injection is therefore generally well tolerated. Almost all tumors smaller than 2 centimeters can be completely ablated in a single session while larger tumors may require several sessions over several weeks. The long-term outcomes are good: the survival rates of percutaneous ethanol injection versus resection are comparable at 1 and 4 years. The downside of percutaneous ethanol injection is that needle-track seeding has occasionally been reported and, thus, is not the preferred method of ablation if orthotopic liver transplant is a consideration.

Radiofrequency ablation is performed in a single session and is well tolerated. The procedure involves introducing a needle into the tumor under radiologic guidance. An alternating current is then generated in the needle resulting in a sharp increase of heat (up to 100 °C). This causes destruction of an area up to 5 centimeters in diameter. The risks include bleeding from the puncture site especially if the hepatocellular carcinoma is near the surface of the liver, fever, abdominal pain, and transient elevation of the serum transaminases. Needle-track seeding of hepatocellular carcinoma has been reported, but this is not a universally observed phenomenon.

Comparisons of percutaneous ethanol injection and radiofrequency ablation have shown that complete tumor necrosis is in the order of 90% with radiofrequency ablation versus 80% with ethanol injection. More sessions may be required with percutaneous ethanol injection while long-term survival rates have not yet been assessed with radiofrequency ablation. Ablation can be considered as a primary mode of therapy in patients who are not surgical candidates, and in surgical candidates while awaiting orthotopic liver transplantation, although the utility of this is not well established. At times, ablative therapy may be technically unfeasible, and a percutaneous approach and a laparotomy may be required to access the lesion. Other described ablative therapies include percutaneous acetic acid injection, cryosurgery, and microwave surgery. Undoubtedly, however, radiofrequency ablation is the procedure that is used most often.

Chemoembolization

Chemoembolization requires catheterization of the segmental hepatic artery supplying the tumor, and performance of an arteriogram. The arteriogram is then followed by the injection of chemotherapeutic agents intra-arterially and the subsequent occlusion of the hepatic artery by injection of material to obstruct flow. In this way, a high concentration of chemotherapy is delivered to the tumor with a marked increase in contact time between the drugs and tumor cells, and high rates of first-pass extraction. The drugs administered are concentrated in the liver and the tumor itself and, thus, systemic side effects are minimized. Drugs commonly used include doxorubicin, cisplatinum, and mitomycin C. These are mixed with a water-soluble contrast as well as lipiodol (iodized poppyseed oil) to form an emulsion. Finally, particulate embolization materials are injected at the end of the procedure to reduce arterial inflow and prevent chemotherapeutic agents from being washed out.

Extensive tumor necrosis can be achieved in more than 80% of patients, albeit with serious potential side effects that include liver failure, severe pain, and the formation of a liver abscess. Randomized controlled trials of chemoembolization versus standard supportive therapy for unresectable hepatocellular carcinoma have shown no enhanced survival in the chemoembolization group over a 4-year period. The contraindications of chemobolization include a diffuse tumor through the liver, the presence of liver failure, and portal vein thrombosis. This therapy is currently used most often as an adjuvant to other forms of treatment, when there are more than three lesions in the background of adequate hepatic function, or as a bridge to orthotopic liver transplant.

Chemotherapy

Chemotherapeutic agents are not generally used in patients with other potentially curative options and their role is largely palliative. There are a variety of chemotherapeutic agents tested against hepatocellular carcinoma. There are two approaches to chemotherapy of hepatocellular carcinoma: systemic or regional. A systemic approach is associated with objective response rates less than 25% and dosing may be limited by the backdrop of cirrhosis. A regional approach includes intra-arterial treatment, the results of which are similar to chemoembolization. Antiangiogenic agents hold considerable promise in the treatment of hepatocellular carcinoma because of the vascularity of the tumor.

Conclusion

There has been a steady increase in the incidence of hepatocellular carcinoma worldwide. From a global perspective, it has had a smaller impact in the US than elsewhere, although it is predicted that this will steady increase over the next 10 to 20 years. This will largely be a consequence of progressive liver disease secondary to hepatitis C virus infection. In areas where hepatitis B virus infection is the predominant predisposing cause for hepatocellular carcinoma, there is actually a decrease in the incidence particularly observed in the pediatric and adolescent population. This is undoubtedly because of public health measures of universal hepatitis B virus vaccination. Unless diagnosed in an asymptomatic state with rigid screening measures, prognosis is likely to be poor in patients who have symptomatic disease. Although the cost-effectiveness of screening for hepatocellular carcinoma is debated, it still appears prudent to periodically screen patients at risk so that the best outcomes can be achieved. Surgical options remain the preferred modes of treatment for hepatocellular carcinoma, although short- and intermediate-term survival has been comparable with both surgical and non-surgical therapies.

The ultimate form of therapy for hepatocellular carcinoma is orthotopic liver transplantation which removes both the tumor and the tumorogenic and cirrhotic liver. There has been an increasing enthusiasm for living donor liver transplantation because of the increasing demand for orthotopic liver transplant and the finite number of available organs.

Unfortunately, orthotopic liver transplantation and living donor liver transplantation are not readily available at most hospitals, especially outside the developed western world. Until the molecular and biochemical basis of the natural history of hepatocellular carcinoma is well known, prognostic indicators such as the CLIP system or the BCLC classification will fall short in helping to stratify patients for treatment. For now, orthotopic liver transplantation remains the preferred treatment regimen for primary hepatocellular carcinoma, but radical therapies such as percutaneous ethanol injection, radiofrequency ablation, and chemoembolization remain for those who fall into the necessary strata to receive such treatment. Further collaboration between oncologists, hepatologists, gastroenterologists, and interventional radiologists remains the best possible approach to the management of hepatocellular carcinoma.

Further reading

Befeler AS, Di Bisceglie AM. Hepatocellular carcinoma: diagnosis and treatment. *Gastroenterology* 2002; 122: 1609–1619.

Bruix J, Llovet JM. Prognostic prediction and treatment strategy in hepatocellular carcinoma. *Hepatology* 2002; 35: 519–524.

Bruix J, Sherman M, Llovet JM, *et al*. Clinical management of hepatocellular carcinoma: conclusions of the Barcelona–2000 EASL conference. *J Hepatol* 2001; 35: 421–430.

Collier J, Sherman M. Screening for hepatocellular carcinoma. *Hepatology* 1998; 27: 273–278.

Fujiyama S, Tanaka M, Maeda S, *et al*. Tumor markers in early diagnosis, follow-up and management of patients with hepatocellular carcinoma. *Oncology* 2002; 62 (suppl 1): 57–63.

Llovet JM, Brú C, Bruix J. Prognosis of hepatocellular carcinoma: the BCLC staging classification. *Semin Liver Dis* 1999; 19: 329–337.

The Cancer of the Liver Italian Program Investigators. A new prognostic system for hepatocellular carcinoma: a retrospective study of 435 patients. *Hepatology* 1998; 28: 751–755.

Trevisani F, D'Intino PE, Grazi GL, *et al*. Clinical and pathologic features of hepatocellular carcinoma in young and older Italian patients. *Cancer* 1996; 77: 2223–2232.

Chapter 11

Non-Viral Hepatic Infections

Kia Saeian

CHAPTER OUTLINE

Invasion of the liver by infectious agents is not surprising when it central role in receiving the portal blood flow is considered. In fact, it is probably the liver's intricate anatomy and elaborate immune system, which preclude a much higher incidence of infectious complications. From the time of Hippocrates (around 40 BC), liver abscesses have been recognized. This chapter covers pyogenic and amebic liver abscesses, as well as parasitic liver infections (Figure 11.1). In the US approximately 85% of liver abscesses are pyogenic, whereas in developing countries 80% to 90% of abscesses are amebic. Of course, ease of migration throughout the world makes it imperative for all physicians to be knowledgeable about all of these entities. Use of radiologic imaging has become an integral part of the diagnostic and therapeutic management of liver abscesses. Computed tomography scanning is the gold standard with an almost 100% sensitivity but ultrasound also provides good sensitivity along with better evaluation of internal structures and at a significantly lower cost. Nevertheless, other lesions may occasionally be confused with liver abscesses including cystic lesions, hypodense liver masses, hemangiomas, pseudoaneurysms of the hepatic or gastroduodenal arteries, and angiomyolipomas.

Pyogenic liver abscesses

In older series, hepatic abscesses accounted for approximately 0.12% of acute hospitalizations, for 8 to 16 cases per 100 000 hospital admissions, and had a prevalence of up to 0.41% in an autopsy series. With the introduction of antibiotic therapy, better diagnostic modalities, and improved therapeutic

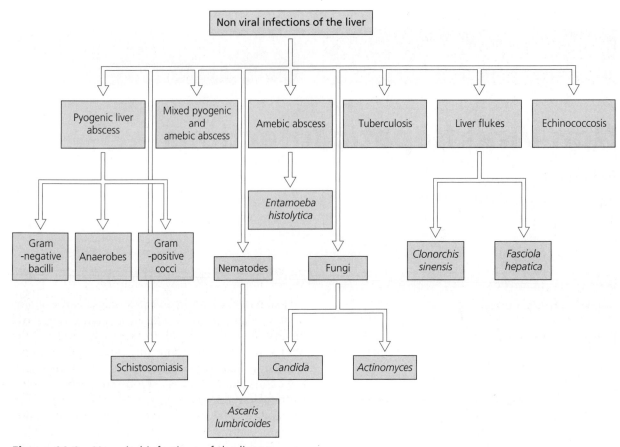

Figure 11.1 Non-viral infections of the liver.

interventions, the prognosis of pyogenic liver abscesses has dramatically improved. Not long ago, mortality rates as high as 40% were encountered, but this rate has diminished remarkably and is now in the range of 10% to 25%. Mortality is now often a reflection of the poor prognosis of the underlying cause rather than the abscess itself.

The etiologies of the abscesses have also undergone a remarkable shift. Previously, appendicitis and associated pyelophlebitis had been the most common cause of pyogenic liver abscesses, but better management of this entity and other abdominal infections has reduced the frequency of pyelophlebitis as a source. The proliferation of hepatobiliary interventions and the increasing age of the population have resulted in biliary sources including cholelithiasis, hepatobiliary surgery, and biliary obstruction (malignant or benign) as the most common causes of pyogenic liver abscesses (up to 42% in some series). A number of other causes have been identified (Box 11.1). Further, in a large number (approximately 15%) of abscesses, a distinct source remains unidentified (cryptogenic).

Pathogenesis and etiology

Bacteria may invade the liver and result in abscesses via direct hematogenous spread (either pyelophlebitis or arterial spread), trauma or direct extension (Figure 11.2). Complete formation of the abscess is a gradual process (Table 11.1). Because of the frequency of biliary involvement, if no other cause is readily discovered, evaluation of the biliary system is warranted. Intra-abdominal sources are most common and the presence of diverticular disease, appendicitis and a rare first presentation of colon adenocarcinoma should be sought. Multiple microabscesses can be seen in patients with sepsis but patients are not considered to have a pyogenic liver abscess unless the abscess is macroscopically visible (Figures 11.3, 11.4).

Diabetics appear to be more susceptible to the development of pyogenic liver abscesses, particularly infection with *Klebsiella pneumoniae*, and diabetes mellitus has been noted in up to 15% of adults with liver abscesses. Cirrhotics are not only more susceptible to developing pyogenic liver abscesses but when they do so, they have a higher 30-day fatality rate (38% in one series).

Box 11.1 Etiology of pyogenic liver abscesses

Biliary disease/obstruction
Caroli's disease
cholelithiasis
malignancy
parasitic obstruction (e.g. *Ascaris lumbricoides*)

Cryptogenic

Direct extension
cholecystitis
Meckel's diverticulum
perinephric abscess
subphrenic abscess
ventriculoperitoneal shunt

Pyelophlebitis
appendicitis
diverticulitis
inflammatory bowel disease
omphalitis
pancreatitis
postoperative infections
Yersinia infection (e.g. hemochromatosis)

Systemic bacteremia
endocarditis

Trauma

Other
foreign-body ingestion with perforation
iatrogenic – post-chemoembolization,
aspiration of amebic abscess
sickle cell disease

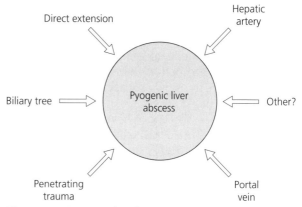

Figure 11.2 Portals of entry in the pathogenesis of pyogenic liver abscess.

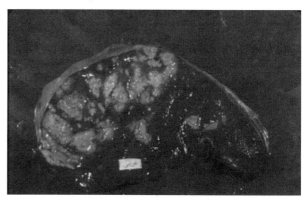

Figure 11.3 Resected specimen containing necrotic pyogenic liver abscess.

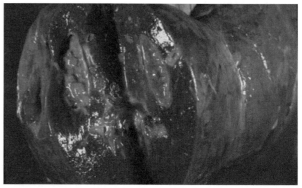

Figure 11.4 Autopsy specimen of pyogenic liver abscess.

A number of more atypical sources of pyogenic liver abscesses have been described. Perforation of the gallbladder with formation of a cholecystohepatic fistula as well as intrahepatic perforation of the gallbladder are rare events but they have been associated with abscess formation. Local factors such as

Table 11.1 Phases of abscess formation

Phase	Duration	Features
Acute phase	Days 1–10	Tissue necrosis with initiation of liquefaction.
Subacute phase	Days 10–15	Formation of abscess cavity with thin walls. Liquefaction and resorption of cellular material.
Chronic phase	Days > 15	Formation of thick fibrotic wall. Possible calcification.

chronic inflammation (e.g. cholelithiasis) and gall-bladder-wall ischemia (e.g. impaired vascular supply) along with predisposing factors such as immunosuppression, malignancy, and trauma, are likely contribute to perforation. The fundus of the gallbladder appears most susceptible because of its relatively poor blood supply.

Pyogenic liver abscesses have been noted not only in those with established Crohn's disease or ulcerative colitis, but also in a number of cases of previously undiagnosed Crohn's disease. Thus, those presenting with a pyogenic liver abscess and without a distinct cause also warrant evaluation for inflammatory bowel disease.

Hepatocellular carcinoma may present as a pyogenic liver abscess because of either tumor necrosis or biliary obstruction predisposing to bacterial infection. Cholangiocarcinoma presenting with a liver abscess has been noted with a particularly high in-hospital mortality rate in those with concomitant hepatolithiasis. The latter is more commonly encountered in the Far East in conjunction with liver-fluke infestation. Colon cancer may also initially present as a hepatic abscess and should be particularly suspected if the abscess cultures grow *Streptococcus bovis*. Pyogenic liver abscesses in the setting of any malignancy portend a particularly poor outcome.

A number of surgical procedures are associated with an increased incidence of liver abscess, these include pancreaticoduodenectomy or liver resection with biliary–enteric anastamosis, anastamosis with subsegmental bile ducts, and concomitant vascular reconstruction. *Streptococcus milleri* has been the causative organism in some of these cases.

An infrequent complication of ventriculoperitoneal shunt placement is pyogenic liver abscess formation presumably via direct trauma or extension from the shunt. Papillon–Lefevre syndrome is an autosomal-recessive disorder associated with palmoplantar keratoderma and severe periodontopathy resulting in loss of deciduous and permanent dentition. A higher incidence of pyogenic liver abscess has been observed in patients with this rare disorder and it is presumed that bacteremia resulting from periodontal disease predisposes to abscess formation.

An unusual presentation has been that of hepatic abscess caused by bowel perforation after ingestion of foreign bodies including fish bones, a sewing needle, a ballpoint pen, and a wooden tooth pick. Mentally ill individuals, from whom it may be difficult to elicit the antecedent history of ingestion, have been most commonly affected. Rarely, pyogenic liver abscess has been associated with a Meckel's diverticulum although it is unclear whether this was from contiguous or hematogenous spread.

Role of parasites

An interesting theory has been put forth which implicates certain parasites in providing either portals of entry or a foothold for bacterial infection of the liver resulting in pyogenic liver abscesses. Some have postulated that chronic helminthic infections (e.g. with *Toxocara* spp.) result in either granuloma formation in the liver, which subsequently enhances localization of bacteria, or induce immunomodulation and thus increase the risk for pyogenic liver abscess. Granuloma formation around the eggs or worms of *Schistosoma mansoni* has been implicated as a possible focus and substrate for pyogenic abscesses caused by *Staphylococcus aureus*. In Brazil, a higher prevalence of antibodies to visceral larva migrans have been noted in patients with pyogenic liver abscess, a much higher prevalence than that seen in the general population. Further study of this issue is warranted.

Microbiology

Overall, 50% to 70% of infective organisms are aerobic gram-negative rods. *Escherichia coli* is the most commonly isolated organism with *Klebsiella pneumonia*, *Streptococcus* spp., enterococci and anaerobes being the next most common organisms. Anaerobes are more difficult to culture and care must be taken when cultures are obtained to avoid under-diagnosis. When properly cultured, a high rate of anaerobic infection has been reported comprising up to 46% of isolated organisms in one series (range 15% to 46%).

The incidence of abscesses due to *Klebsiella pneumonia* appears to be on the rise and is particularly high in diabetic patients, even in the absence of a biliary or any other intra-abdominal source. *Streptococcus milleri* infection may present with a longer duration of illness and may often be dormant. If *S. milleri* bacteremia is encountered, up to a third of the cases will be associated with hepatic abscesses and thus appropriate investigations should be performed. A proteobacteria of the genus *Desulfovibrio* has also been implicated as an opportunistic pathogen resulting in pyogenic liver abscess.

Clinical presentation

Whereas fever is present in the majority of cases, the classic presentation of fever, jaundice, right upper quadrant tenderness and hepatomegaly is seen in only a minority. On examination, right upper quadrant tenderness, hepatomegaly, and splenomegaly are frequently, but not universally, encountered (Figures 11.3, 11.4). Jaundice is typically seen in those with underlying biliary disease. Leukocytosis with a left shift is noted along with anemia in approximately three quarters of patients. The alkaline phosphatase (elevated in approximately two thirds of patients) and bilirubin tend to predominate the hepatic biochemical test abnormalities. The presence of eosinophilia should raise the suspicion of parasitic or echinococcal infection. The prodrome appears to be longer in patients with pyelophlebitis as opposed those with systemic bacteremia.

Pyogenic liver abscesses are more commonly single than multiple, more frequent in males, occur more often in the right lobe although those in the left lobe are more commonly associated with intrahepatic stones and have the potential for rupture (Table 11.2). The radiologic findings of liver abscesses are delineated in Table 11.3. Air in the abscess may reflect gas-forming organisms or communication with the biliary tree, including cases of emphysematous cholecystitis. In one series, up to 15% of patients with liver abscesses had gas detectable by CT. Cases of patients presenting with spontaneous pneumoperitoneum due to the rupture of a gas-containing liver abscess have been reported.

Liver abscesses are encountered more frequently in older individuals with the highest incidence occurring in the sixth and seventh decades of life. In a study comparing the clinical presentation of abscesses in patients over 70 years of age to those 70 years of age or younger, those over 70 were more likely to be women, had less abdominal tenderness on examination, and fewer positive blood cultures. The presence of abdominal pain, nausea and vomiting, and temperature above 101°F, or hematologic or hepatic biochemical test abnormalities did not differ between the groups in this small study.

Treatment

Experience with ultrasound or CT-guided aspiration with catheter drainage indicates that this technique is the optimal treatment modality with surgery being reserved for those in whom operative intervention is warranted for other reasons. Broad antibiotic coverage including coverage of gram-negative bacilli, streptococci and anaerobes should be used adjunctively, but drainage by some means is the key to success. Drainage itself may be associated with complications (Box 11.2). The majority of patients achieve resolution with antibiotics and adequate drainage but approximately 5% (up to 30% in some series) may eventually require surgical intervention. Surgery is advocated as the initial therapy in some cases, not only for the treatment of the underlying source of the abscess but also where

Table 11.2 Characteristics of single versus multiple liver abscesses

Single	Multiple
Higher incidence of abdominal pain.	Higher hepatic biochemical tests. Higher creatinine.
Higher hemoglobin.	Higher white blood cell count.
Usually larger than 5 cm.	Usually smaller than 5 cm.
More common in the right side.	
More *Klebsiella pneumoniae*.	More *Escherichia coli*.
More *Staphylococcus aureus*.	More enterococci and *Streptococcus viridans*.
Streptococci.	
More cryptogenic?	Higher treatment failure.
Higher operative rate and mortality.	
More likely to be amebic.	More likely to be fungal.

Table 11.3 Radiologic findings in liver abscesses

Medium	Findings
Abdominal plain films[1]	Presence of right upper quadrant air–fluid levels (indicates a fistula or gas-producing organisms). Ileus (particularly seen with rupture and peritonitis).
Chest X-ray	Elevation of right hemidiaphragm. Right pleural effusion (sympathetic versus rupture/fistula). Atelectasis. Loss of pulmonary vessels beyond the diaphragm.
Ultrasound	Hypoechoic. Hyperechoic border reflecting fibrosis. More useful than CT in demonstrating internal structure. May miss early lesions.
CT scan	Hypodense (120–140 Hounsfield units after IV contrast). Cluster sign (smaller, less than 2-cm lesions surrounding a central large abscess). Rim enhancement in approximately 20% of cases. Highly sensitive but may miss early lesions.
MRI scan	Decreased intensity on T1 images. Increased intensity on T2 images.
Scintigraphy	Gadolinium-labeled leukocytes localize in the periphery of the abscess; particularly good for early lesions. Sulfur colloid particles labeled with ^{99m}technetium are typically taken up by Kuppfer cells but absence of cells in the abscess produces a defect. Iminodiacetic acid derivatives: absence of hepatocytes and biliary excretion also produces a defect.

[1] Chilaiditi Syndrome, in which part of the large intestine (or occasionally small intestine) is trapped between the liver and the diaphragm, can be confused with this.
[1] Note: typically because of their smaller size, fungal abscesses less commonly produce these findings.

there is severe disease and systemic signs of sepsis, abscess rupture, and where prompt and adequate drainage may preclude higher morbidity and mortality.

Although, generally, percutaneous catheter drainage is the preferred approach over needle aspiration alone, the latter can be successfully performed in the majority of patients, with approximately half the patients requiring only one session and approximately three quarters requiring two or fewer sessions. In a series from Japan, ultrasound-guided percutaneous needle aspiration without catheter placement has been shown to be effective with an overall cure rate of 98.3% (113 of 115 cases) although approximately half of the

patients required more than one puncture. Recurrence and significant complications were not encountered.

There have been attempts to treat liver abscesses of biliary origin endoscopically with endoscopic biliary sphincterotomy and local antibiotic lavage via an endoscopically placed nasobiliary catheter. Excellent rates of success with only 5% requiring percutaneous drainage have been reported. Because of the small amount of experience, however, further validation is required before this modality can be widely advocated.

The role of ERCP in the evaluation of patients with cryptogenic pyogenic liver abscesses is well established. This is illustrated by the fact that approximately half of the patients are found to have a biliary abnormality ranging from biliary obstruction (stones or stricture), ductal dilatation alone, choledochoduodenal fistula, to direct communication between the abscess and the biliary tree.

Factors associated with the failure of non-operative management include renal impairment, multiloculated abscesses, unresolving jaundice, rupture on presentation, and biliary communication. Thus, in addition to advocating operative management as the initial therapy for correcting underlying pathology (e.g. cholecystitis), operative intervention may

Box 11.2 Complications of percutaneous drainage

Fistula formation
Hemorrhage
Infection (superimposed)
Laceration of vessels or small bowel
Potential anaphylactic reaction from drainage of echinococcal cysts

be required for abscesses inadequately drained by percutaneous means, particularly when they are multiloculated.

Complications

The most ominous complications are related to rupture of the abscess. Lesions located peripherally or in the left lobe are more susceptible to rupture. Pericardial abscess has also been seen with pyogenic liver abscesses and carries a high mortality, which can be reduced to less than 20% by early surgical and medical intervention. Other potential complication of pyogenic liver abscesses include the occurrence of emboli, including septic pulmonary emboli, uncomplicated pleural effusions (due to local pleural reaction), and fistulas, including gastric fistulas. Overall, more of these complications are seen with amebic than with pyogenic liver abscesses. One exception is endophthalmitis, which has been reported in up to 8% of those with *Klebsiella pneumonia* bacteremia complicating liver abscesses. It has also been noted with the fastidious anaerobe *Eikenella corrodens*. The infection is rapidly progressive and frequently results in visual loss. In the setting of *Klebsiella pneumonia*-associated abscess, and particularly if any visual deterioration occurs, urgent ophthalmologic evaluation is warranted and if necessary intravitreal antibiotics should be instituted in order to achieve adequate intraocular antibiotic concentrations.

Prognosis

Hyperbilirubinemia, presence of malignancy, and an elevated activated partial thromboplastin time are commonly associated with a higher rate of mortality. Other poor factors include rupture on presentation, female gender, older age, anemia, leukocytosis, concomitant pleural effusion at presentation, high serum urea nitrogen and creatinine, an elevated prothrombin time, emergency laparotomy, high APACHE II (Acute Physiological And Chronic Health Evaluation II) score, management without aspiration or catheter drainage, and hyperglycemia. A complicated clinical course is predicted by the presence of hemodynamic compromise or shock, a low hemoglobin level, elevated prothrombin time, multiple abscesses, and polymicrobial infection.

Although infrequent (range 5.4% to 15%), ruptured pyogenic liver abscesses present in a similar fashion to unruptured abscess, except for more diffuse abdominal pain and a higher likelihood of septic shock. Another group with a high mortality are those presenting with rupture (up to 43.5%) even in the setting of operative intervention (27.8%). Operative intervention is the modality of choice in these patients.

Previously high mortality rates were reported, but more recently significantly decreased mortality rates (0.5% to 12.5%) have been reported. The one group of patients who still have a high mortality rate are those with underlying malignancy. The severity of their underlying disease is often the responsible factor. For instance, in one series 84% (16 of 19) of those with cholangiocarcinoma presenting with pyogenic liver abscess were dead within 6 months of diagnosis.

Amebic liver abscesses

Although infection with *Entamoeba* spp. is very common, it is now known that only *Entamoeba histolytica* and not *Entamoeba dispar* causes invasive disease. Interestingly, colonization with *E. dispar* is up to 10 times as common as that with *E. histolytica*, and the two are identical on microscopic evaluation. The lack of tissue invasiveness of *E. dispar* precludes an immunologic reaction, and therefore does not induce antibody formation, and there is no known disease as a result of *E. dispar* infection. Thus, the presence of antibodies indicates invasive *E. histolytica* infection. Using serologic positivity, approximately 10% of the world's population is infected with *E. histolytica*, particularly in areas with poor sanitation. Up to 40 000 people a year die from its complications including colitis and amebic liver abscesses. In developed countries such as the US, the prevalence is significantly lower (approximately 4%) outside high-risk groups such as homosexual men. Although amebic liver abscess is the most common extraintestinal form of invasive amebiasis, it only occurs in about 4% of patients with invasive amebiasis.

Pathogenesis

A commensal in the human colon, *E. histolytica* exists in one of two forms: the trophozoite and the cyst. The trophozoite is the vegetative form and is the pathogenic entity, the cyst or ova is the form in which the parasite is transferred from one host to the next.

Most infected individuals are not affected by the disease, but simply transmit the cyst. Recent studies suggest that there may be pathogenic isolates of *E. histolytica* which can be differentiated, based on their surface antigens. The typical latency period of infection in humans is 3 to 4 weeks with a broad range from 2 days to 4 months. Invasion of the intestinal mucosa by the trophozoite form, subsequent migration via the portal vein, and eventual invasion of the liver parenchyma leads to an inflammatory reaction around the ameba. This inflammatory reaction, as opposed to direct toxicity, appears to be responsible for hepatic necrosis. The classic anchovy-paste appearance of the material aspirated from amebic abscesses is the result of liquefaction of hepatocytes and surrounding tissue.

Clinical presentation

Initial manifestations are usually right upper quadrant abdominal pain, tender hepatomegaly, leukocytosis, and a mildly elevated alkaline phosphatase. When fever is present, it is abrupt in onset. Children are more commonly affected, as are men in their second and third decades of life. In the west, homosexual men are clearly at higher risk for amebic colitis, but it is unclear whether they are at any increased risk for amebic liver abscesses. Interestingly, only about 50% of those with amebic liver abscess report a history of diarrhea and only about 50% will still have trophozoites in their stool. The right lobe is preferentially involved (in approximately 75% of cases) and single lesions are more common than multiple ones.

Diagnosis

The combination of the proper clinical scenario, epidemiologic factors, and radiologic appearance of the lesion make the diagnosis likely. A positive serology, particularly in a non-endemic area, supports the diagnosis of amebic liver abscess. There are no radiologic findings that definitively distinguish amebic from pyogenic liver abscesses.

The sensitivity of serology is reported to range from 90% to 100% with lower sensitivities reported in luminal disease, particularly in endemic areas. A caveat is that the antibody may be negative early in

the course of infection, particularly with luminal disease, and that if there is a high index of suspicion, repeat serologic testing 5 to 7 days later may be warranted. If stool examination is carried out, the sample must be examined fresh and a careful search for trophozoites should be carried out. The yield is best when carried out prior to the administration of antidiarrheals, antacids, or antimicrobials and barium sulfate, all of which may diminish the yield. Positive serology, by ELISA or immune hemaglutination, indicates that there has been tissue invasion at some point in time but does not distinguish acute from chronic disease. However, a positive result in a symptomatic patient from a non-endemic area is specific and is usually sufficient evidence. Although titers are typically higher in acute infections, the level does not correlate with disease activity or preclude recurrent disease.

In patients with intestinal amebiasis, organisms are not shed in a uniform pattern and thus single stool specimens may miss evidence of intestinal carriage and have only a 33% sensitivity. By increasing the number of stool specimens to three, the sensitivity is increased up to 85% to 95% for luminal disease. Furthermore, on routine microscopy, *E. histolytica* and *E. dispar* cannot be distinguished from one another. Definitive culture and DNA-based testing which distinguish these organisms have been developed but remain research tools only. Of course, because *E. dispar* remains non-invasive, seroconversion does not occur with it and amebic serology is only positive with *E. histolytica* infection. In any case, because of the high miss rate in patients with amebic liver abscess, stool studies are not typically rewarding.

The suspicion of an amebic liver abscess warrants an imaging study with the available radiologic modalities. Because of its high sensitivity and low cost, abdominal ultrasound is typically the first investigation. There are no specific radiologic features for amebic liver abscess and the diagnosis is made on the basis of a constellation of clinical features, epidemiology, serology, and radiologic presence of an abnormality indicative of an abscess.

Treatment

The introduction of emetine in 1912 provided the first effective form of medical therapy for amebiasis and the therapy of this disease was further improved with the introduction of metronidazole in 1966. Currently, over 95% of cases respond to a 10-day course of metronidazole therapy at dose of 750 mg three times a day. For those intolerant of metronidazole, dehydroemetine (1.0 to 1.5 mg kg^{-1} day^{-1} IM for 5 days) is an option. In the US, this medication is only available through the Centers for Disease Control. Aspiration is typically not required except in cases of failure of medical treatment, suspected pyogenic or mixed abscess, imminent rupture, or large left lobe or complicated abscesses. If aspirated, the classic anchovy-paste material is derived. Of note, it is rare to recover *E. histolytica* from the aspirated material.

It must be kept in mind that despite successful, ongoing therapy, the abscess cavity may actually enlarge for the first 3 to 5 days after initiation of treatment. When treated appropriately, mortality rates of less than 1% have been reported. Surgical drainage is typically only necessary if complications have taken place.

Currently it is also recommended to give a course of additional specific therapy with either iodoquinol (650 mg three times a day for 20 days) or paromomycin (10 mg/kg three times a day for 7 days) to eradicate concurrent luminal amebiasis. Some evidence indicates that administration of metronidazole alone may be sufficient for luminal eradication.

Complications

Peripheral location or occurrence in the left lobe predispose to rupture. Some of the complications are associated with rupture of the abscess into the abdominal cavity, thoracic cavity, extension to the skin, or rarely into the pericardial cavity. Rupture of amebic abscesses with communication with the bronchial tree results in a cough producing thick bilious sputum with a metallic taste. These fistulas typically resolve on their own with appropriate antibiotic therapy. Prior to the availability of antibiotic therapy, these fistulas actually afforded a route for drainage and were associated with a better prognosis. Uncomplicated pleural effusions resulting from a local pleural reaction have also been noted. Pleuropulmonary involvement is the most common complication seen in up to 20% to 30% of amebic liver abscesses. Empyemas clearly require drainage.

Rupture into the pericardial cavity has the greatest mortality and should particularly be suspected if the chest X-ray reveals elevation of the hemidiaphragm along with a pleural effusion and enlargement of the cardiac silhouette. Left lobe or centrally located abscesses are more commonly implicated and a mortality rate of up to 60% has been reported. Further imaging with CT or ultrasound can confirm continuity of the abscess with the pericardial sac and possibly even visualize the fistulous tract. Aggressive supportive care, prompt initiation of metronidazole, and surgical drainage should be undertaken. If anchovy-paste fluid is found in the pericardium, pericardiectomy is recommended with placement of a pericardial drain for at least 72 hours. Some clinicians have attempted therapy by solely draining the hepatic abscess but this appears to be a risky proposition. Sympathetic effusions can be managed conservatively.

Cerebral involvement is rarely encountered clinically and portends a poor prognosis. It has been seen in up to 2.5% of autopsy series. Genitourinary involvement is also rare but responds well to treatment.

Parasitic infections

In areas where parasitic infestation is endemic, involvement of the intra- and extrahepatic biliary tree by parasites with resultant biliary obstruction and concomitant complications is a cause of significant morbidity. The most commonly encountered parasites include hydatid disease and *Ascaris lumbricoides*, followed by *Clonorchis sinensis*, and less frequently *Fasciola hepatica* and *Opisthorcic felineus*. Conventional abdominal imaging modalities may be insufficient in making the correct diagnosis and cholangiography, most often via ERCP, may provide the means of visualization and has the potential of therapy. The role of the nascent technology of magnetic resonance cholangiopancreatography in this setting remains to be evaluated. Schistosomal and malarial infection are quite common in endemic areas. It is worth noting that in endemic areas schistosomal infection is a frequent cause of presinusoidal portal hypertension.

Cystic liver disease

A wide variety of entities result in cystic liver disease (Figure 11.5). A true cyst is defined by the presence of an epithelial lining whereas false cysts have no such lining. Although not common, pyogenic and amebic infection of the cysts in polycystic liver disease does occur.

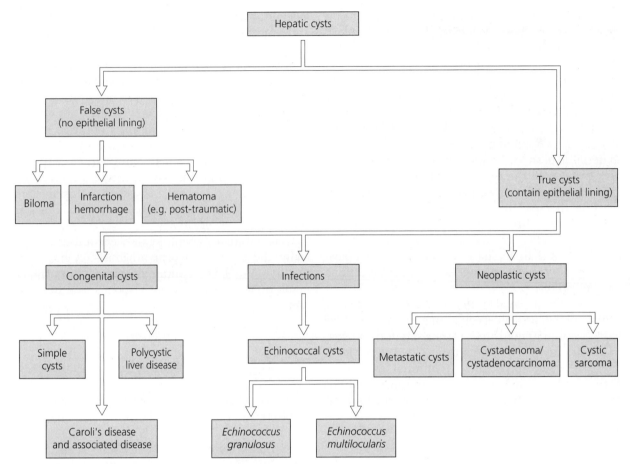

Figure 11.5 Differential diagnosis of hepatic cysts.

Hydatid cysts (echinococcal infections)

Endemic in the Middle East, Mediterranean region, and South America, hydatid disease is a term used to describe infestation of humans by the canine tapeworms *Echinococcus granulosus* or *Echinococcus multilocularis*. It commonly involves the liver (up to three quarters of cases) with formation of cysts (Figures 11.6, 11.7) and is often asymptomatic. Rarely, a third tapeworm, *Echinococcus vogeli*, causes disease predominantly in Central and South America. The tapeworm multiplies as a larval scolex within the cysts formed in solid organs of the infected host.

When symptoms do occur, they may arise from mechanical effects resulting in right upper quadrant or epigastric pain, biliary obstruction, or toxic and potentially anaphylactic reactions due to the parasite itself. The majority (more than 95%) of hydatid cysts are caused by *E. granulosus*, which is significantly less virulent than *E. multilocularis*. The latter organism is more invasive, results in more diffuse and less well-delineated cysts, and causes the highly lethal entity of alveolar echinococcosis.

On examination, hepatomegaly and/or a palpable abdominal mass may be found. Communication with the biliary tract is seen in up to 25% of cases.

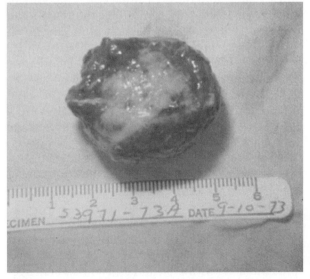

Figure 11.6 An intact, resected hydatid cyst due to *Echinococcus granulosus* infection.

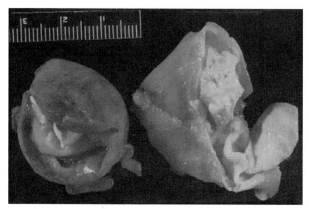

Figure 11.7 Large cysts demonstrating the contents of individual hydatid cysts due to *Echinococcus granulosus* infection.

On imaging with CT scan, calcification of the cyst wall and the presence of daughter cysts may be observed. In the presence of the typical radiologic appearance, serology (either ELISA or indirect hernagglutination) can confirm the presence of echinococcal disease in over 90% of cases. Although eosinophilia is typically present, stool studies are not useful. Complications include rupture into surrounding structures, secondary infection of the cysts, and cholangitis due to infection of the biliary tree.

Traditionally, concerns about spillage of viable scolices and contamination have made careful surgical resection the therapeutic option of choice. Adjunctive medical therapy with albendazole or mebendazole may decrease the risk of spillage and simplify resection, particularly in alveolar echinococcosis. By itself, medical therapy is effective in less than 30% of cases. During the operation, care must be taken to remove the entire cyst plus lining and avoid spillage of the fluid or daughter cysts. Liver resection may or may not be required. Surgeons advocate perioperative instillation of agents such as hypertonic saline into the cysts in order to kill the scolices and avoid spillage of material that may cause anaphylaxis. This practice has been questioned, however, since it may result in secondary sclerosing cholangitis, when there might be communication of the cyst with the biliary tree. Recently, percutaneous aspiration with the introduction of albendazole and subsequent re-aspiration has been shown to be as effective as surgery with a negligible risk of anaphylaxis. Further study of this technique appears warranted. Because of the potential recurrence of cysts, serology may be used to monitor patients.

Ascaris lumbricoides

Poor sanitation, a warm climate, and wet soil all promote the development of *Ascaris lumbricoides*. This parasite can frequently cause abdominal pain. While it predominates in the jejunum, it may also migrate proximally and invade the biliary tree with individuals who have had compromise of the sphincter of Oddi being more susceptible. Biliary colic may result because of obstruction (as can pancreatitis) but also reported are hepatic abscesses, ascending cholangitis, and acute cholecystitis. The remnants of the dead organisms within the bile ducts may serve as a nidus for pigment-stone formation, a process which may be accelerated by the high glucuronidase activity of *A. lumbricoides* resulting in deconjugation of bilirubin. In those with biliary colic, and hailing from an area endemic for *A. lumbricoides*, stool studies looking for its ova should be performed and treated appropriately. Imaging with ultrasound or cholangiography may demonstrate the worm itself and ERCP also provides a therapeutic option with extraction of the worm or of associated stones.

Clonorchis sinensis

This flat, leaf-shaped, gray liver fluke is endemic in the Far East, and eating raw freshwater fish predisposes individuals to infection. These flukes may be up to 1.5 cm long and 4.0 mm wide. Chronic infestation (up to 20 years) of the intrahepatic bile ducts is the rule with resultant chronic inflammation. This evolves into adenomatous or papillary hyperplasia, fibrosis, and also likely plays a role in the association of this entity with cholangiocarcinoma arising in any portion of the biliary tree.

Either the flukes themselves, the inflammatory reaction, or the accompanying intrahepatic biliary ductal stones may result in biliary obstruction. Complications may range from biliary colic, jaundice, recurrent ascending cholangitis, and abscess formation, or, as already mentioned, cholangiocarcinoma. Imaging studies show evidence of dilation of the bile ducts and discrete filling defects, which may reflect the flukes or biliary stones. Pancreatic involvement has also been reported. On cholangiography, it may be difficult to distinguish this entity from primary sclerosing cholangitis, cholangiocarcinoma, Caroli's disease, *Fasciola hepatica* infestation, or choledocholithiasis.

Treatment with chloroquine diphosphate at a dose of 250 mg three times a day for a 6-week course is highly successful. Praziquantel (25 mg/kg three times a day also for 6 weeks) provides an alternative regimen.

Fasciola hepatica

This is a large fluke measuring up to 3.0 cm long and 1.5 cm wide. Rare in the US and Europe, *F. hepatica* is particularly frequent in the Nile delta, northern Iran and the Andean region of South America. It is a zoonotic disease in which humans are incidental hosts typically infected by ingestion of uncooked aquatic plants including watercress. The organisms, in the form of metacercariae, burrow through the intestinal wall and take up residence in the peritoneal cavity from where they can invade the liver and biliary tree by perforating the capsule.

The clinical presentation may take on two stages. In the initial stage, the fluke is in the process of invading the liver by perforating the capsule and migrating through the liver parenchyma. In this stage, patients exhibit fever, pain, hepatomegaly, hypergammaglobulinemia, and eosinophilia. In the biliary stage of the disease, the adult worms reside in the bile duct and, either by themselves or because of an inflammatory reaction similar to *Clonorchis sinesis*, cause fibrosis, inflammatory and adenomatous change, and biliary obstruction. The symptoms include biliary colic and jaundice and may be associated with cholangitis. Involvement of the gallbladder has also been noted. The diagnosis is made by recovery of oval, large, yellowish-brown ova from the feces and in bile from duodenal aspiration. An ELISA test is available and can help confirm the diagnosis. Treatment with prior agents had been less than optimal until the use of single-dose of triclabendazole (at 10 to 20 mg/kg body weight) which has been shown to be very effective. Occurrence of biliary colic approximately 3 to 7 days after initiation of therapy typically reflects expulsion of dead or damaged parasites.

Miscellaneous infections

Tuberculosis

Hepatic involvement has been reported in approximately 10% to 50% of cases of pulmonary tuberculosis and is most often noted in individuals with miliary tuberculosis. The latter entity typically results in diffuse hepatic involvement with characteristic caseating granulomas ranging from 0.6 to 2.0 mm in size. Focal hepatic involvement (with a lesion larger than 2.0 mm) is rare but may result in abscess formation in about 0.3% of those with elevated liver enzymes and miliary tuberculosis. Abscess formation appears to be more common in the immunosuppressed and in particularly those with AIDS. Interestingly, immunocompromised hosts often exhibit more necrotic and less well-formed granulomas. Biliary obstruction with a picture suggestive of sclerosing cholangitis, pseudotumors, pyelophlebitis, and abdominal lymphadenopathy has also been noted. The diagnosis of hepatic infection is particularly problematic in the HIV population because they often present with an atypical picture and/or without typical features of tuberculosis.

In those who remain refractory to conventional therapies for pyogenic liver abscesses, in addition to amebic etiology, tuberculosis as well as malignancy, actinomyces, and syphilitic gummas should be considered. Diagnosis of tuberculosis is made by demonstration of acid-fast bacilli on examination of the smear, culture of aspirated material, or wall of the abscess cavity. There is often a time delay in appropriate diagnosis in part due to the non-specific nature of presenting symptoms and failure to consider tuberculosis in the initial differential diagnosis. Clinical clues that raise the possibility of tuberculosis include the typical risk factors (alcoholism, immunosuppression, persons from endemic areas) as well as a relatively mild leukocytosis and anemia, malnutrition, and a disproportionately elevated alkaline phosphatase over bilirubin level. The clinical picture of tuberculous hepatic abscess in 23 patients was characterized in one study. Abdominal pain (87%), fever (70%), weight loss (55%), and anorexia (52%) were the most common symptoms. When there is a known extrahepatic focus of tuberculosis, up to 63% of liver biopsies reveal abnormal histology. Liver involvement in the absence of overt splenic or lung involvement is rare but has been reported.

Besides direct infection, long-standing tuberculosis may result in amyloidosis with hepatic involvement, fatty liver secondary to weight loss, or drug-induced hepatitis particularly due to isoniazid. Other complications in the liver have included a case of hepatic artery mycotic aneurysm of tubercular etiology in a 13-year-old boy with epigastric pain and a hepatic bruit who subsequently developed hematemesis and succumbed to massive bleeding.

Treatment of hepatic tuberculosis should include triple anti-mycobacterial therapy with isoniazid and rifampin for 6 months and pyrazinamide for 2 months. If an abscess is present, drainage with catheter placement is more effective than simple aspiration.

Fungal infections

Fungal spread is usually via an arterial route and is more common in immunocompromised individuals, particularly those undergoing chemotherapy for hematologic malignancies. Multiple microabscesses, most often due to candidiasis, particularly with concomitant splenic abscesses should raise suspicion of a fungal etiology. Rarely, aspergillosis presents as a liver mass with a low attenuation lesion with rim enhancement on CT scan. Other rarely encountered fungal infections include cryptococcosis, histoplasmosis, and mucormycosis.

Hepatic actinomycosis is rare but has been reported in 36 English-language reports, and liver involvement has been reported in approximately 5% of all patients with actinomycosis and in 15% of patients with abdominal actinomycosis. Diagnosis is established via anaerobic culture of *Actonimyces* spp. or identification of sulfur granules, which reflect microcolonies of the organism. Standard treatment is appropriate drainage accompanied by a prolonged course of initially high-dose intravenous and subsequently oral penicillin G.

Further reading

Bernhard JS, Bhatia G, Knauer CM. Gastrointestinal tuberculosis: an eighteen-patient experience and review. *J Clin Gastroenterol* 2000; 30(4): 397–402.

Bhargava DK. Endoscopy and biliary parasites. *Gastrointest Endosc Clin N Am* 1996; 6(1): 139–152.

Chu KM, Fan ST, Lai EC, Lo CM, Wong J. Pyogenic liver abscess. An audit of experience over the past decade. *Arch Surg* 1996; 131(2): 148–152.

Corredoira J, Casariego E, Moreno C, *et al*. Prospective study of *Streptococcus milleri* hepatic abscess. *Eur J Clin Microbiol Infect Dis* 1998; 17(8): 556–560.

Dull JS, Topa L, Balgha V, Pap A. Non-surgical treatment of biliary liver abscesses: efficacy of endoscopic drainage and local antibiotic lavage with nasobiliary catheter. *Gastrointest Endosc* 2000; 51(1): 55–59.

Fujihara T. Nagai T, Kkubo T, Seki S, Satake K. Amebic liver abscess. *J Gastroenterol* 1996; 31(5): 659–663.

Hashimoto L, Hermann R, Grundfest-Broniatowski S. Pyogenic hepatic abscess: results of current management. *Am Surg* 1995; 61(5): 407–411.

Johannsen EC, Sifri CD, Madoff LC. Pyogenic liver abscesses. *Infect Dis Clin N Am* 2000; 14(3): 547–563, vii.

Molle I, Thulstrup AM, Vilstrup H, Sorensen HT. Increased risk and case fatality rate of pyogenic liver abscess in patients with liver cirrhosis: a nationwide study in Denmark. *Gut* 2001; 48(2): 260–263.

Perkins M, Lovell J, Gruenewald S. Life-threatening pica: liver abscess from perforating foreign body. *Australas Radiol* 1999; 43(3): 349–352.

Rayes AA, Teixeira D, Serufo JC, *et al*. Human toxocariasis and pyogenic liver abscess: a possible association. *Am J Gastroenterol* 2001; 96(2): 563–566.

Rintoul R, O'Riordan MG, Laurenson IF, *et al*. Changing management of pyogenic liver abscess. *Br J Surg* 1996; 83(9): 1215–1218.

Sugano S, Matuda T, Suzuki T, *et al*. Hepatic actinomycosis: case report and review of the literature in Japan. *J Gastroenterol* 1997; 32(5): 672–676.

Teichmann D, Grobusch MP, Gobels K, *et al*. Acute fascioliasis with multiple liver abscesses. *Scand J Infect Dis* 2000; 32(5): 558–560.

Yeh TS, Jan YY, Jeng LB, *et al*. Pyogenic liver abscesses in patients with malignant disease: a report of 52 cases treated at a single institution. *Arch Surg* 1998; 133(3): 242–245.

Chapter 12

Liver Transplantation

Kim M. Olthoff, Peter L. Abt and Abraham Shaked

CHAPTER OUTLINE

Introduction

Since the first human liver transplant was carried out by Thomas Starzl in 1963 liver transplantation has evolved as an effective therapy for acute and chronic liver failure. The introduction of cyclosporine in the 1980s and the refinement in operative techniques, as well as increasing experience in donor and recipient selection, have increased the success of this procedure so that it is the gold standard for the treatment of patients with end-stage liver disease. As a testament to this success, current 1- and 3-year patient survival rates are 82% and 76% respectively, according to United Network of Organ Sharing data.

Indications for liver transplant

The indications for liver transplant are numerous, however patients with cirrhosis who develop signs and symptoms of end-stage liver failure are most often evaluated for transplantation (Table 12.1). Complications of end-stage liver disease include portal hypertension which is manifested by variceal hemorrhage, hypersplenism, and ascites. Inadequate liver cell mass is reflected by poor synthetic function with associated coagulopathy, encephalopathy, and malnutrition. A smaller number of patients require transplantation for fulminant liver failure, development of malignancy within a cirrhotic liver, and inborn errors of metabolism. A discussion of some of the more common indications for transplantation is presented.

Hepatitis C

Hepatitis C virus is an RNA virus of the flavivirus family which can lead to chronic inflammation of the liver in approximately 85% of infected individuals. As many as 20% of these patients, over the next 20 years, will progress to cirrhosis. Despite the fact that the number of new infections has decreased dramatically, approximately four million Americans are infected with HCV, and cirrhosis secondary to HCV or to a combination of HCV and alcohol has become the leading indication for hepatic transplant in adults in the US. Hepatocellular carcinoma may develop in between 1% and 4% of patients with cirrhosis every year. Post-transplant, virtually all donor livers are re-infected with HCV. While single-center studies indicate that survival is comparable to survival following liver transplantation for other indications, data from the United Network of Organ Sharing registry indicate that recurrent HCV shortens patient and graft survival.

Alcoholic liver disease

Cirrhosis secondary to alcohol ingestion is the second most common indication for liver transplantation in adults. Liver injury results from the toxic effects of ethanol on the hepatocytes and the intensity of the inflammatory process is directly related to the amount consumed. The co-existence of HCV can accelerate the process and development of cirrhosis. Potential recipients are carefully screened to assess the status of their abuse and dependence on alcohol prior to transplant. Many centers and insurance companies require 6 months of abstinence, but there is no strong evidence that this period of sobriety correlates with recidivism or outcome. This length of time may be important for patients with acute alcoholic injury in a cirrhotic liver, and allow for recovery of some residual liver function, thereby eliminating the need for transplantation in compensated cirrhotics. In general, with careful selection, recidivism is generally low and outcomes are equivalent to other disease processes.

Hepatitis B

Hepatitis B virus (HBV) belongs to a family of DNA viruses called *Hepadnavirus*. Chronic HBV infection affects approximately 1.25 million people in the US. Patients progressing to cirrhosis are also at high risk for the development of hepatocellular carcinoma. Early experience with transplantation for HBV infection was dismal, as all grafts became re-infected and patients developed a unique entity of fibrosing cholestatic hepatitis that led to high morbidity and mortality. With the introduction of high titer post-operative hepatitis immune globulin (HBIg) and long-term nucleoside analogues such as Epivir®, results have improved dramatically and are now equivalent to other indications.

Primary sclerosing cholangitis

The chronic inflammatory process of primary sclerosing cholangitis produces strictures of the intra-

Table 12.1 Indications for liver transplantation, OPTN (1994–1999)

Children	%
Non-cholestatic cirrhosis	9.2
Cholestatic liver disease/cirrhosis	4.0
Biliary atresia	42.7
Acute hepatic necrosis	13.0
Metabolic diseases	11.7
Malignant neoplasms	3.1
Other	16.3
Adults	**%**
Non-cholestatic cirrhosis	67.3
Cholestatic liver disease/cirrhosis	15.4
Acute hepatic necrosis	7.0
Metabolic diseases	3.5

and extra-hepatic biliary system with associated cholestasis, giving rise to signs and symptoms of chronic biliary tract disease such as jaundice and pruritus. Synthetic function of the liver is usually maintained until there is significant decompensation manifested by hyperbilirubinemia and malnutrition. There is a high association with inflammatory bowel disease, which occurs in approximately 70% of these individuals. There is an increased incidence of cholangiocarcinoma in primary sclerosing cholangitis patients and during the transplant evaluation, distinguishing strictures from cholangiocarcinoma can be difficult. Liver transplantation is highly successful in this group of patients and recurrence of the disease is rare. Interestingly, post-transplant immunosuppression does not affect the progression of inflammatory bowel disease.

Primary biliary cirrhosis and autoimmune hepatitis

Similar to primary sclerosing cholangitis, primary biliary cirrhosis is a chronic cholestatic disease characterized by an inflammatory process that destroys the intrahepatic bile ducts. It is a slowly progressive disease, eventually resulting in cirrhosis and hyperbilirubinemia. Hepatic transplantation represents the only effective long-term therapy. As with primary sclerosing cholangitis, the results of liver transplantation are excellent.

Autoimmune hepatitis is a chronic inflammatory disease, usually seen in women. Several antibodies have been associated with this process. The disease is often treated with steroids and other immunosuppressant therapies to control the inflammation and hopefully avoid transplantation. Transplantation is indicated for individuals who develop decompensated cirrhosis. Recurrent disease has been described in the allograft.

Hepatocellular carcinoma and other malignancies

Indications for transplantation among patients with primary and metastatic hepatic tumors have become refined in recent years as subsets that may benefit from transplantation have been identified. The rationale for transplantation in patients with hepatocellular carcinoma developing within a cirrhotic liver is a logical extension of surgical oncologic principles, with the potential for complete removal of the tumor as well as curing the underlying cirrhosis. Patients with tumor limited to the liver and with a single lesion less than 5 cm in size, or up to three lesions each less than 3 cm, are generally considered the best candidates for transplantation. Using these criteria, 5-year survival equivalent to non-malignant indications can be obtained and recurrence rates below 15% may be expected. In general, the outcome following transplantation in well-selected patients is better than that achieved with resection or other ablative techniques with regard to tumor recurrence and long-term survival. It has yet to be determined if the addition of pre- or postoperative adjuvant therapy is of any benefit in the prevention of tumor recurrence.

Transplantation for cholangiocarcinomas remains controversial. Early series demonstrated virtually 100% recurrence and poor outcome, the result being that many programs considered cholangiocarcinoma to be a contraindication to transplantation. More recent protocols with preoperative adjuvant chemoirradiation and aggressive staging with laparotomy or laparoscopy have resulted in improved results, but still much lower than with other indications for transplantation.

Neuroendocrine tumors with metastases limited to the liver are the only metastatic tumor for which transplantation is generally considered. This is generally considered in patients with carcinoid syndrome and can be an effective palliative procedure.

Budd–Chiari syndrome

Budd–Chiari syndrome describes obstruction of hepatic venous drainage by various causes. The end result is liver damage leading to fibrosis and portal hypertension. Hematological disorders associated with a hypercoagulable state are the most common causes. Tumors compressing the hepatic veins and membranous webs in the vena cava are additional causes of this syndrome. Early portosystemic shunting may provide the liver with an excellent outflow tract, and prevent the development of fibrosis and cirrhosis. Transplantation is indicated for the development of signs and symptoms compatible with end-stage liver disease.

Fulminant hepatic failure

Acute liver failure can result from drug toxicity (e.g. acetaminophen), viral hepatitis B or A, or other uncertain etiologies. The expression of fulminant hepatic failure is marked by the development of encephalopathy, coagulopathy, and hypoglycemia progressing to hepatic coma. Progression from a state of confusion to unresponsiveness is associated with an increased risk for irreversible brain injury. At this stage monitoring must include brain imaging using CT or MRI prior to considering liver transplant, and consideration of intracranial pressure monitoring. Unrecoverable injury is associated with persistent elevation of intracranial pressure leading to the development of severe brain edema and herniation. It is crucial to transplant these patients prior to this stage otherwise the patient may not achieve full recovery.

In most cases the diagnosis is a clinical one. Liver biopsy can have an increased risk because of severe coagulopathy, and should only be utilized to determine non-transplant treatment options for other etiologies for liver failure such as autoimmune hepatitis, Budd–Chiari syndrome, or tumor. In fulminant hepatic failure, liver biopsy has not been shown to accurately predict outcome because the injury may be heterogeneous, and the sample may not be representative of the state of the remaining liver. Areas of severe hepatocellular necrosis and collapse may be directly adjacent to areas of regenerating or viable cells. Careful assessment of clinical variables that reflect the extent of liver injury, such as the severity of hepatic encephalopathy, changes in prothrombin time and levels of Factor V, persistence of hypoglycemia, and increasing jaundice, may help to predict prognosis and possible recovery or need for transplantation. Correction of severe coagulopathy is best treated with fresh frozen plasma, although it may be difficult to achieve significant improvements. Plasmapheresis may be beneficial in the pediatric population where volume is an issue. If transplanted quickly, survival can be excellent, but prolonged stays in the intensive care unit or progressive cerebral edema can significantly affect outcome.

Of all patients who present with acute liver failure, approximately 40% recover spontaneously, 30% undergo transplantation, and 30% expire. One-year survival following transplantation for fulminant hepatic failure ranges between 60% and 70%, slightly lower than that observed with other etiologies.

Biliary atresia

Biliary atresia is the most common indication for hepatic transplantation in children. Biliary atresia is an obliterative cholangiopathy that may affect the intrahepatic and the extrahepatic biliary tree. It occurs in 1:10 000 neonates. The diagnosis is usually suggested in neonates who remain jaundiced for 6 weeks or more after birth and who have pale stools and dark urine. By then, the liver is enlarged and firm or hard, a reflection of the presence of underlying portal fibrosis. Kasai hepatic portoenterostomy for resecting the obliterated bile ducts and re-establishing biliary drainage to the intestine successfully increases survival rates at the early stage. However, progressive intrahepatic bile duct destruction by chronic inflammation, fibrosis, and cirrhosis is common. Failure of the Kasai surgical procedure is expressed by hyperbilirubinemia, ascites, portal hypertension, failure to thrive and poor growth, as well as recurrent cholangitis, and should be the indications for transplantation.

Inherited metabolic disorders

These disorders can be grouped into those with enzyme deficiencies that cause chronic liver problems and those that cause problems in organs other than the liver. Examples of the former include tyrosinemia, type 1 glycogen storage disease, Wilson's disease and alpha–1-antitrypsin deficiency. Liver transplantation treats the failing liver as well as the enzyme deficiency. Examples of the latter include oxalosis, amyloidosis, and hemophilia A and B. In this case liver transplantation corrects an enzyme deficiency. Metabolic disorders are the second most common indication for liver transplantation in children.

Exclusion criteria and contraindications

Contraindications for transplantation are an evolving process. There remain extremely few "absolute" exclusion criteria that automatically eliminate a recipient from consideration for transplantation. These have generally included extrahepatic malignancy, AIDS, active substance abuse, uncontrolled systemic infection, inability to comply with the immunosuppression regimen, and advanced cardiopulmonary disease. Even these require careful individual consideration prior to denying a dying patient an opportunity for evaluation. There are very few "relative" contraindications, such as positive HIV status or recent prior malignancy, and even these patients are considered appropriate for transplantation by certain programs if the patient meets specific criteria and the disease is well controlled. There are few, if any, technical reasons to withhold transplant evaluation. Obese patients tend to have an increased morbidity, but there are no definitive data to bar them from receiving a liver. Anatomic findings such as portal vein thrombosis or prior shunt surgery, make the operation technically complex, but are not contraindications to transplant.

Indications for referral, evaluation, and listing criteria

When a patient is being evaluated for liver transplantation there are three core questions that are asked.

1. What is the severity and prognosis of the patient's liver disease?
2. Are there confounding medical, surgical, or psychological factors which would reduce the expectation of a successful liver transplant?
3. What are the wishes of the patient in regard to liver transplantation?

The answers to these questions are best addressed in a multi-disciplinary process at a liver transplant center. It is the role of the primary care physician and the referring specialist to identify which patients may indeed qualify for liver transplantation, currently or in the future. The liver allocation scheme in the US has changed significantly in the past 5 years, in that it was previously designed to give priority to those patients who had the most accumulated time on the waiting list. Variations existed in deaths on the waiting list and waiting times for transplantation, suggesting regional/center differences for listing patients and differing policies on who was a candidate for transplantation. There was agreement between centers that any patient with fulminant hepatic failure, or any cirrhotic patient who had experienced an episode of decompensation, or was in Child's Class B, met minimal criteria for placement on the transplant waiting list. There was less consensus on the minimal criteria for chronic cholestatic disorders or special cases such as hepatocellular carcinoma, Budd–Chiari syndrome or polycystic liver disease.

Until recently, the listing criteria were based upon the Child–Turcotte–Pugh classification. A Child–Turcotte–Pugh score of 7, which reflected a 1-year survival rate of 90%, was selected as the minimum score. Patients were assigned to one out of four United Network of Organ Sharing statuses

based upon the Child–Turcotte–Pugh score and either the in-patient or out-patient status. Status 3 required a Child–Turcotte–Pugh score greater than 7, status 2B a Child–Turcotte–Pugh score greater than 10, status 2A a Child–Turcotte–Pugh score greater than 10 and admission to the intensive care unit with an expected survival of less than 7 days. Status 1 was reserved for those with fulminant failure, or post-transplant primary non-function or hepatic artery thrombosis. Consequently, liver allocation was based on patient status as well as accumulated waiting time on the list.

The Model for End-stage Liver Disease (MELD) arose from the desire to allocate organs to those candidates in most urgent need of transplantation and to minimize the impact of waiting time, as time on the list did not correlate with the risk of dying. It is a continuous disease severity score ranging from 6 to 40 calculated from bilirubin, international normalized ratio, and creatinine. It predicts the probability of death among patients with liver disease from a variety of etiologies and with varying severity. The MELD score offers advantages over the Child–Turcotte–Pugh score in predicting mortality as it uses variables that are readily available, standardized, reproducible, and objective. In several studies MELD has proven better at predicting the risk of death than the Child–Turcotte–Pugh score. The score is recalculated at varying times after listing based upon the previous score. Those patients with a high MELD score require frequent blood work for recalculation. There are also certain additional "exception" points given to patients with special circumstances, such as development of hepatocellular carcinoma or hepatopulmonary syndrome.

It is important to remember that patients on the waiting list require constant re-evaluation by the transplant team during the pre-transplant period in order to determine their continued appropriateness for transplantation, and to increase their MELD score if they deteriorate. This should also include screening for hepatocellular carcinoma with alpha-fetoprotein and imaging, as this can increase their score, and early transplantation with small tumors can improve survival.

Donor evaluation

Cadaveric donors

Most liver grafts are obtained from cadaveric donors who meet brain-death criteria. To determine if an individual is suitable for organ donation, a detailed evaluation is performed by the local organ procurement organization staff regarding donor demographics, medical and surgical history, hospital course, cause of death, hemodynamics, social history, laboratory data and serologies. This information is relayed to the transplant surgeon who decides whether the liver is appropriate for transplantation.

Management of the potential donor is extremely important in maximizing the quality of the organs that can be used. The effects of brain death can cause profound hypotension, acidosis, hypoxia, hypernatremia, and renal insufficiency, and poor donor management can cause a potential donor to be eliminated. It is critical to have an on-site coordinator experienced in donor management for minute-to-minute critical care decisions.

The success of liver transplantation has placed greater demands on a limited supply of organs. With these demands, transplant surgeons have sought to increase the donor pool by accepting organs that previously were thought to be associated with an increased risk of poor graft function or primary non-function, or transmission of donor-related disease. These "expanded criteria" donors traditionally have included older donors, those with fatty livers, positive serologies for HCV or HCB, history of central nervous system malignancy, and non-heart-beating donors. The concept of the "expanded criteria" donor, however, has changed with increasing experience and improved outcomes. Many organs from these donors are used safely and routinely at large experienced centers and are found to have excellent post-transplant hepatic function in the appropriate recipient.

Most transplant centers will use HCV-positive donors in recipients with decompensated chronic hepatitis C. Under these circumstances, there is no documented difference in patient and graft survival at 5 years in grafts infected with hepatitis C. However, a baseline liver biopsy at the time of recovery demonstrating severe active hepatitis and/or fibrosis is a contraindication to donation.

Other expanded-criteria donors are those that test positive for hepatitis B core antibody (anti-HBc). These donors have been found to have a significant transmission rate into naïve recipients regardless of the donor hepatitis B surface antibody (HBsAb) status. Data indicate that the risk of viral transmission may be lower for recipients who are immune from previous infection (HBsAb+/HBcAb+) compared to recipients who are immune from vaccination (HBsAb+/HBcAb–). It is not known whether the presence of antibody to hepatitis B surface antigen alone in the recipient may protect from infection, and if the recipient with anti-HBc alone can become re-infected. Although treatment with antivirals or hyperimmune globulin (HBIg) may prevent infection, there is always the risk of drug resistance and mutant infections. Therefore, these livers should only be used routinely in hepatitis B surface antigen-positive recipients, and selectively in others who have evidence of previous exposure or immunization. If they are to be used in patients with anti-HBc or anti-HBs, then HBV prophylaxis should be instituted with antivirals and/or HBIg, and the recipient should be informed of the possible risk.

Other ways of expanding the donor pool include surgical techniques that split the liver into two parts in both cadaveric and living donors. *In situ* splitting of the cadaveric liver has been established as a method of obtaining two partial liver grafts from a cadaveric donor. The procedure is performed during procurement, and involves dissection of the left lateral segment from the remaining liver. The left lateral segment is used in a child and the remaining tri-segment is used in an adult. The surgical procedure has been mastered by many adult and pediatric liver surgeons and has not been associated with adverse effects on either the donor or the procurement of other organs. The procedure has greatly benefited child recipients since it increases the number of grafts available for transplantation. The tissue mass of the reduced right tri-segment is capable of supporting a recipient of adult size without signs of liver failure. Interestingly, the refinement of this procedure has been associated with a decrease in the number of living donor, left-lateral segment transplants done in major transplant centers, whereas waiting time on the pediatric list has been minimized. Recently, the initiation of adult living donor liver transplantation that has resulted in successful transplantation of either a full-size left lobe or right lobe into an adult recipient, has prompted the interest in the development of a similar split-liver technique for cadaveric donors, allowing for a cadaveric liver to be split into right and left segments for transplantation into two adults. Very few donors are appropriate for this procedure, and these hemi-livers have increased biliary complications and a higher incidence of poor postoperative liver function, so recipient selection is extremely important.

Living donors

For the past two decades, living donors have been utilized to overcome the dramatic organ shortage that faces patients awaiting transplantation. The concept of utilizing a living donor liver segment for children awaiting hepatic transplantation was first entertained in the 1980s, and increased utilization of this technique decreased the mortality of small children on the waiting list. The procedure was shown to have excellent recipient results with a low risk for morbidity and mortality in the donor. The success of the living donor and *in situ* split liver experience led to the adaptation of this technique for adults. The first series of adult-to-adult living donor liver transplantations in the US was presented in 1998 and the enthusiasm for this procedure escalated, not only within the transplant community, but in patients and their families who either wanted to undergo this procedure or to offer themselves as donors.

The surgical expertise required to perform living donor liver transplantation in adults has evolved from advances in hepatobiliary and transplant surgery. Although some centers originally utilized the left lobe for this procedure, it was felt that its smaller size and anatomic positioning increased the risk of graft failure. As a result, nearly all centers currently performing living donor liver transplantation in adults now utilize the right lobe except in select situations where the adult recipient is considerably smaller than the donor.

The donor evaluation is designed to determine appropriate anatomy and to identify any medical issues that might increase morbidity or mortality related to major hepatic resection. To be consistent with ethical principles the donation must be voluntary and free of coercion, and most programs prefer there to be a significant established relationship between the donor and the recipient. The great majority of donors are emotionally related to their recipient, however some centers have utilized anonymous donors.

The donor evaluation is divided into several phases as summarized in Box 12.1. Initially, the potential donor undergoes a short interview to ascertain their medical history, body size, general condition, psychosocial circumstances, and compatibility of blood type. The risks and complications of the surgery are also discussed. Many potential donors are excluded during this phase. During the second phase the potential donor undergoes a complete history and physical examination by an internist or hepatologist, a psychosocial and a cardiovascular evaluation, laboratory studies, and imaging studies to assess the size of the right lobe, the remaining liver mass, and vascular supply; MRI with MRA and/or MRC and CT have been utilized for these purposes at various centers. The final

---

Box 12.1 Living donor evaluation

Phase 1
Initial discussion of the procedure and risks
Demographic data
Blood type
    screening laboratory tests: liver function tests, CBC, PT/PTT

Phase 2
Medical evaluation (surgeon, hepatologist)
Volumetric CT or MRI (± MRA and MRCP)
Social and/or psychiatric evaluation
Serology (HCV, RPR, VZV, HCV, HBV, HAV, EBV, CMV, HIV)
EKG, ECHO
CXR
Other tests and consultations as deemed necessary by the medical team (i.e. cardiac, endocrine, pulmonary, coagulation)

Phase 3
Splanchnic arteriography (±)
Liver biopsy (±)
    autologous blood donation
    final surgical/medical review
    final consent.

---

phase includes invasive procedures that are required to complete the evaluation and prepare the patient for surgery. These may include liver biopsy, angiography, ERCP, or additional consultations and procedures. Most centers place an upper limit on the age of the potential donor, although this may vary considerably between centers.

Complications that are reported to occur in living liver donors may be significant and include bile leaks, re-operation, infection, bleeding that requires a blood transfusion, and even liver failure of the donor's remaining segment requiring transplantation. There are also complications that may occur later such as biliary strictures and hernias. Bile-duct strictures may increase the lifetime risk of the donor for developing secondary biliary cirrhosis, the significance of which may not be realized for several decades. The overall risk of death to the donor from this procedure is felt to be low but is not insignificant. Donor deaths have been reported in Europe and the US.

There is much discussion within the transplant community regarding the ethics of a healthy patient undergoing the risk of a partial hepatectomy, the issue of informed consent, and psychosocial effects upon the donor. It is estimated that the risk of mortality to the donor undergoing right hepatectomy is about 0.2% to 0.5%, the risk of a complication around 30%, and the risks of long-term complications are not yet known. There have been single-center reports regarding complications and outcomes, but no studies have been done in a systematic controlled fashion. The development of a national living donor database and more detailed multi-center cohort studies will provide valuable information regarding actual morbidity and mortality, as well as the long-term outcome in the liver donor.

Complications encountered in the recipient of an adult-to-adult living donor liver transplantation are similar to those observed following cadaveric transplantation (see p. 251), but bile-duct strictures and leaks appear to be encountered more often after transplantation of partial grafts. Septic complications appear to be more frequent when patients with advanced decompensated cirrhosis undergo adult-to-adult living donor liver transplantation and this is the major factor leading to mortality following this procedure. It has also been reported that hepatitis C appears to recur at a more rapid pace in adult-to-adult living donor liver transplantation recipients.

The transplant procedure

Almost all liver transplants follow a similar procedure, although each surgeon has his or her own unique style and each institution has specific protocols. The first portion of the operation is the recipient hepatectomy, which can be the most complex part of the procedure because of the presence of significant portal hypertension and coagulopathy, and it is made more difficult by previous abdominal surgery. The second phase is the anhepatic phase during which the patient is without a liver and the new liver is being sewed in. Some centers utilize veno–venous bypass during this phase to maintain hemodynamic stability, normothermia, and prevent mesenteric congestion. The anastomoses usually (in order) include suprahepatic vena cava, infrahepatic vena cava (if not placed in a piggy-back fashion), the portal vein, and the hepatic artery. The final phase is the neohepatic phase following reperfusion of the new liver. Significant cardiovascular instability can occur in this period and it depends on the function of the new liver, and hemostatic problems due to coagulopathy and fibrinolysis. It is essential for a program to have a specialized anesthesia team that understands the metabolic complexities of a patient with end-stage liver disease, and with the ability to correct severe coagulopathy and manage the hemodynamic changes occurring during the transplant operation. The biliary anastomosis is done in this final phase and is usually a duct-to-duct anastomosis with or without stenting or T-tube, or a Roux-en-Y hepaticojejunostomy, which is usually performed in small children, or in patients with primary sclerosing cholangitis.

Postoperative management

The postoperative liver transplant patient usually requires a short stay in the intensive care unit. Many patients return to the intensive care unit still intubated because of the severity of their disease preoperatively, however, an increasing number of patients are being extubated in the operating room if they meet certain extubation criteria with an uncomplicated procedure and a well-functioning graft. The stay in the intensive care unit can be brief, but is helpful to observe the function and recovery of the graft, ensure hemodynamic and respiratory stability, rule out any acute technical complications, and monitor renal function. Cardiac monitoring, evaluation of fluid status with measurement of central venous pressure and urine output, assessment of liver function with liver function tests, coagulation factors and bile output (if T-tube is in place), are all critical in the early postoperative period. Immunosuppression is started in the operating room or within hours of the transplant, which renders the care of these patients more complex than other critically ill intensive care unit patients. The preoperative state of the patient significantly affects the course of their postoperative recovery, as does the initial graft function, with several factors having an impact in outcome. Patients that are mechanically ventilated or who have renal failure have a much worse outcome than those who have been living at home. Prolonged stays in the intensive care unit pre-transplant are associated with an increase in the incidence of infections that may impair recovery.

Once the patient is known to be stable with a functioning graft, they can be transferred to a transplant ward where daily liver function tests are reviewed with appropriate changes made in immunosuppression management. Postoperative studies and imaging are kept to a minimum and performed only when indicated. A T-tube cholangiogram is performed around postoperative day 5 or 6, if one is present. Percutaneous or transjugular liver biopsies may be performed if liver function tests become elevated. Nutritional assessment and supplementation is extremely important in these debilitated patients, and physical therapy is started in the first few days after transplant. The length of stay varies depending on the patient's preoperative status, graft function, complications, immunosuppression monitoring, and the need for rehabilitation. Early discharge planning is encouraged to ensure adequate teaching and physical therapy is provided prior to discharge home or to a rehabilitation facility, this can significantly reduce the length of stay. The patients are then followed with weekly laboratory studies and clinic visits in the outpatient setting.

Intraoperative complications

Intraoperative complications include bleeding, portal vein thrombosis, and the need for hepatic artery reconstruction. Excessive bleeding from significant portal hypertension may occur during hepatectomy, aggravated by the severity of coagulopathy, as well as adhesions from previous upper abdominal surgery. Skillful efficient removal of the cirrhotic organ, transplantation of a functioning graft, and aggressive correction of coagulopathy by the appropriate use of platelets and fresh frozen plasma provide hemostasis during hepatectomy and after reperfusion.

Portal vein thrombosis can increase the complexity of the dissection. The presence of a chronic thrombus in the portal vein often results in inflammatory scarring in the portahepatis as well as development of large delicate collaterals. In most cases the thrombus extends up to the bifurcation of the splenic/superior mesenteric vein confluence and can be removed using endarterectomy techniques while preserving an intact main portal vein. The placement of a transjugular intrahepatic portosystemic shunt that extends into the main portal vein may also increase the technical difficulty of portal vein dissection. Rarely, a vein graft obtained from the donor iliac vessels may need to be placed to the superior mesenteric vein. Complete occlusion of the portal venous system is not an absolute contraindication for transplantation, since the infrahepatic vena cava or a large collateral such as the coronary vein, may be used for inflow.

More frequently the surgeon is faced with a very small hepatic artery, intimal dissection of the celiac axis, arcuate ligament syndrome, or other pathologies which necessitate the careful dissection of the entire celiac axis and possible placement of an allogeneic vascular graft to the supraceliac or infrarenal aorta. The potential need for venous or arterial grafts for revascularization mandates that the procuring team obtains adequate vessels from the donor during every procedure. Unused grafts should be refrigerated for a few days after transplantation in preservation solution, in case of emergent need for vascular reconstruction at a later date.

Postoperative complications

Primary non-function

Occasionally, the new graft fails to function at all, resulting in the term "primary nonfunction". This clinical manifestation is seen in 2% to 5% of liver grafts, and is characterized by extremely high transaminases, severe coagulopathy, poor bile output, deepening encephalopathy, onset of renal failure, acidosis, and progressive hemodynamic instability, eventually resulting in death. The development of primary non-function is a surgical emergency that is successfully corrected by early retransplantation, aided by the fact that patients with primary non-function get the highest priority on the waiting list as a Status 1. The failure to find a suitable graft within a few days is associated with a very high morbidity and mortality.

The mechanisms for immediate graft failure following successful implantation are not completely understood, but they may relate to donor variables such as steatosis and age, prolonged cold ischemia, severe preservation injury, or a combination of these factors. Many variables have been shown to be associated with an increased incidence of primary non-function or poor initial function, however the studies identifying these factors were retrospective in nature, and there was no consistency in the definition of poor graft function. There are very few tests performed before procurement that can determine liver function following transplantation, and nothing may be more accurate than an experienced donor surgeon's visual evaluation at the time of recovery. Liver biopsies at the time of procurement have not been reliable predictors of function.

Not as dramatic as primary non-function, delayed non-function of a liver graft is characterized by progressive poor early graft function and failure to recover completely. This pathology is expressed with coagulopathy and the development of severe persistent hyperbilirubinemia. Liver biopsies often show cholestatis and ischemic injury despite intact vasculature. The low residual reserve cannot support other system failures or the presence of infection, and in most cases it results in high mortality secondary to bacterial or fungal sepsis. Retransplantation in this setting has a much worse prognosis than primary non-function, and may not be indicated if there are any signs of infection.

Postoperative bleeding

The failure to correct post-transplant coagulopathy, ongoing fibrinolysis, and the presence of multiple vascular anastomoses contributes to the possibility of post-operative bleeding. Important intraoperative measures, including warming the patient with veno–venous bypass and/or warming blankets, appropriate use of fresh frozen plasma and platelets, and meticulous surgical technique can help prevent this complication. Coagulopathy should also self-correct in the presence of recovering liver graft function. A persistent drop in hemoglobin and the need for the transfusion of five or more units of packed red blood cells are usually indications for re-exploration and evacuation of the hematoma. In most cases removal of the clot will be sufficient to arrest further fibrinolysis, and will stop bleeding. Occasionally, it will be necessary to repair bleeding sites.

Hepatic artery thrombosis

Vascular complications such as hepatic artery thrombosis following liver transplantation are more common among children, and are directly related to the small size of the vessels that are used for reconstruction. It can also been seen in the transplantation of partial liver grafts, such as adult-to-adult living donor liver transplantation where just the right hepatic artery is used without the celiac axis. The use of loupe magnification and microsurgical techniques has greatly reduced the incidence of hepatic artery thrombosis. Acute arterial thrombus can present with rapid and/or progressive worsening of graft function, marked elevation liver function tests, or necrosis of the bile ducts with dehiscence of the biliary enteric anastomosis and resultant bile leak. Early recognition with duplex sonography, MRA, or angiogram, as well as immediate exploration and successful thrombectomy may salvage the graft. However, deteriorating liver function and bile-duct necrosis usually results in the need for immediate retransplantation, and these patients are given priority status.

Biliary leak

Bile-duct reconstruction with either duct-to-duct anastomosis (choledochocholedochostomy) or Roux-en-Y hepaticojejunostomy may be complicated by an early bile leak, usually secondary to technical error or ischemic injury of the donor duct. Early leaks can be diagnosed by the appearance of bile in the drains, and are confirmed by a T-tube cholangiogram or hydroxy iminodiacetic acid (HIDA) scan. Some minor leaks may resolve with T-tube decompression and drainage, or placement of an endoscopic stent with ERCP. A persistent leak or development of bile peritonitis mandates immediate surgical exploration and revision of the anastomosis. Ischemic bile-duct injury secondary to early hepatic artery thrombosis is an indication for retransplantation.

Infections

Infectious complications continue to be responsible for most of the early mortalities in liver transplantation. There is a direct correlation between the preoperative status of the recipient, the pattern of recovery after transplantation, and the incidence of serious bacterial and fungal infections. Patients who require an intensive care unit setting while awaiting transplantation have a high probability for the development of such complications and poor outcome. These are chronically ill and malnourished patients who are exposed to and acquire the resistant hospital flora prior to surgery, and who are then placed on high-dose immunosuppression immediately after the procedure. If these patients develop organ system failure or graft malfunction, this further contributes to the morbid outcome. The spectrum of infection appears to be evolving, leading to more common infections by resistant gram-positive bacteria (such as vancomycin-resistant enterococcus, and methicillin-resistant *Staphylococcus aureus*) rather then those caused by gram-negative bacteria. The deliberate use of broad-spectrum antibiotics in the debilitated immunosuppressed patient contributes in part to the development of systemic fungal infection (candidiasis, aspergillosis). Invasive fungal infections in an immunocompromised patient have an extremely high mortality, and successful outcome requires careful surveillance so treatment should be started early. It is recommended that antibiotic treatment against common bacteria and fungi is started when the clinical status suggests the presence of infection, before the cultures may become positive. The treatment can be further modified when the results of the cultures are known.

Immunosuppression

The purpose and goals of immunosuppression therapy are to prevent rejection of the graft, avoid complications and side effects of the medications, maximize long-term survival, and treat acute rejection when it occurs. Although there are standard immunosuppressive protocols, it is important to realize that the regimen prescribed should be tailored to the patient, depending on their disease, general medical status, age, renal function, and the development of side effects.

The relatively low immunogenicity of the liver allograft and its ability to regenerate and recover from injury are probably the main reasons for the excellent long-term function following transplantation. These results are achieved when graft and recipient are ABO blood group compatible, and without the necessity for preoperative human HLA matching. Although each patient requires an individualized approach, most recipients are treated with combination therapy, which includes a calcineurin inhibitor (cyclosporine or tacrolimus), along with prednisone, with or without mycophenolate mofetil. The recent introduction of sirolimus offers another option besides a calcinuerin inhibitor (Table 12.2). If the postoperative recovery is smooth and there is no episode of acute rejection, efforts are made to minimize the dose and avoid long-term complications of immunosuppressant therapies. Most programs utilize a protocol for the rapid taper of steroids within the first 3 to 6 months after surgery, and significant reduction in the calcineurin inhibitor. Patients with autoimmune-type diseases, such as autoimmune hepatitis or primary sclerosing cholangitis, tend to stay on steroids and higher levels of immunosuppression. Long-term maintenance immunotherapy is necessary in most recipients, as complete cession of immunosuppression carries significant risk for the development of acute and chronic rejection, although there may be a subpopulation of patients who can maintain their graft without immunosuppression in the long term.

Unfortunately, there is no good immunologic test to indicate which recipients fall into this category.

Acute cellular rejection is seen at a rate of 20% to 50% within the first 6 months after transplantation, most occurring within the first 10 days. The patient may present with the development of fever, jaundice, or abdominal pain, but most early rejections are asymptomatic and picked up by routine laboratory studies. The diagnosis is confirmed by a liver biopsy that will demonstrate the presence of periportal lymphocytic infiltrate that extends into the liver parenchyma, as well as the invasion of inflammatory cells into the vascular endothelium. The great majority of rejection episodes are responsive to the administration of high-dose steroids or simply to an increased dose of calcineurin inhibitor and the addition of another agent, such as mycophenolate mofetil. More potent monoclonal or polyclonal anti-T-cell antibodies are effective against steroid-resistant rejection, leading to the reversal of the acute episode in nearly all of the recipients. Less response in seen when the acute episode occurs long after transplant and/or in the presence of chronic rejection.

Diagnosis and treatment of acute rejection is complicated in patients with chronic hepatitis C. Mild-to-moderate elevation in transaminases may be reflective of either HCV re-infection, or signs of early rejection. Even experienced pathologists may have difficulty distinguishing between the two on biopsy, and viral titers may not be reflective of the graft pathology. Often acute rejection is treated with bolus steroids, only to have significant recurrent HCV infection develop within the graft. It is believed that avoidance of high-dose steroids is beneficial in this patient population.

Chronic rejection is seen months or years after transplantation, and is usually expressed with paucity of the bile ducts, often being described as "vanishing bile-duct syndrome". Chronic rejection may present with poor synthetic liver function and hyperbilirubinemia. The etiology for this phenomenon is not well understood, and may be related to a humoral reaction involving antibodies and fibrogenic cytokines. The treatment for chronic rejection is limited, and some patients may be considered as candidates for retransplantation if it progresses to liver failure.

Recurrent disease

The reappearance of the primary disease within the transplanted liver can be a source of much controversy as well as frustration for the clinician. It is

Table 12.2 Immunosuppressive agents

Immunosuppressant (Commercial name)	Class	Mechanism	Dosing target levels
Azathioprine (Imuran®)	antimetabolite	Purine synthesis inhibition.	1–3 mg kg^{-1} d^{-1} i.v. or p.o.
Mycophenolate mofetil (CellCept®)	antimetabolite	Purine synthesis inhibition – *do novo* synthesis inhibited more than salvage pathway.	500–1000 mg p.o. b.i.d.
Prednisone and methylprednisolone	glucocorticoid	Multiple effects on immune system, most important is blocking lymphocyte proliferation.	Induction: 2–5 mg/kg i.v. Maintenance: 20 mg/d p.o. Taper to 5 mg/d, or discontinue. Rejection: 500–1000 mg/d i.v., with or without taper.
Cyclosporine (Neoral® among others)	calcineurin inhibitor	Blocks transcription of early T-cell activation genes.	1–8 mg/kg p.o. b.i.d. Initial target level 250–300.
Tacrolimus/FK506 (Prograf®)	calcineurin inhibitor	Blocks transcription of early T-cell activation genes.	0.05–0.15 mg/kg p.o. b.i.d. Initial target level 10–15.
Sirolimus/rapamycin (Rapamune®)	TOR inhibitor	Blocks the downstream events initiated by IL-2 production.	2–5 mg/d p.o. Initial target level 10–15.
Atgam	antibody	Polyclonal antibody directed against thymocytes.	10–30 mg kg^{-1} d^{-1} i.v. for 5–14 days.
Thymoglobulin	antibody	Polyclonal antibody directed against thymocytes.	1.25–2.5 mg kg^{-1} d^{-1} i.v. for 3–14 days.
Muromonab-CD3 (OKT3®)	antibody	Monoclonal antibody to CD3 molecule on T-cells.	2.5–10 mg/d i.v. for 5–14 days.
Basiliximab (Simulect®)	antibody	Binds to IL-2 receptor.	20 mg i.v. pre-operatively and day 4 post-transplant.
Daclizumab (Zenapax®)	antibody	Binds to IL-2 receptor.	1 mg/kg i.v. pre-operatively and then post-transplant at 2 week intervals for 4 weeks.

recognized that hepatitis B and C, as well as certain autoimmune-related diseases, reoccur within the allograft. In addition, malignancies such as hepatocellular carcinoma can also reappear in the liver.

In the past, re-infection with hepatitis B often led to an accelerated path of graft failure with up to 20% of recipients developing a picture of fibrosing cholestatic hepatitis within weeks to months of transplant. The dismal results seen with hepatitis B have essentially been eliminated with the administration of long term HBIg in combination with nucleoside analogs. Recipients who are hepatitis B positive may now expect to attain survival rates similar to patients transplanted for other indications.

The clinical picture following transplantation for hepatitis C is very different to that for hepatitis B. Essentially all allografts are re-infected, often manifested by elevated transaminases and histologic evidence of recurrence within the first year following transplant. However, in most recipients the disease is mild, with only about 5% of individuals developing fibrosing cholestatic hepatitis progress-

ing to liver failure. Little data exists to support the use of chemoprophylaxis with interferon and/or ribavirin. Furthermore most transplant recipients tolerate this therapy poorly. Retransplantation for recurrent hepatitis C is controversial, as the disease appears to recur even sooner in the retransplanted graft. Given the large number of transplants being performed for hepatitis C, attention is being directed toward the development of therapeutic and prophylactic protocols, and several multicenter trials are in progress.

The autoimmune-related diseases, including primary biliary cirrhosis, primary sclerosing cholangitis, and autoimmune hepatitis, are also thought to recur in the transplanted liver. It is often difficult to make a clinical diagnosis as elevated liver enzymes and biliary strictures are non-specific findings and may have several etiologies. In addition, autoimmune markers often persist following transplant. In all cases exclusion of preservation injury, rejection, viral infection, and hepatic arterial occlusion are mandatory before a diagnosis of recurrent disease can be entertained. In general, patient and graft survival does not appear to be adversely impacted by disease recurrence.

Long-term outcome

With advances and progress in surgical technical innovations, perioperative care, tailoring of immunosuppression, and a better understanding of recurrent disease, liver transplantation has become very successful. Overall long-term survival for adults now approaches 75% at 5 years and 60% at 10 years as determined by the United Network of Organ Sharing database (Figure 12.1), with pediatric results even higher. Future areas of study that may further impact outcome include the development of immunosuppression protocols that reduce significant side effects, treatment of recurrent hepatitis C, expansion of living donor transplantation, and methods to support hepatocyte recovery in injured grafts.

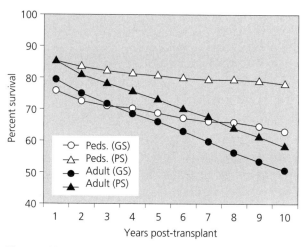

Figure 12.1   Long-term survival: United Network of Organ Sharing database.

Further reading

Bucuvalas JC, Ryckman FC. Long-term outcome after liver transplantation in children. *Pediatr Transplant* 2002; 6: 30–36.

Carithers RL. Liver transplant practice guidelines. *Liver Transpl* 2000; 6: 122–135.

Cattral MS, Lilly LB, Levy GA. Immunosuppression in liver transplantation. *Semin Liver Dis* 2000; 20: 523–531.

Faust TW. Recurrent primary biliary cirrhosis, primary sclerosing cholangitis, and autoimmune hepatitis after transplantation. *Semin Liver Dis* 2000; 20: 481–495.

Markmann JF, Markowitz JS, Yersiz H, Morrisey M, Farmer DG, Farmer DA. Long-term survival after retransplantation of the liver. *Ann Surg* 1997; 226: 408–418.

McDiarmid SV, Millis MJ, Olthoff KM, So SK. Indications for pediatric liver transplantation. *Pediatr Transplant* 1998: 2; 106–116.

Olthoff K. Cadaver liver donor selection criteria. In: Norman and Turka (eds) *Primer on Transplantation*. American Society of Transplantation. Mt Laurel, NJ. 2001: pp. 536–539.

Sheiner PA. Hepatitis C after liver transplantation. *Semin Liver Dis* 2000; 20: 201–209.

Shiffman ML, Brown RS, Olthoff KM, Everson G, Miller C, Siegler M, Hoofnagle JH. Living donor liver transplantation: Summary of a conference at the National Institutes of Health. *Liver Transpl* 2002; 8: 174–188.

The recipient hepatectomy and grafting. In: Busuttil and Klintmalm (eds) *Transplantation of the Liver*. WB Saunders Co., Philadelphia, PA 1996: pp. 405–418.

Wiesner RH, McDiarmid SV, Kamath PS, Edwards EB, Malinchoc M, Kremers WK. Meld and PELD: application of survival models to liver allocation. *Liver Transpl* 2001; 7: 567–80.

Chapter 13

Etiologies of Acute and Chronic Pancreatitis

Jeremy Schwartz

CHAPTER OUTLINE

Etiologies of acute pancreatitis

Biliary disease

Biliary disease is the most common cause of acute pancreatitis in the US and is responsible for 50% to 70% of cases. The main forms of biliary disease include macroscopic gallstone-induced pancreatitis and microlithiasis. The presence of congenital bile duct cysts is another form of biliary disease associated with the development of acute pancreatitis.

Gallstones

The presence of gallstones increases the relative risk for developing acute pancreatitis 14-to 35-fold in men and 12- to 25-fold in women. However, acute pancreatitis develops in only a small percentage of people with gallstones, with one large cohort study reporting the cumulative incidence of acute pancreatitis as 0.17% per year. Even so, the presence of gallstones is the most common cause of acute pancreatitis. Women are affected more frequently than men and have a peak incidence between the ages of 50 and 60 years. Estimated population incidences for acute gallstone pancreatitis in the USA range from 45 to 65 per 100 000 person years depending on the criteria used to definitively diagnose gallstone pancreatitis. In western countries gallstone disease accounts for 34% to 54% of cases of acute pancreatitis.

Gallstone size less than 5 mm increases the risk of developing pancreatitis approximately four to fivefold. However, the number and total weight of gallstones does not influence the incidence of acute pancreatitis. Gallstone shape, with the exception of mulberry-shaped stones, does not appear to increase the risk of acute pancreatitis. Mulberry-shaped stones have been found to increase the risk by more than twofold. Finally, a larger diameter of the common bile duct has been shown to be associated with an increased incidence of acute gallstone pancreatitis. Gallstone pancreatitis has a high rate of recurrence if underlying biliary disease is not corrected.

Microlithiasis

An increasing body of data suggests that many patients with acute idiopathic pancreatitis may indeed have biliary sludge or biliary microcrystals (microlithiasis) as the underlying etiology for their pancreatitis. Most series in the literature on the subject are small. However, they reveal that in selected patients with suspected biliary disease based on biochemical or ultrasonographic data, examination of the bile reveals evidence of microlithiasis (mostly calcium bilirubinate granules and occasionally cholesterol monohydrate) in approximately 80% of cases.

Congenital bile duct cysts

Hyperamylasemia and repeated attacks of acute pancreatitis are common features in patients with choledochal cysts, particularly in childhood, with a wide range of estimated occurrences from 0% to 70%. Although there are five subtypes of congenital bile duct cyst, types I (diffuse dilatation of the extrahepatic bile duct) and III (dilatation of the intraduodenal segment of the biliary system, also known as a choledochocele) are most often described in association with acute pancreatitis. Recently, the first case of acute pancreatitis associated with type IV congenital bile duct cyst (intrahepatic and extrahepatic biliary tract cystic dilatation) has been reported. There are only unpublished anecdotes regarding possible associations of types II (diverticulum of the common bile duct) and V (cystic dilatation of the intrahepatic biliary tract) congenital bile duct cyst with acute pancreatitis.

Alcohol

Slightly less than one quarter of cases of acute pancreatitis are caused by ethyl alcohol. Most cases are associated with heavy, long-term use of ethanol averaging approximately 100 to 150 g/day. However, acute pancreatitis can also follow after only one or two exposures to ethanol, usually of a large quantity, or "binge drinking." The actual type of ethanol consumed (i.e. wine, beer, or spirits) does not appear to make a difference. Recent evidence suggests that certain genetic predispositions toward developing ethanol-induced acute pancreatitis exist. Specifically, certain human leukocyte antigen types (B40, Aw23, Aw24, B13), blood groups O and Le have been implicated. Furthermore, in Chinese alcoholic patients, certain liver alcohol dehydrogenase (ADH) and acetaldehyde dehydrogenase (ALDH) alleles have been studied, and it has been shown that certain alleles are present in those patients who develop acute alcoholic pancreatitis. There is evidence from these genetic studies to suggest that there is a subpopulation of alcoholic patients who never develop acute pancreatitis no matter how much they drink. Acute alcohol-induced pancreatitis can resolve completely or it can, in a significant percentage of patients, go on to chronic pancreatitis (see Etiologies of chronic pancreatitis, p. 262). Methanol ingestion can also lead to acute pancreatitis.

Iatrogenic causes

Acute pancreatitis can be caused iatrogenically either through endoscopic or surgical procedures.

Endoscopic procedures

Pancreaticobiliary endoscopy, also known as endoscopic retrograde cholangiopancreatography (ERCP), is the main endoscopic procedure associated with acute pancreatitis. The incidence of ERCP-induced acute pancreatitis is approximately 5%. Approximately 500 000 ERCPs are performed each year in the USA with approximately 25 000 associated cases of acute pancreatitis. Factors associated with an increased risk of inducing pancreatitis following ERCP include female sex, younger age, smaller distal bile-duct diameter, biliary and/or pancreatic sphincter hypertension or dysfunction, performance of sphincter of Oddi manometry, performance of biliary and/or pancreatic sphincterotomy, and pancreatic duct injection. The incidence of pancreatitis increases with the number of pancreatic injections performed as well as the total quantity of contrast injected into the pancreatic duct. Following ERCP, pancreatitis develops in about 20% of patients with biliary dyskinesia. The incidence of pancreatitis following ERCP varies inversely with the skill and experience of the endoscopist as well as the frequency with which that endoscopist performs ERCP. Use of low-osmolar contrast or premedication with steroids has no effect on the incidence of pancreatitis following ERCP. There is evidence that stenting the pancreatic duct in patients with sphincter of Oddi dysfunction undergoing sphincterotomy may lessen the risk of developing acute pancreatitis. Some evidence suggests that balloon sphincter dilatation performed instead of sphincterotomy may carry a lower risk for developing acute pancreatitis.

Acute pancreatitis has also been reported following endoscopic ultrasound with fine needle aspiration of the pancreas as well as following endoscopic ampullectomy for adenomatous polyps and other lesions.

Surgical procedures

Postoperative acute pancreatitis occurs after a variety of procedures including those that involve direct manipulation of the pancreas itself or structures contiguous to the pancreas, as well as after procedures on organs at distant sites. Specific procedures associated with postoperative pancreatitis include common bile duct exploration, sphincteroplasty, distal gastrectomy, renal surgeries, and cardiovascular surgeries. Postoperative acute pancreatitis is a documented but rare complication of obstetric and gynecological surgery, with an overall incidence of approximately 1 case per 17 000 procedures. Many of these cases were noted to be associated with biliary disease.

It had formerly been thought that intraoperative cholangiography was an independent risk factor for acute pancreatitis. However, a recent, large, retrospective study failed to find any cases of acute pancreatitis attributable to intraoperative cholangiography amongst the patients they reviewed. Therefore, intraoperative cholangiography without subsequent common bile duct exploration is not considered a likely cause of acute pancreatitis.

Papillary stenosis

Papillary stenosis, which is usually caused by scarring of the papilla, can lead to recurrent bouts of acute pancreatitis. The incidence of papillary stenosis varies from 0.04% to 0.12% in postmortem studies. The majority of cases, 61% in one large study, were associated with choledocholithiasis.

Papillary stenosis can also develop as a long-term complication of endoscopic sphincterotomy. Repeated cannulation attempts and excessive use of coagulation current during endoscopic sphincterotomy are associated with an increased risk of scarring leading to papillary stenosis. Other iatrogenic manipulation, especially pancreaticobiliary surgery, can also lead to papillary stenosis. Altogether, iatrogenic causes account for approximately 7% of cases of papillary stenosis.

Papillary carcinoma accounts for an additional 14% and juxtapapillary duodenal diverticula and celiac disease account for an additional 1% to 2% of cases of papillary stenosis. Finally, some cases of papillary stenosis are idiopathic and are termed primary papillary stenosis.

Traumatic causes

An estimated 1% to 3% of patients who experience significant abdominal trauma (e.g. assault, motor-vehicle accident) can sustain pancreatic ductal disruption or pancreatic parenchymal injury, resulting in acute or, less frequently, chronic pancreatitis.

Medications

Drugs are a relatively uncommon cause of acute pancreatitis in adult patients, but should be considered when other, more common, causes have been excluded. Definitive proof that a particular medication causes acute pancreatitis requires that acute pancreatitis develops during treatment with that drug, that the pancreatitis resolves when the medication is withdrawn, and that the pancreatitis often recurs with re-administration of the drug. Because of ethical considerations, rechallenge with a particular drug is a relatively uncommon event, occurring only when re-administration of that drug is medically necessary. As such, many medications have been implicated only as potential and not definitive causative agents for acute pancreatitis (Table 13.1). Medications listed as having strong association with acute pancreatitis are those shown to produce pancreatitis on rechallenge or having a significant association in controlled trials.

Table 13.1   Medications potentially causing acute pancreatitis

Strong association	Weak association	Uncertain association
L-asparaginase	ACE-inhibitors	Alpha-methyl-dopa
Azathioprine	Acetominophen	Amino-salicylic acid
Didanosine	Cytarabine	Ceftriaxone
6-mercaptopurine	Ergotamine	Cimetidine
Pentamidine	Estrogens	Clomiphene
Vinca alkaloids	Furosemide	Clozapine
	Isotretinoin	Corticosteroids
	Sulfasalazine	Cyclosporine
	Sulfonamides	Erythromycin
	Tamoxifen	Interferon-alpha
	Tetracycline	Metolazone
	Thiazide diuretics	Metronidazole
	Valproic acid	Morphine sulfate
		Nitrofurantoin
		NSAIDs
		Octreotide
		Olanzapine
		Piroxicam
		Procainamide
		Propofol
		Ranitidine
		Ritonavir
		Zalcitabine

The medications most likely to cause acute pancreatitis are didanosine (incidence of up to 23%), and pentamidine, as well as azathioprine and mercaptopurine (incidence 3%–5%).

Whether or not corticosteroids cause acute pancreatitis is controversial. Reports of corticosteroids causing pancreatitis are difficult to interpret because most of these patients had other potential causes of pancreatitis. It is probable that corticosteroids may directly precipitate pancreatitis, but this appears to be an extremely rare event.

Infectious causes

Many different infectious agents, including viruses, parasites, and bacteria, have been implicated in the etiology of acute pancreatitis.

Viruses

Infrequently, viral hepatitis, even if not fulminant, has been associated with the development of acute pancreatitis. Pancreatitis has been reported most commonly with acute hepatitis A and B; however, acute non-A non-B viral hepatitis is also associated. Recently, the first case of hepatitis E associated with acute pancreatitis was reported.

It is thought that human immunodeficiency virus (HIV) is associated with acute pancreatitis with a 1-year incidence rate of 14% in a recent, large, retrospective study. The risk for developing acute pancreatitis in HIV is inversely related to the number of CD4 lymphocytes in the patient's blood. No patient with a CD4 count greater than 500 per mm^3 developed pancreatitis. In patients with a low CD4 count, pancreatitis was associated with gallstones, active intravenous drug abuse, pentamidine intake, and *Pneumocystis carinii* and *Mycobacterium avium* complex infections. It is, therefore, unclear whether HIV infection itself can cause acute pancreatitis.

Other viral infections, such as mumps, rubella, coxsackie B, Epstein–Barr virus, and cytomegalovirus, have also been linked to acute pancreatitis.

Parasites

Both macroscopic and microscopic parasitic diseases can cause acute pancreatitis. The *Echinococcus* tapeworms are the cause of hydatid liver disease. There are multiple case reports of hydatid cysts (unilocular or multi locular) gaining access to the pancreaticobiliary system and leading to bouts of acute recurrent pancreatitis, or less commonly, to chronic pancreatitis. The nematode, *Ascaris lumbricoides*, can access the pancreaticobiliary system via the small bowel and lead to pancreatitis. Another macro-parasite implicated in pancreatico-biliary infection and associated acute pancreatitis is *Clonorchis*.

Plasmodium falciparum (the cause of falciprum-type malaria) has been implicated in causing acute pancreatitis with about 10 cases reported in the world-wide literature.

Bacteria

Many species of bacteria have been found to cause acute pancreatitis, including *Mycoplasma pneumoniae*, *Campylobacter jejuni*, *Mycobacterium tuberculosis*, *Mycobacterium avium* complex, and *Legionella* species.

Metabolic causes

Lipid abnormalities

Triglyceride levels over 1000 mg/dL are associated with acute pancreatitis. Type V hypertriglyceridemia is the predominant cause of the illness, but types I and IV also contribute. Cases of acute pancreatitis related to hypertriglyceridemia have been reported in patients with uncontrolled gestational diabetes mellitus. Moreover, a recent large review of patients with diabetic ketoacidosis found that 11% developed acute pancreatitis. Hypertriglyceridemia was the most common co-existing etiologic factor in these patients. However, alcohol and medications were also cited as potential etiological factors in some patients. Furthermore, a significant portion of cases were labeled as idiopathic. It is unclear whether diabetes mellitus is also an independent etiologic factor in the development of acute pancreatitis.

Clomiphene has also been reported in a few cases to cause hypertriglyceridemia-induced acute pancreatitis.

Hypertriglyceridemia can also occur transiently because of an attack of acute pancreatitis (usually in alcoholics), and in those cases is not thought to play an etiologic role in the disease.

Hypercalcemia

Acute pancreatitis has been reported with hypercalcemia of various etiologies (hyperparathyroidism, multiple myeloma, T-cell leukemia, and milk alkali syndrome). It should be noted, however, that hypercalcemia in general, and hyperparathyroidism in particular, are very infrequently associated with acute pancreatitis. One recent large study found that only 0.23% of patients with acute pancreatitis had documented hyperparathyroidism.

Pregnancy

Biliary causes

Most cases of gestational acute pancreatitis are due to cholelithiasis. This includes macroscopic gallstones and microlithiasis as described above (see p. 257).

Hypertriglyceridemia

Pregnancy can lead to phenotypic hypertriglyceridemia through several potential factors. These etiologies of hypertriglyceridemia during gestation can be secondary to metabolic conditions such as diabetes mellitus, or can be due to genetic mutations. A mutation in the lipoprotein lipase gene involving the substitution of glutamine for glycine at amino acid residue 188 has been found in two sisters who developed gestational hypertriglyceridemia-induced acute pancreatitis. Other work suggests an association with the apolipoprotein E4/2 genotype. However, a significant amount of work still needs to be done to fully establish the genetics involved in hypertriglyceridemia-induced gestational pancreatitis.

Hereditary causes

Although patients with hereditary pancreatitis do suffer attacks of acute pancreatitis, it is felt that these are often recurrent acute attacks of what will evolve into chronic pancreatitis. Therefore, hereditary pancreatitis will be discussed at length in the section on chronic pancreatitis (see p. 262). The reader should be aware, however, that about half the patients with hereditary pancreatitis who develop acute attacks of pancreatitis will never go on to develop chronic pancreatitis.

Duodenal diverticula

Intraluminal diverticula

Intraluminal diverticula are rare and result from the presence of congenital webs or membranes within the second part of the duodenum. Recurrent acute pancreatitis may be present in 20% of cases.

Extraluminal diverticula

Extraluminal diverticula are more common and occur with a prevalence of 3% to 23% on various autopsy and ERCP series. It is thought that they are due to a combination of a weak area and a pulsion mechanism. This likely explains the increased age of patients in whom they are found. Patients with these peri-ampullary extraluminal duodenal diverticula have a significantly higher rate of choledocholithiasis, possibly related to bacterial infection due to biliary stasis. Acute pancreatitis may be related to this higher incidence of biliary stones, however, one recent study did not find statistically different rates of biliary acute pancreatitis in these patients versus controls without diverticula. Instead, a significantly higher incidence of idiopathic pancreatitis was found in these patients. Finally, as discussed above (see p. 259), duodenal diverticula can also be associated with papillary stenosis.

Other causes

There are multiple other potential etiologies for acute pancreatitis (Table 13.2). It is presently unclear if pancreas divisum is truly an etiologic factor in acute pancreatitis. Finally, it is important to point out that even after exhaustive evaluations for an underlying etiology, a significant percentage of acute pancreatitis cases (perhaps 10%–20%) truly remain idiopathic.

Table 13.2 Other potential etiologies of acute pancreatitis

Crohn's disease	Ischemia
Scorpion venom	Organophosphate insecticides
Pancreatic carcinoma	Translumbar aortography
Duodenal amyloid deposition	Penetrating peptic ulcer
Brunner's gland hyperplasia of ampulla	

Etiologies of chronic pancreatitis

Alcohol

The most common etiology for chronic pancreatitis in adults is long-term ethanol abuse, accounting for approximately 70% to 80% of cases. In general, an intake of more than 80 g/day for at least 5 years is necessary to cause chronic pancreatitis. Studies have shown that the risk for developing chronic pancreatitis increases with increasing ethanol intake.

As in acute alcoholic pancreatitis, genetic factors also play a role. In Japan, specific alleles of the ADH and ALDH genes are found in patients with chronic alcoholic pancreatitis. Other alleles for these genes are not found in any patients with chronic alcoholic pancreatitis. This evidence supports a genetic predisposition for developing chronic alcoholic pancreatitis.

Racial factors may be important in the risk of chronic alcoholic pancreatitis. One recent study found that black patients who abused alcohol were two to three times more likely to develop chronic pancreatitis than white patients who abused alcohol. The explanation for this finding is unclear but may be related to differences in diet, body habitus, type or quantity of alcohol consumed, smoking, or genetic differences in detoxification capabilities.

Smoking

Many patients with chronic pancreatitis, regardless of its etiology, smoke cigarettes. A recent case-control study found highly significant odds ratios for the development of chronic pancreatitis in smokers. These findings were significant even for those consuming fewer than 20 cigarettes per day. Other work has shown that cigarette smoking is highly associated with the development of pancreatic calcifications in patients with late onset chronic pancreatitis. However, this same study found that calcification was not associated with smoking in patients with early onset chronic pancreatitis.

Hereditary causes

Cationic trypsinogen mutations

Chronic pancreatitis develops in approximately half of patients with hereditary pancreatitis who suffer acute attacks of pancreatitis. These acute attacks usually begin in childhood around the age of 10 to 12 years, and nearly 75% of patients will be symptomatic by 20 years of age. Approximately 100 families with hereditary pancreatitis have been studied. The mode of inheritance has been found to be autosomal dominant with 80% penetrance. Evidence suggests that those individuals who are asymptomatic carriers are truly unaffected at the histological level. Discordance of penetrance in monozygotic twins suggests that environmental factors are likely to play a significant role in determining phenotypic penetrance in individual cases of hereditary pancreatitis. Multiple phenotypic expressions were also identified relating to the age of onset of disease, disease severity, and type of pancreatitis (i.e. hemorrhagic, calcific, etc.).

Genetic linkage studies with microsatellite markers in large families revealed a linkage between hereditary pancreatitis and the long arm of chromosome 7 (7q35). Further work discovered that eight trypsinogen genes are located on chromosome 7q35. Through the evaluation of many of these hereditary pancreatitis families, three specific mutations in the cationic trypsinogen gene have been identified: (HP1) ARG117 HIS mutation, (HP2) ASP21 ISO mutation (a clinically less severe disease), and (HP3) ALA16 VAL mutation. Recently, several other new mutations to this gene have reportedly been identified.

Cystic fibrosis transmembrane regulator gene mutations

In one study, approximately one third of patients with idiopathic chronic pancreatitis had mutations in the cystic fibrosis transmembrane regulator gene, identified at locus 7q31. Furthermore, the frequency of cystic fibrosis transmembrane regulator gene gene mutations in idiopathic chronic pancreatitis patients was found to be increased sixfold. The genotypes observed in patients with idiopathic chronic pancreatitis were combinations of severe and mild mutations rather than two mild or two severe mutations. The phenotypic expression of cystic fibrosis in these patients is therefore generally mild. The most common mutations in the cystic fibrosis transmembrane regulator gene gene of idiopathic chronic pancreatitis patients are deletion of phenylalanine at residue 508, arginine-to-histidine substitution at residue 177 (R177H), and the 5T genotype of the polythymidine tract of intron 8. As the incidence of chronic pancreatitis in the parents of these patients with cystic fibrosis does not

appear to be significantly increased compared to the general population, it would appear that both alleles must be mutated in order for the risk of chronic pancreatitis to be increased. Therefore it is felt that this is, in all likelihood, an autosomal recessive disorder.

Serine protease inhibitor, kazal type 1

The serine protease inhibitor, kazal type 1 (SPINK1), also known as pancreatic secretory trypsin inhibitor, plays a major role in protecting the pancreas against prematurely activated trypsin. The SPINK1 gene codes for a 56-amino acid sequence. The SPINK1 gene is located in the region of chromosome 5q31, and two mutations of this gene have been identified (N34S, P55S). Available evidence suggests that SPINK1 mutations are associated with hereditary chronic pancreatitis and may even help to promote it. SPINK1 mutations are found at substantially higher levels (34%) in patients with idiopathic chronic pancreatitis as opposed to the general population (1%). However, the data suggest that SPINK1 mutations alone do not cause chronic pancreatitis but may lead to earlier presentation.

Other genetic considerations

Several families with autosomal dominant hereditary pancreatitis were found without linkage between the HP gene and a locus on chromosome 7. Subsequent studies have suggested that this form of hereditary pancreatitis was linked to a gene on the short arm of chromosome 12. It is likely that this gene will be identified in the near future.

Medications

Chronic abuse of the analgesics paracetamol and phenacetine is associated with the development of calcific chronic pancreatitis. One study found a 10% incidence of chronic pancreatitis attributed to analgesic abuse in patients with chronic nephropathy.

Autoimmune and inflammatory causes

Autoimmune causes

Autoimmune chronic pancreatitis can be primary or secondarily associated with other autoimmune disorders. Primary autoimmune pancreatitis is an extremely rare form of chronic pancreatitis which presents in the same manner as other types of autoimmune-associated pancreatitis, however, patients with this disorder are not affected by other immunologic disorders.

Approximately one third of patients with primary biliary cirrhosis will have morphological changes on pancreatography consistent with chronic pancreatitis. While many of these patients will also have evidence of pancreatic exocrine insufficiency on testing, few have clinically apparent chronic pancreatitis. Similar findings have also been noted in primary sclerosing cholangitis.

Sjögren's disease is an autoimmune syndrome that induces impairment of salivary and lacrimal glands. Recently, Sjögren's disease has been related to pancreatic exocrine involvement and chronic pancreatitis. A prospective case-control study has shown significant impairment of pancreatic exocrine function in patients with Sjögren's disease compared with controls.

Finally, while the CREST (calcinous, Raynaud's phenomenon, esophageal dysfunction, sclerodactyly and telangiectasia) syndrome and systemic lupus erythematosis have been found to be associated with chronic pancreatitis, these connective tissue disorders are more frequently associated with acute pancreatitis.

Inflammatory bowel disease

Numerous cases of pancreatitis occurring during the course of either Crohn's disease or ulcerative colitis have been described. However, in the overwhelming majority of cases, another cause, usually biliary-lithiasis or medication, is readily discovered. A very small minority of inflammatory bowel disease patients have idiopathic chronic pancreatitis. It is unclear whether idiopathic pancreatitis in these patients is merely coincidental or a very rare extraintestinal manifestation of inflammatory bowel disease.

Behçet's disease

Behçet's disease is a chronic, systemic disease characterized by relapsing iridocyclitis, orogenital lesions, and frequent involvement of the visceral organs (cardiovascular, pulmonary, neurological, articular, and gastrointestinal). Both acute and chronic pancreatitis have been reported in patients with Behçet's disease with acute pancreatitis being noted in approximately 2% to 3% of patients in one large autopsy series.

Antioxidants

Antioxidant levels have been measured in patients with recurrent acute pancreatitis, patients with chronic pancreatitis, and in healthy controls. It has been noted that certain antioxidant levels (selenium, vitamin A, vitamin E, beta-carotene, xanthine, beta-cryptoxanthine, and lycopene) are significantly lower in patients with chronic pancreatitis, particularly during painful exacerbations of the condition. This has led some to speculate that oxidative stress may be an etiological factor in chronic pancreatitis. However, antioxidant levels may be lower in patients with chronic pancreatitis, because of pancreatic exocrine dysfunction in these patients. No differences in antioxidant levels were noted between patients with recurrent acute pancreatitis and healthy controls.

Pancreas divisum

Pancreas divisum occurs when fusion between the ventral pancreatic duct of Wirsung and the dorsal pancreatic duct of Santorini is partial or absent. When such non-communication of the ducts occurs, a relatively larger proportion of pancreatic exocrine secretions must drain via the relatively small duct of Santorini through the accessory papilla. Pancreas divisum has also been noted in some patients with idiopathic chronic pancreatitis, and there are reports of pancreatitis limited to the dorsal pancreas. Furthermore, isolated ventral pancreatitis has also been reported in patients with pancreas divisum. This evidence has led some to conclude that this anatomic variant may predispose to pancreatitis. Pancreas divisum has a reported incidence of approximately 5% to 10% at autopsy and 2% to 7% at ERCP. One study found pancreas divisum present in approximately 25% of patients with idiopathic acute recurrent pancreatitis. However, subsequent studies have not confirmed an increased incidence of pancreas divisum in idiopathic pancreatitis. Therefore, at present it is not clear what etiologic role, if any, pancreas divisum plays in the development of pancreatitis.

Sphincter of Oddi dysfunction

In patients with manometrically confirmed sphincter of Oddi dysfunction, an association has been found with chronic pancreatitis. Specifically, one recent study found that patients with sphincter of Oddi dysfunction were more than four times as likely to have chronic pancreatitis as those without sphincter of Oddi dysfunction. Of note, the investigators found that those patients with sphincter of Oddi dysfunction who did not have pancreatitis were significantly younger than those with chronic pancreatitis (43 years versus 55 years). It is likely that risk of developing chronic pancreatitis increases with age and duration of sphincter of Oddi dysfunction in these patients.

Tropical pancreatitis

Tropical pancreatitis (also referred to as tropical calcific/calculous pancreatitis, juvenile tropical pancreatitis, and nutritional pancreatitis) was first described in 1995 in a report describing 18 cases of diffuse pancreatic calcification in young non-alcoholic individuals in Indonesia. This form of chronic pancreatitis occurs mostly in children and young adults in developing countries. The highest incidence of tropical pancreatitis appears to occur in the southern Indian state of Kerala with a reported prevalence of 1 in 500 to 800 people. The disease is seen less frequently in northern and western India, Sri Lanka, and Bangladesh. There are reported cases of this disease from southeast Asia (Indonesia, Thailand, Malaysia), Africa (Nigeria, Uganda, Burundi, Zaire, and Malawi), and South America (Brazil).

The exact etiology of tropical pancreatitis is unknown. Factors implicated include malnutrition, dietary toxins, and possible genetic disposition. Early observations of patients with tropical pancreatitis described a state of emaciation and severe malnutrition leading some to conclude that protein-calorie malnutrition is a causative factor in this disorder. However, others, citing evidence that Kerala has one of the highest health standards and lowest infant mortality rates within India, feel that malnutrition is actually an effect rather than the cause of tropical pancreatitis. Furthermore, the pancreatic fibrosis and calculi seen in tropical pancreatitis rarely occur in patients with malnutrition. Finally, it has been postulated that a low dietary fat intake may predispose to pancreatic calcification, but dietary surveys have shown no significant difference in diet between patients with tropical pancreatitis and controls.

Another potential etiologic factor for tropical pancreatitis is the cyanogenic glycosides (linnamarin and methyl linnamarin) present in cassava roots (e.g. tapioca) that are the major source of diet in many of the high-incidence countries. Consumption of large quantities of cassava, especially if it is improperly cooked or stored, can lead to chronic cyanide poisoning. Other plant species (e.g. millets) also contain cyanogenic glycosides. These glycosides are thought to cause pancreatic damage by a number of mechanisms. A case-control study, however, failed to find a relationship between cassava consumption and tropical pancreatitis. Furthermore, the disease has been seen in patients who have never consumed cassava, and chronic cassava ingestion does not lead to acute or chronic pancreatitis in a rat model.

Finally, a genetic predisposition to this disease has been postulated because of reported familial clustering and the development of tropical pancreatitis in the children of immigrants from Kerala to western countries. However, human leukocyte antigen studies have not identified any specific predisposition, nor have any specific genetic mutations been found. Therefore, the precise etiology for tropical pancreatitis is yet to be elucidated.

Pediatric chronic pancreatitis

In contrast to adults, alcohol is a rare cause of chronic pancreatitis in children. Pediatric chronic pancreatitis takes two forms, obstructive (non-calcific) and calcific. Obstructive pancreatitis may be due to trauma resulting in focal chronic scarring, duct disruption, or duct compression. Traumatic pancreatic injuries in children, as in adults, may also be acute and self-limited. Congenital duct anomalies such as pancreas divisum, choledochal cysts, pancreatic duct duplication, or renal cysts, may cause chronic obstructive pancreatitis.

Sclerosing pancreaticocholangitis is a rare disorder that can cause chronic pancreatitis in children. It is characterized by stricturing of the pancreaticobiliary tree remarkably similar to that seen in primary sclerosing cholangitis, however, this disorder is not associated with ulcerative colitis or Crohn's disease.

Chronic calcific pancreatitis in the pediatric population can be due to tropical pancreatitis, hypercalcemia, hypertriglyceridemia, and hereditary factors. These specific etiologies are each discussed in more detail in earlier sections. Finally, it should be noted that the cause of chronic pancreatitis in children is often idiopathic.

Further reading

Chwistek M, Roberts I, Amoateng-Adjepong Y. Gallstone pancreatitis. A community teaching hospital experience. *J Clin Gastroenterol* 2001; 33(1): 41–44.

Gottlieb K, Sherman S. ERCP and endoscopic biliary sphincterotomy-induced pancreatitis. *Gastrointest Endosc Clin North Am* 1998; 8: 87–114.

Kohut M, Nowak A, Nowakowska-Dulawa E, Kaczor R, Marek T. The frequency of bile duct crystals in patients with presumed biliary pancreatitis. *Gastrointest Endosc* 2001; 54(1): 37–41.

McArthur KE. Review article: drug-induced pancreatitis. *Aliment Pharmacol Ther* 1996; 10: 23–38.

Perrault J. Hereditary pancreatitis, historical perspectives. *Med Clin North Am* 2000; 84(3): 519–529.

Runzi M, Layer P. Drug-associated pancreatitis: facts and fiction, *Pancreas* 1996; 13(1): 100–109.

Sakorafas GH, Tsiotou A. Etiology and pathogenesis of acute pancreatitis, *J Clin Gastroenterol* 2000; 30(4): 343–356.

Topazian M, Gorelick FS. Acute pancreatitis. In: Yamada T, Alpers DH, Laine L, Owyang C, Powell DW (eds) *Textbook of Gastroenterology* 3rd edn. Lippincott Williams & Wilkins, Philadelphia, 1999; pp 2124–2132.

Whitcomb DC. Genetic predispositions to acute and chronic pancreatitis. *Med Clin North Am* 2000; 84(3): 531–547.

Chapter 14

Pathophysiology of Pancreatitis

William B. Long

CHAPTER OUTLINE

Acute pancreatitis

For the past century acute pancreatitis has been regarded as an "autodigestive" disease initiated by inappropriate activation of trypsin in the pancreas. The pathophysiology of acute pancreatitis now appears to be more complicated. Acute pancreatitis is a multiorgan illness. Initial activation of trypsin may occur within acinar cells, rather than in the pancreatic interstitium or ducts as previously thought. Acinar-cell injury is followed by a local inflammatory cascade that potentially leads to pancreatic necrosis, systemic inflammatory response syndrome, and sys-temic organ dysfunction. During the first several days of disease, systemic repercussions, including shock and acute respiratory distress, rather than pancreatic injury *per se*, cause much of the morbidity and mortality. After the first week, superimposed infection with augmentation of systemic inflammatory response may occur, adding to morbidity and mortality. The pathologic events of acute pancreatitis may be separated into four sequential, but overlapping and interacting, phases

- trypsin activation in acinar cells
- cytokines, inflammation and necrosis in the pancreas
- systemic inflammatory response
- infection.

Unless there is extensive necrosis complete resolution of pancreatic injury usually occurs. Although necrotizing pancreatitis is more lethal than non-necrotizing pancreatitis, deaths in the first week from the systemic inflammatory response can occur without marked pancreatic necrosis. Why some patients develop only limited inflammatory response and others severe systemic inflammation is poorly understood. Current therapy for acute pancreatitis is empiric but when vigorous appears to have improved outcomes. Therapies designed to correct the underlying pathology of pancreatitis have shown much promise in animal models, but need careful evaluation in humans. Clinical trials must consider the complex pathology of pancreatitis and its time course. Treatments that work prophylactically may be totally ineffective several hours after onset or later in the course of the disease. Great care must be taken since some therapies are two-edged swords. Anti-inflammatory therapy such as interleukin-10 (IL-10) might be beneficial early, but may later reduce the immune response and aggravate infection.

Progress in understanding the pathophysiology of pancreatitis has involved clinical observations, application of molecular biologic techniques, and the development of animal models. The two most common animal models are pancreatitis produced in mice or rats by supramaximal cerulein stimulation or by bile-salt injection into the pancreatic duct. Cerulein is an analog of cholecystokinin and at lower doses stimulates pancreatic secretion. Intraperitoneal or intravenous injections of doses several times those required for maximal secretory response produces acute pancreatitis. Paradoxically, such supramaximal stimulation inhibits normal apical acinar cell secretion of enzymes. Pancreatitis in the cerulein model is relatively mild with only spotty necrosis. Intraductal injection of bile-salt solution produces a more severe necrotizing pancreatitis. Pancreatitis can also be produced in animal models by choline-deficient and ethionine-supplemented diet, and by obstruction of the pancreatic duct.

The animal species used in experimental pancreatitis can affect outcome. For instance, bile-duct obstruction in rats leads to edema, mild inflammatory cell infiltration, and apoptosis followed by atrophy. In contrast, obstruction of the pancreatic duct in the opossum produces necrotizing pancreatitis. There is greater infiltration of the pancreas by neutophils in the opossum than in the rat and differences in the type of cell death in the two models may reflect differences in inflammatory cell infiltration. Other experimental conditions may affect the severity of pancreatitis. For example, feeding or intravenous cholecystokinin exacerbate the pancreatitis in rats with ligation of the pancreatic duct.

Once initiated, pancreatitis of different etiologies may have similar pathophysiology. There is little understanding of the earliest molecular events through which diverse etiologies such as alcoholism, gallstones, medications, hypercalcemia, hypertriglyceridemia, or the various animal models initiate pancreatitis.

Inappropriate trypsin activation

The pancreas synthesizes and secretes large amounts of enzymes but is protected against autodigestion by several mechanisms. Proteolytic enzymes are synthesized and secreted as inactive proenzymes. Sequestering the enzymes in secretory zymogen granules provides further protection. A trypsin inhibitor in the secretory granules (SPINK1 or PSTI) is capable of inactivating inappropriately activated trypsin. SPINK1 is secreted with trypsinogen into the acinar lumen. There is sufficient SPINK1 to inactivate 10% of the total potential trypsin activity in acinar cells. If trypsin becomes activated within an acinar cell in excess of the amount that SPINK1 can inhibit, there are cytosolic proteases that can lyse limited amounts. In addition, there are non-specific protease inhibitors (alpha-1-antitrypsin and alpha-2-macroglobulin) in the interstitium and blood.

Under physiologic stimulation, proenzymes are secreted at the apical portion of the acinar cell and are activated in the intestine. Activation is initiated by the intestinal brush border enzyme enterokinase splitting off a portion of the proenzyme trypsinogen producing a peptide fragment called trypsin-activating peptide and trypsin. Trypsin then can activate trypsinogen or other proteolytic proenzymes. If other substrates are not abundant in the intestinal lumen trypsin digests itself.

Several lines of evidence indicate that inappropriate activation of trypsin in pancreatic acinar cells is a major, and probably the major, initiating event of acute pancreatitis. Active trypsin is found in the pancreas consistently during the earliest stages of acute clinical or experimental pancreatitis. Trypsinogen activation occurs within 10 minutes of supramaximal cerulein stimulation in rats. Trypsin production is detected as early as morphologic injury.

The earliest ultrastructural changes include dilation of endoplasmic reticulum and formation of cytoplasmic vacuoles containing fragments of organelles. Apical secretion of zymogen granules is interrupted and enzymes leak abnormally from the basolateral portion of the cell into the acinar interstitium. *In vitro*, acinar cells stimulated supramaximally with cerulein manifest similar colocalization of zymogen granules and lysosomal hydrolases, trypsinogen activation, and cell injury. *In vivo*, enzymes or proenzymes are found in high concentration in lymph and portal blood draining the pancreas. Trypsin-activating peptide appears in acinar cells, serum and urine, within hours of onset. Although they may not have a pathologic role, other enzymes such as lipase and amylase are also elevated in serum at this very early stage.

Intracellular activation of trypsin may be triggered by colocalization of zymogen granules and lysosomes containing hydrolases, such as cathepsin B. Cathepsin B has been shown to activate trypsinogen *in vitro* and electron microscopy has demonstrated colocalization with trypsinogen in organelles in experimental pancreatitis. The role of

Table 14.1 Experimental acute pancreatitis

Noxious agent/event	Therapeutic benefit
Trypsin activation	antitrypsin (gabexate)
	cathepsin B knockout
Inflammatory cytokines	interleukin-1 receptor antagonist
	anti-tumor necrosis factor antibody
	tumor necrosis factor, interleukin-1, and interleukin-6 knockouts
	veno-venous hemofiltration
	glucocorticoids
Platelet activating factor	platelet activating factor inhibitors
Kinins	bradykinin inhibitor
Neutrophils	anti-neutrophil antibody
Inadequate anti-inflammatory	interleukin-10 and interleukin-10 gene therapy
	induction of heat shock proteins
Nuclear transcription factor	nuclear transcription factor inhibitor
Intercellular adhesion molecule	intercellular adhesion molecule knockout/antibody
Reactive oxygen species	antioxidants
	vitamin E
	N-acetyl cystine
Microcirculatory injury	hyperbaric oxygen
	intravenous dextran
Phospholipase A2	phospholipase A2 inhibitor
Matrix metalloproteinases	matrix metalloproteinases inhibitor
Bacterial translocation	prophylactic antibiotics
	enteral feeding
	epidermal growth factor
	veno-venous hemofiltration
Autoimmune activity	glucocorticoid
Capillary leakage	endothelin receptor antagonist
	intercellular adhesion molecule antibody
	thromboxane A2 antagonist

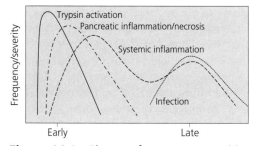

Figure 14.1 Phases of acute pancreatitis.

cathepsin B has been studied in mice genetically deficient in cathepsin B. These mice, which are phenotypically indistinguishable from wild-type mice, have been studied with the cerulein suprastimulation model of pancreatitis. In cathepsin B-deficient mice subjected to supramaximal cerulein, intracellular trypsin activity is reduced by 80% and pancreatic necrosis by 50%. Nevertheless, since a small amount of intracellular trypsin is activated in these deficient mice, it appears that cathepsin B is not the only factor involved in premature trypsinogen activation. Furthermore, the rate of apoptosis (about 9% of cells), neutrophil infiltration into pan-

creas and lung, and pulmonary edema did not differ in normal and cathepsin B-deficient mice. The findings suggest that substantial trypsin activation may not be necessary for the systemic and pancreatic inflammatory responses.

In the cerulein model less than 1% of the total trypsinogen in the pancreas is converted to active trypsin. The amount of trypsinogen in the thoracic duct in the first few hours of stimulation markedly exceeds the amount of trypsin-activating peptide, indicating that there has been only limited activation of trypsin even though trypsinogen is leaking from the basolateral cell membrane. Further activation of interstitial trypsinogen by infusing enterokinase intravenously produces severe necrotizing pancreatitis. These experiments indicate that trypsin activation may be a multi-stage process with varying outcomes and that greater activation of trypsin will produce more severe disease.

Inactivation of trypsin can prevent or ameliorate pancreatitis but this occurs only if the inhibitors are administered before disease is established. Gabexate mesilate is a potent protease inhibitor that can penetrate acinar cells because of its small molecular size. Given prophyllactically it reduces ERCP-induced and experimental pancreatitis, but has questionable benefit if given following onset of pancreatitis in animals or human trials.

Genetic influences (cationic trypsinogen and SPINK)

Minimal colocalization of zymogen granules and lysozomes has been observed in normal acinar cells. Presumably SPINK1 can inactivate the small amounts of trypsin produced by such colocalization. Genetic abnormalities in SPINK1 have been identified in about 2% of healthy subjects, indicating that such abnormalities alone do not cause disease. However, earlier onset of chronic idiopathic pancreatitis in patients with SPINK1 mutations indicates that such mutations are disease modifying. One group of investigators found mutations in the SPINK1 gene in 12% of chronic pancreatitis patients. No role for SPINK1 mutations in acute pancreatitis has yet been shown.

In 1996 genetic linkage studies of families with hereditary pancreatitis revealed an abnormality in the long arm of chromosome 7. A single point mutation was shown to result in an arginine (R) to histidine (H) substitution at residue 117 in the amino acid sequence of cationic trypsinogen, the residue where autolysis of trypsin would normally begin. The R117H mutant trypsin appears resistant to autolysis. Mutant trypsin that escapes inactivation by SPINK1 may, therefore, cause cell injury. Other mutations including N29I, A16V, and K23R have been identified. The mechanism of pancreatitis associated with these mutations is debated. Mutations R117H and N29I have a high penetrance dominant pattern of pancreatitis, but not all patients with these mutations develop disease.

Pancreatic inflammation

Immediately following the initial disruptive changes in acinar cells, edema develops in the pancreatic interstitium, cytokines are released and inflammatory cells invade the pancreas. These inflammatory processes may further aggravate the pathologic changes in acinar cells.

Interstitial edema and disruption of tight junctions

The initial stages of acute pancreatitis are characterized by proteolytic degradation of cytoskeleton of acinar cells. Similar destruction occurs at cell-to-cell contacts known as tight junctions at the intersection of the apical and basolateral domains of acinar cells. Extravasation of protein-rich fluid from abnormally permeable pancreatic blood vessels distends the interstitial space creating pancreatic edema within the first hour of cerulein hyperstimulation. Concurrent with edema is a nearly complete interruption of ductal secretion and a significant increase in levels of pancreatic enzymes in peripheral blood. Under healthy conditions the tight junctions restrict molecular movement from the acinus and pancreatic ducts. Disruption of these junctions contributes to interstitial edema and interruption in pancreatic secretion. Enzymes that leak into the interstitial fluid enter the peripheral blood via portal blood drainage and via the marked increase in pancreatic lymph drainage noted in acute pancreatitis. In mild cerulein pancreatitis repair of tight junctions and resorption of interstitial fluid begins within several hours. Restoration of cell-to-cell contacts is one of the earliest detectable signs of repair.

Cytokines

Increased cytokines appear within the pancreas in the earliest stages of experimental pancreatitis and within peripheral blood shortly after pain onset in humans. Cytokine production is induced by activation of the nuclear transcription factor-kB (NF-kB) that translocates from the cytoplasm into the nucleus and stimulates cytokine promoter genes.

Cytokines are a group of low molecular weight proteins that communicate between cells by interacting with specific cell surface receptors. Multiple cell types, including acinar cells, leukocytes, and macrophages, produce cytokines. Some cytokines are pro-inflammatory and others anti-inflammatory. One cytokine may enhance production of others and even of itself, leading to an amplification of the inflammatory response. Cytokines are not constitutively expressed, but when produced in response to stress they are effective in minute (fentomolar) concentrations. Pro-inflammatory cytokines include TNFα, IL-1, IL-6, IL-8, and platelet activating factor. Interleukin-10 and IL-1 receptor antagonists are anti-inflammatory. Pro-inflammatory cytokines attract and activate neutrophils and promote neutrophil adhesion to vascular endothelium, diapedesis, and migration into tissue. Associated with production of cytokines is increased generation of cytokine receptor proteins on cells. Although tissue levels are responsible for most of the biologic effects of cytokines, elevated serum levels cause fever, hypotension, and disseminated intravascular coagulation.

Experimental pancreatitis models implicate IL-1 and TNF as major initial cytokines in pancreatic and systemic injury. Production occurs within 30 minutes of induction of pancreatitis and concentrations in the pancreas are several times those seen in the blood. Tumor necrosis factor is actively cleared from portal blood by the liver and this may explain the relatively low levels appearing in peripheral blood. Although acinar cells produce some IL-1 and TNF, invading leukocytes and macrophages are the predominant sources. Transgenic animals devoid of receptors for IL-1 and TNF do not develop as severe pancreatitis as wild type animals. About 70% of knock-out mice lacking TNF survive for 6 days after initiation of pancreatitis compared with 25% of wild-type animals. Blocking TNF with specific antibodies also decreases pancreatic edema, necrosis, inflammation, and mortality. Although IL-1 and TNF intensify the severity of pancreatitis they do not, in themselves, initiate pancreatitis. Perfusion of isolated pancreas with IL-1 or TNF does not result in colocalization of zymogen granules and lysosomes, or induce pancreatitis.

Interleukin-6 and IL-8 and platelet activating factor are other important inflammatory mediators. Interleukin-6 induces pyrexia and stimulates synthesis of acute phase proteins, including C reactive protein, from hepatocytes. Interleukin-1, TNF, and endotoxin stimulate production of IL-6, and serum IL-6 in clinical pancreatitis correlates with disease severity. Interleukin-8 is a potent chemokine (a type of cytokine which attracts and activates leukocytes) and increased levels in clinical pancreatitis also predict morbidity. Early administration of hydrocortisone has been reported to reduce inflammatory cytokines, arachidonic acid breakdown products, and improve survival in animals.

Platelet activating factor is a low molecular weight phospholipid that binds to cell surface receptors of numerous cells including platelets, leukocytes, and endothelial cells. Intravascular or intraperitoneal injection of platelet activating factor in animals increases the severity of pancreatitis and platelet activating factor inhibitors given early in animal models have been beneficial. Nevertheless, a potent platelet activating factor inhibitor (Lexipafant®) given within 48 hours of pain onset in a large randomized human trial was completely ineffective.

Elevations of kinins are reported to play a role in the local and peripheral circulatory disturbances of acute pancreatitis. In experimental pancreatitis bradykinin is elevated in peritoneal exudates, lymph, and plasma. Exogenously administered bradykinin causes vasodilation, hypotension, and increased vascular permeability. Urinary trypsin-activating peptide and mortality of pancreatitis are significantly lower in animals pretreated with a new potent inhibitor of bradykinin (Icatibant®). Decreased urinary trypsin-activating peptide after Icatibant® indicates that kinins may augment trypsinogen activation in pancreatitis.

Anti-inflammatory factors: cytokines and heat shock protein

Anti-inflammatory events may compensate for some of the inflammatory factors described above. Early or prophylactic treatment with anti-inflammatory cytokines (IL-10 and IL-1 receptor antagonist) or induction of heat shock protein decreases the severity of experimental pancreatitis. A study published in 2002 describes marked reduction in mortality of rats transfected with the gene for human IL-10 30 minutes after bile-salt induction of severe pancreatitis. Interleukin-10 production in pancreas, liver, and lung persisted for 3 days but was not increased over baseline at 1 week. This late decline in IL-10 production is thought to be important since IL-10 could suppress an immune response to infection. There is also human data suggesting a protective effect of IL-10. Survival correlates with the level of IL-10 in bronchoalveolar lavage fluid of patients with adult respiratory distress syndrome. Serum IL-10 is increased in parallel with inflammatory cytokines IL-6 and IL-8 during the first several days of severe clinical pancreatitis. Patients who are genetically unable to mount as vigorous an IL-10 response tend to develop more severe pancreatitis. Conflicting results have been reported regarding the effectiveness of a single prophylactic dose of IL-10 before ERCP. Since the half-life of IL-10 is short, one wonders if repeated doses are needed.

Heat shock proteins are a group of proteins that are increased in many cell types in response to stress. In non-stressed cells these proteins are believed to act as "molecular chaperones" accompanying newly synthesized proteins through various intracellular compartments. Stressed cells translate heat shock proteins to the exclusion of other messages and the heat shock proteins produced exert a protective effect against cellular injury. Prophylactic induction of heat shock proteins by water immersion reduces intracellular activation of trypsin and ameliorates the severity of cerulein-induced pancreatitis. Whether heat shock proteins are involved as a defense mechanism after induction of pancreatitis is unknown.

Nuclear factor-kB

Nuclear factor-kB (NF-kB) activation in acinar cells appears to be an important pathologic event in acute pancreatitis. Nuclear factor-kB is a family of proteins that bind to DNA and activate a multitude of cellular stress-related genes including genes for cytokines and adhesion molecules. In the nonstressed cell NF-kB is kept inactive in the cytoplasmin by inhibitory proteins. Certain cytokines or trypsin injury can activate NF-kB. The feedback link of cytokines and NF-kB provides a pathway by which an inflammatory response may be amplified. Pancreatitis produced by both cerulein superstimulation and intraductal bile salt is characterized by synchronous activation of NF-kB and trypsin. The similar time course and requirement of calcium for both NF-kB and trypsin activation suggest that the two processes are mechanistically linked. But inhibition of NF-kB activation does not prevent trypsinogen activation and supraphysiologic CCK can stimulate NF-kB production in cells lacking trypsinogen. Therefore, it appears that trypsinogen and NF-kB can be activated independently. On the other hand, trypsin in the cell causes cell stress and, like other stressful stimuli, would be expected to activate NF-kB. Furthermore, inflammatory cells recruited by NF-kB-induced cytokines can lead to greater trypsin activation. In acute pancreatitis, as in other inflammatory conditions, there is the possibility of numerous interactive damaging events.

Activation of NF-kB occurs in two phases in rats suprastimulated with cerulein. The first phase peaks within 30 minutes and before inflammatory cells infiltrate the pancreas. The second phase occurs a few hours later when inflammatory cells are abundant in the pancreas. Interleukin-1, TNF, and platelet activating factor released by inflammatory cells appear to contribute to this second phase of NF-kB production. Antioxidants such as N-acetylcysteine block this late activation of NF-kB, indicating that reactive oxygen intermediates are involved. These treatments that inhibit NF-kB production lessen the severity of cerulein pancreatitis. Similar findings are reported in the more severe bile-salt infusion model of pancreatitis.

Inflammatory cells, intercellular adhesion molecule-1, and reactive oxygen species

Although the trigger for the cascade of inflammatory mediators is in acinar cells, inflammatory cells including macrophages, neutophils, and lymphocytes amplify cytokine release and cause much of the injury to the pancreas and other organs. Microscopic and nuclear medicine studies show marked pancreatic invasion by macrophages and leukocytes in the early stages of human and experimental pancreatitis. Neutrophils are attracted by cytokines and transverse vascular endothelium in which intercellular adhesion molecule-1 (ICAM-1) has been induced. Under physiologic conditions ICAM-1 is minimally expressed but is upregulated in pancreatitis by cytokines such as IL-1. Mice that have a homozygous deficiency in production of ICAM-1 develop less severe cerulein pancreatitis than do wild-type mice, as measured by pancreatic necrosis, edema, and mortality. A similar reduction in severity is noted in mice depleted of neutrophils by anti-neutrophil serum.

Platelet activating factor is one of the factors that activates and attracts neutophils in experimental pancreatitis. Platelet activating factor increases in the pancreas and systemically during acute pancreatitis. Prophylactic use of antagonists of platelet activating factor markedly reduces pancreatic inflammation and acinar cell necrosis experimentally. In a large clinical study, however, a potent inhibitor of platelet activating factor did not improve the outcome of pancreatitis even though used within the first 48 hours of the attack; it is possible that 48 hours is too late for an inhibitor to be effective.

Activated neutrophils may injure acinar cells by discharge of reactive oxygen species such as superoxide, hydrogen peroxide, and nitric oxide. Neutrophils infiltrating the pancreas have been shown to augment intracellular trypsin activation, and this trypsin activation is reduced in rats genetically lacking in enzymes that produce reactive oxygen species. Reactive oxygen species oxidized trypsinogen is more susceptible to activation by intracellular serine proteases.

Microscopic studies employing antibodies against trypsin-activating peptide show that the trypsin activation mediated by neutrophils occurs within the acinar cell. Neutrophils are responsible for most intrapancreatic trypsin activation in the cerulein model. Rats, depleted of neutrophils before cerulein stimulation, increase pancreatic trypsin to levels only 20% and 33% of levels seen in animals with normal levels of neutrophils. These investigations suggest that trypsin activation in acute pancreatitis is a two-phase event mediated initially by neutrophil independent mechanisms, and subsequently by neutrophil dependent mechanisms.

Microcirculatory injury

Microcirculatory vasoconstriction, stasis, increased vascular permeability, and ischemia may amplify pancreatic injury in acute pancreatitis and promote necrosis. These changes have been attributed to a host of noxious factors including reactive oxygen metabolites, cytokines, platelet activating factor, adhesions molecules, kinins, endothelin, prostaglandins, and proteolytic enzymes. Many of the harmful effects are mediated by leukocytes. Increased capillary permeability in the pancreas and systemically probably contributes to hemoconcentration which has been identified as a prognosticator of adverse outcome. Capillary permeability has been significantly decreased in experimental pancreatitis by use of antibody against ICAM and by antagonists against platelet activating factor, endothelin receptors, and thromboxane. Hyperbaric oxygen improved pancreatic pathology caused by intraductal bile salts. Normalization of circulatory volume with intravenous dextran reduces acinar necrosis, counteracts the impairment of pancreatic microcirculation caused by intravenous radiographic contrast, and improves survival in animal models.

Systemic inflammatory response

Approximately 80% of patients with acute pancreatitis have a rather mild disease. The others have severe and often, but not always, necrotizing pancreatitis with a 20% to 50% mortality. The inflammatory response in the pancreas initiates a systemic inflammatory response syndrome mediated by pancreatic enzymes (especially trypsin, phospholipase, and elastase), cytokines, kinins, and activated neutrophils. The systemic inflammation, rather than pancreatic disease *per se*, accounts for most of the mortality in the first several days of disease. Systemic complications including fever, shock, renal failure, pleural effusions, and acute respiratory distress syndrome often become apparent many hours after the onset of clinical disease. This lag between onset of pain and development of complications may provide a potential therapeutic window.

Continuous veno-venous hemofiltration recently was reported to improve survival and reduce serum TNF in necrotizing porcine pancreatitis. Continuous veno-venous hemofiltration was begun after a 30% fall in peripheral resistance, presumably when pancreatitis is quite advanced.

Trypsin-activating peptide levels were no different in treated and control animals suggesting that either continuous veno-venous hemofiltration did not reduce continued trypsin activation, or it was begun when trypsin activation had ceased. Attenuation of serum TNF was related to removal of TNF in the hemofiltrate.

Acute respiratory distress syndrome

Acute respiratory distress syndrome is the most common cause of death in the first several days of clinical and experimental pancreatitis. The lung injury is characterized by infiltration of inflammatory cells, especially neutrophils, increased alveolar capillary permeability, interstitial edema, and hyalinization of alveolar membranes. It is pathologically indistinguishable from acute respiratory distress syndrome of sepsis. In the lung, as in the pancreas, migration of neutrophils into the parenchyma is associated with an increase in ICAM-1 and the process causing injury is oxygen radical mediated. Depletion of neutrophils or blockage of neutrophil adhesion with antibodies against ICAM-1 reduces lung injury.

After transversing the capillary endothelium neutrophils must also penetrate the alveolar basement membrane before entering the alveolar space and causing hyalinization of alveolar membranes. Penetration of basement membrane matrix is associated with production of specific matrix metalloproteinases by polymorphonuclear granulocytes. Matrix metalloproteinases are endopeptidases with specificities for collagens, fibronectins, and gelatin of the extracellular matrix. Matrix metalloproteinases are not found in normal lung but are highly expressed in lungs of animals with severe pancreatitis and to a lesser degree in animals with mild pancreatitis. Levels of matrix metalloproteinases increase significantly by 6 hours and peak by 12 hours after induction of pancreatitis. Matrix metalloproteinases are found in the supernatant of neutrophil cultures in pancreatitis. *In vitro*, trypsin, IL-1B, and TNF stimulate matrix metalloproteinase release from human neutrophils. Treatment of animals with an inhibitor of matrix metalloproteinases significantly reduces alveolar capillary leakage and exudation into the alveolar space.

Other factors may be involved in acute respiratory distress syndrome associated with acute pancreatitis. Pancreatic elastase injected intraperitoneally in mice activates pulmonary NF-kB and TNF with subsequent neutrophil infiltration and pulmonary vascular leakage. This lung injury is markedly reduced in TNF knock out animals.

Platelet activating factor may also play a role. In a model of severe pancreatitis produced in the opossum by ligation of the biliopancreatic duct, administration of a platelet activating factor inactivating enzyme prevented lung injury. But, as mentioned previously, a potent inhibitor of platelet activating factor had no beneficial effect in a large human trial. These variable effects emphasize that experimental findings must be carefully evaluated in patients.

Another agent of injury may be phospholipase A that digests lecithin, a component of lung surfactant. Increased serum phospholipase A is reported in human and experimental pancreatitis, and correlates with the degree of respiratory failure in some studies. An inhibitor of phospholipase A2 has been shown to prevent experimental pancreatitis-associated lung injury. But levels of phospholipase A2 may not correlate with survival.

Other systemic complications

Other systemic complications of acute pancreatitis have not been as well evaluated as acute respiratory distress syndrome. Hypotension and shock are attributed to hypovolemia, vasoactive peptides, and possibly to a myocardial depressant. Hypovolemia reflects loss of volume caused by increased vascular permeability into "third spaces" such as pleural effusions, ascites, and peripancreatic edema. Marked vascular endothelial apoptosis has been reported with the systemic capillary leak syndrome in acute pancreatitis. Oxidative injury of endothelial cells may be a cause of the apoptosis. Elevated bradykinin is reported to contribute to hypotension in experimental models by increasing vascular permeability and dilation.

Hypertension is noted on admission to hospital in about 30% of patients. Speculations as to the cause of hypertension include increased sympathetic response to pain or a vascular response to an unidentified vasoactive substance. Expanded blood volume is certainly not a factor and medication to lower blood pressure should generally be avoided. Patients with hypertension are somewhat more likely to have a complicated course than those patients whose blood pressure is normal on admission. The hypertension resolves in most patients with improvement in the pancreatitis.

Acute tubular necrosis may result from hypotension, hypovolemia, or systemic toxins. Patients with acute pancreatitis have a marked increase in renal clearance of amylase and other small proteins, thought to reflect tubular dysfunction. The cause of the tubular dysfunction is unclear.

Hypocalcemia reflects hypoalbuminemia, binding of calcium by free fatty acids, and possibly inadequate parathyroid response. Diabetes and pancreatic exocrine insufficiency can be induced by extensive pancreatic necrosis. *De novo* hyperglycemia is an indicator of severe disease in humans.

Infection

About a third of patients with severe necrotizing pancreatitis develop superimposed infection of necrotic pancreas or other serious systemic infection. The highest risk is in the second and third week and infection is the cause of most fatalities after the first week of pancreatitis. Sepsis can induce a systemic inflammatory response similar to that of uninfected severe pancreatitis. Infecting organisms include gram-negative species (*Escherichia coli*, *Proteus*, *Pseudomonas* and *Klebsiella*), other aerobes (enterococci, *Staphyloccci aureus*) and a variety of anaerobes. Fungal infections are increasing in frequency with more widespread use of antibiotics. Most infections are polymicrobial. The probable source of bacteria is the intestine, with bacteria reaching the pancreas by translocation into lymphatics or blood, or by spreading directly to contiguous pancreas. It is unclear if the large or small bowel, or both, is the major source of bacteria. A study in which enclosing the colon in an impermeable bag reduced pancreatic infection suggests that the colon may be a source of bacteria.

Bacterial translocation, defined as the passage of viable bacteria from the gastrointestinal tract to mesenteric lymph nodes, has been found in shock, burn patients, bile-duct obstruction, intestinal obstruction, and acute pancreatitis. Bacterial translocation is attributed to an alteration in intestinal microflora, increased intestinal permeability, and impairment of host immunity. Each of these defects has been described in acute pancreatitis. Increased intestinal gram-negative organisms have been identified in clinical and experimental pancreatitis. Intestinal propulsion is dramatically reduced and this altered motility is associated with overgrowth of small bowel bacteria. Although not usually associated with overt ischemia, splanchnic hypoperfusion has been demonstrated in acute clinical pancreatitis by monitoring gastric mucosal pH. Mucosal pH is lower in patients developing organ failure. Such hypoperfusion may lead to increased permeability to endotoxin as well as bacteria. Villous height is diminished in acute pancreatitis and decreased mucus production has been associated with bacterial translocation. Alterations in immune response have been identified and include depression of phagocytosis by monocytes, lymphopenia, and a decrease in T helper cells. Effects of cytokines and alterations in gut-associated lymphoid tissue are potentially important.

The previously mentioned study of continuous veno-venous hemofiltration in porcine pancreatitis indicates that this therapy may reduce bacterial translocation and improve immune response in severe pancreatitis. The therapy reduced bacteremia from 100% to 31% of animals at 24 hours. Endotoxin levels and phagocytosis by neutrophils were also improved in treated animals.

Whole gut washout with polyethylene glycol has been shown to reduce translocation and improve survival in rats with bile-duct ligation pancreatitis.

Epidermal growth factor, prophylactic antibiotics, and enteral feeding have been suggested as therapies to prevent bacterial translocation and infection in acute pancreatitis. Epidermal growth factor is a peptide in mucosal fluids such as saliva, bile pancreatic juice, and duodenal secretions. It increases villous height and decreases bacterial translocation in experimental pancreatitis. Prophylactic antibiotics reduce infection in animal models and may have been beneficial in human trials. Unfortunately, the clinical trials have been small and unblinded and their results should be interpreted with caution. Enteral feeding has been proposed as a way to correct intestinal flora and atrophy but clinical trials suffer from the same defects as the trials of prophylactic antibiotics.

Specific etiologies

Gallstones

Gallstones are found consistently in the stools of patients during the recovery phase of gallstone pancreatitis. It is unclear, however, if the passage of stones through the papilla of Vater provokes or ameliorates the pancreatitis. Endoscopic identification of stones lodged in the papilla early in acute pancreatitis suggests that impaction of stones rather than their passage causes disease. Anecdotal reports that endoscopic removal of such impacted stones improves pancreatitis also favor impaction as a cause. Impaction has been postulated to cause pancreatitis either by obstructing the pancreatic duct or by allowing bile to reflux into the pancreas if obstruction occurs in the distal portion of a common bile and pancreatic channel. The common channel theory is suspect since a common bile and pancreatic channel is not present in all patients and is only a few millimeters long in others. Furthermore, pancreatic secretory pressure is as great as biliary secretory pressure and significant bile reflux into the pancreatic duct would not be expected.

Gallstones passing through the papilla might render it incompetent, allowing duodenal enterokinase to reflux into the pancreas and activate trypsin. The lack of recurrent pancreatitis after pancreatic sphincteroplasty argues against this theory.

Obstruction of the distal pancreatic duct by stone or edema seems the most plausible theory. Resistance to flow would increase intraductal pressure, especially under secretory stimulation. The molecular mechanism relating increased ductal pressure and intra-acinar activation of trypsin is unclear.

ERCP

As in gallstone pancreatitis, obstruction of the ampullary portion of the pancreatic duct increasing pancreatic duct pressure may be the precipitating event in ERCP-induced pancreatitis. Several pieces of evidence support this hypothesis. The frequency of acute pancreatitis following ERCP increases with the number of cannulation attempts, performance of "pre-cut" sphincterotomy, presence of sphincter spasm ("dyskinesia") and inexperience of the endoscopist. Stenting of the pancreatic duct reduces post-procedure pancreatitis when pre-cut sphincterotomy or sphincterotomy for sphincter dyskinesia are performed. Patency of the accessory duct (which could decompress the main pancreatic duct) is reported to decrease post-sphincterotomy pancreatitis. Acinarization of contrast by excessive injection increases risk of pancreatitis, and drainage of perfusate during biliary manometry decreases risk. Introduction of a guidewire into the pancreatic duct without contrast injection or cholangiogram alone may infrequently produce pancreatitis, perhaps by traumatizing the papilla.

The composition of pancreatic injectate appears to have little influence on the incidence of post-ERCP pancreatitis. Non-ionic contrast injection causes pancreatitis about as often as standard ionic contrast and saline perfusion during biliary manometry is associated with a high incidence of pancreatitis.

It is unclear on a molecular or cellular level what initiates the pancreatitis. One wonders if increased pressure in the ducts and acinar lumen inhibits cellular enzyme secretion. Serum cholecystokinin increases about fivefold in the first several hours of ERCP-induced pancreatitis but not in patients that do not develop pancreatitis. Perhaps events on a molecular level parallel those seen in the experimental cerulein model in which pancreatitis develops because of excess stimulation of the pancreas by a cholecystokinin analog. After this early increase, plasma cholecystokinin becomes almost immeasurable by the second day of symptoms. Reduction in incidence of pancreatitis by infusion of the potent protease inhibitor gabexate indicates that activation of trypsin in the pancreas is involved. A randomized, placebo-controlled trial of octreotide or corticosteroids showed no reduction in post-ERCP pancreatitis; the pathophysiologic implications of these findings are speculative.

Hyperamylasemia occurs within 2 hours following more than half of ERCPs but only a minority of patients develops clinical pancreatitis. Do patients with amylase elevation but no pain have subclinical pancreatitis that is aborted by unknown factors? Are induction of NF-kB, ICAM-1, inflammatory cytokines, or neutrophils involved? The propensity for activation of neutrophils may be important since pre-ERCP neutrophil CD11b receptor status (which is involved in neutrophil activation) correlates with post-ERCP pancreatitis in a small study.

Since ERCP pancreatitis is the only common pancreatitis in which prophylactic or very early therapy is possible, it is ideal for clinical investigation.

Alcohol

Although most patients with alcohol-related pancreatitis have chronic changes in the pancreas, some develop acute pancreatitis that is pathologically and clinically indistinguishable from other forms of acute pancreatitis. The mechanism of ethanol injury is obscure but a recently described animal model provides clues. Rats fed a diet containing alcohol for 2 or 6 weeks developed pancreatitis at doses of intravenous cholecystokinin that are harmless in rats fed regular chow. This effect is associated with increased pancreatic NF-kB, IL-6 and inducible nitric oxide synthase. See the discussion below (p. 278) regarding pathophysiology of alcohol in chronic pancreatitis.

Hypercalcemia

Hypercalcemia has been associated with pancreatitis. Short-term elevations, such as those that have occured with infusion of calcium during cardiopulmonary bypass, are more likely to cause disease. Similar infusion of calcium in rats to produce a threefold increase in ionized serum calcium with return to baseline levels within 3 hours increases serum amylase, tissue trypsinogen activation peptide, pancreatic edema, and neutrophil infiltration within 1 hour. The alterations are dose dependent.

Calcium is a key intracellular messenger controlling enzyme secretion. Binding of cholecystokinin to acinar receptors causes a release of calcium from intracellular stores and oscillations in cytosolic calcium concentration. Calcium release in the secretory pole of acinar cells comes from zymogen granules. Each spike of calcium in the secretory pole is associated with secretion of enzyme. Supramaximal doses of secretagogues (CCK or cerulein) generate a sustained non-oscillating increase in cytosolic calcium, paradoxically inhibit apical enzyme secretion, and induce pancreatitis. The importance of intracellular calcium to enzyme secretion suggests that hypercalcemia might trigger pancreatitis by increasing intracellular calcium.

Hyperlipidemia

Severe hypertriglyceridemia, with serum triglyceride over 1000 mg/dL (11.3 mM), is associated with an increased risk of acute pancreatitis. It is unknown if the increased risk reflects a direct toxic effect of triglyceride or an increased susceptibility to other etiologic factors. Pancreatitis is seen with primary hypertriglyceridemia and with hypertriglyceridemia associated with alcoholism, drugs, pregnancy, or diabetes. The mechanism by which hypertriglyceridemia causes acute pancreatitis is not established. One concept is that free fatty acids produced by lipase from triglycerides in the interstitium of the pancreas damage acinar cell membranes. Acinar cells isolated *in vitro* can be damaged by free fatty acids. Two other hypotheses are that free fatty acids activate trypsinogen by producing interstitial acidosis, and that free fatty acids disturb pancreatic microcirculation by damaging vascular endothelium.

Hypertriglyceridemia induced in rats intensifies acute pancreatitis produced by supramaximal cerulein or by intraductal bile salts. The role of elevated triglyceride in clinical pancreatitis is indicated by lipid plasmapheresis benefiting severe acute pancreatitis and preventing recurrent acute pancreatitis.

Chronic pancreatitis

As its name implies, chronic pancreatitis is a persistent, usually inflammatory, disorder of the pancreas. It has many etiologies. The most common pathological type is characterized by chronic inflammatory cell infiltration, fibrosis, variable loss of exocrine and endocrine parenchymal cells, and irregular ductal strictures and dilation. Protein may precipitate and calcify in ducts. The lesions are often patchy and do not resolve. These pathologic changes are seen in alcoholic, hereditary, and idiopathic chronic pancreatitis. In contrast, in severe cystic fibrosis the pancreas is atrophic, not fibrotic, and not calcified. The recently identified autoimmune type of chronic pancreatitis is manifest by lymphocytic inflammation and response to steroid treatment.

Various theories have been advanced to explain chronic pancreatitis including

- ductal obstruction
- fibrosis produced by pancreatic stellate cell activation
- recurrent acute pancreatitis, the necrosis–fibrosis hypothesis
- autoimmune damage.

The oldest theory is the ductal obstruction theory. Increased protein and decreased bicarbonate concentration has been found in the ductal secretions in alcoholic pancreatitis. Precipitation of protein with formation of plugs in the smaller and major ducts is thought to be a relatively early event. Transient relief of symptoms by endoscopic removal of plugs has suggested that obstruction of ducts by plugs might be a primary cause of parenchymal disease. A protein called GP2 that is related to the Tamm–Horsfall mucoprotein forming the matrix of renal casts has been identified as the major constituent of ductal plugs. The protein GP2 originates from the zymogen granule and is secreted into pancreatic juice. Although total protein concentration in secretions is high, the concentration of another protein, lithostatin, released from the acinus is low. Lithostatin is thought to retard calcium precipitation in pancreatic secretion and its low concentration may contribute to calcification of protein plugs.

Cystic fibrosis is the result of mutations in the cystic fibrosis conductance regulator gene and resultant abnormal chloride channels. These secretory abnormalities produce inspissations in various organs including the lung, liver, and pancreas. Over 800 different mutations causing disease of variable severity have been reported. The classic childhood cystic fibrosis causes pancreatic exocrine insufficiency but rarely acute or painful pancreatitis. More recently, less severe abnormalities in the cystic fibrosis conductance regulator gene have been identified in patients with recurring or chronic painful pancreatitis. These patients often do not have steatorrhea and are referred to as "pancreatic sufficient". The reason for pancreatitis in patients with abnormal cystic fibrosis conductance regulator genes is unclear but obstruction of pancreatic ducts by thick mucus may be involved.

Stellate cells

An exciting line of investigation involves the role of pancreatic stellate cells in human and experimental chronic pancreatitis. The recent identification of hepatic stellate cells as the major source of hepatic fibrosis prompted investigators to search, successfully, for similar cells in the pancreas. These pancreatic cells are termed pancreatic stellate cells. Stellate cells are myofibroblast-like cells that express smooth muscle actin and secrete collagen, laminin, and fibronectin. Pancreatic stellate cells can be grown from rodent pancreas transiently after induction of acute cerulein pancreatitis and are abundant in chronic pancreatitis.

Vitamin A-storing cells are the precursors of stellate cells in the pancreas, as in the liver. The retinoid-storing cells are found in small numbers in the interacinar region of the normal pancreas. When activated, precursor cells lose the vitamin A-containing lipid droplets, enlarge, proliferate, and express cytoplasmic alpha smooth muscle actin characteristic of myofibroblast cells. The cytokines transforming growth factor, platelet derived growth factor and TNF activate pancreatic stellate cells in cell culture and *in vivo*. Although minimally expressed in normal pancreatic tissue, these cytokines are present in significant amounts in pancreatic tissue of patients with chronic pancreatitis. Transforming growth factor and platelet derived growth factor stimulate pancreatic stellate cells to secrete collagen and fibronectin. Platelet thrombi in pancreatic capillaries may be the first source of transforming growth factor and platelet derived growth factor in pancreatitis. Macrophages, neutrophils, and acinar cells also release TNF and transforming growth factor.

Recurrent acute pancreatitis (the necrosis–fibrosis theory)

Unless there is significant necrosis, acute pancreatitis is a self-limited disease and pancreatic architecture and function return to normal. Acute biliary and experimental cerulein pancreatitis usually resolves completely. Nevertheless, it has been proposed that recurrent acute pancreatitis might lead to chronic pancreatitis. It is unclear if necrosis must occur to produce fibrosis, but a possible link between recurrent acute and chronic pancreatitis has been established. Transient collagen production by activated pancreatic stellate cells occurs in acute cerulein pancreatitis. The fibrogenic cytokine response peaks in a few days and then normalizes and does not lead to scarring. By repeating supramaximal cerulein stimulation twice weekly (presumably before pancreatic stellate cells become inactive) investigators have produced progressive fibrosis and atrophy of acinar cells similar to that of human chronic pancreatitis. Stromal matrix producing pancreatic stellate cells are found in these experimental animals.

Alcoholic and hereditary cationic trypsinogen gene mutation pancreatitis may be examples of repetitive acute injury leading to chronic disease. Alcohol causes clinically evident injury to the pancreas after many years of high consumption. Although only a minority of heavy drinkers develops pancreatitis, there is increasing incidence with increasing consumption. Most patients with alcoholic pancreatitis have chronic changes, including scarring and loss of acinar tissue, when first seen. However, a few patients present with acute pancreatitis and no evidence of chronic injury. This variable clinical picture suggests that factors in addition to alcohol toxicity are involved in "alcoholic" pancreatitis.

Oxidative stress appears to be a factor in the development of alcohol-induced pancreatic disease. High doses of alcohol given acutely to rats deplete the antioxidant glutathione in the pancreas; such a reduction in antioxidant status renders the pancreas susceptible to oxidative stress. Heightened free radical activity and increased levels of lipid peroxides have been described in the serum and pancreas of patients with chronic alcoholic pancreatitis. Histologic study of the pancreas of a patient with acute exacerbation of chronic alcoholic pancreatitis revealed oxidative stress in acinar cells and neighboring capillaries. These changes were associated with ICAM upregulation and adherent oxygen free radical-producing neutrophils.

A link has been proposed between oxidative stress, activation of pancreatic stellate cells, and chronic pancreatitis. Acetaldehyde produced by oxidation of ethanol stimulates pancreatic stellate cells to produce collagen in experimental animals. In addition, pancreatic tissue obtained from patients undergoing surgery for chronic pancreatitis reveals increased lipid peroxidation in acinar cells adjacent to active pancreatic stellate cells. It remains unclear if fibrosis reflects induction of fibrogenesis by non-necroinflammatory or necroinflammatory stimuli.

Cationic trypsinogen mutation is postulated to cause chronic pancreatitis by intermittent activation of trypsin in acinar cells. If the trypsin exceeds the binding capacity of SPINK1, autoactivation of trypsin will begin because the mutation prevents autolysis. Necrosis of cells in turn may activate pancreatic stellate cells and produce fibrosis. The attacks of pancreatitis begin between 1 and 13 years of age and are similar to acute attacks from other causes. They may follow large fatty meals, alcohol, and emotional stress but frequently no precipitating event is identified. Occasionally, patients develop pancreatic insufficiency with no history of pain. Perhaps necrosis limited to only a few cells at a time could eventually produce severe scarring without intervening pain.

Autoimmune damage

An unusual form of chronic pancreatitis thought to be of autoimmune etiology has been reported, mainly in Japan. In these patients the pancreas is diffusely enlarged, the main pancreatic duct is irregularly narrowed, there is extensive lymphocytic infiltration, and most have improvement with steroid therapy. Hypergammaglobulinemia, immune complexes, and various autoantibodies are found in nearly all patients. Immunoglobulin G4 (IgG4) is especially elevated and responds to glucocorticoid therapy. Other autoimmune diseases such as rheumatoid arthritis, Sjögren's syndrome, and sclerosing cholangitis may be associated with autoimmune pancreatitis.

Immune mechanisms may be involved in alcoholic pancreatitis as well. Mononuclear cell infiltration is a constant finding, with predominance of T lymphocytes and macrophages, in the pancreas of patients. Activated CD8 T cells adjacent to acini have been implicated in a cytotoxic process. Immunoglobulin E-positive mast cells are increased in alcoholic pancreatitis tissue and such cells are capable of inducing collagen formation by fibroblasts.

understanding of the pathophysiology of pancreatitis will be more successful.

Comments

As is evident from this review, pancreatitis is a very complex disease. Multiple therapies show promise, but most have not been extensively investigated in animal models and may not be effective in human pancreatitis. Evaluation in large numbers of patients will be required to reach reliable conclusions. Several questions must be addressed in designing trials. How ill should patients be? Which of the many therapies should be tried? What doses should be used? When in the course of pancreatitis should they be applied? The problem is exemplified by the Lexipafant® (anti-platelet activating factor) story. Results were encouraging in animals, and even in a relatively small clinical trial, but the drug was without any benefit in a costly multi-center trial involving 500 patients in each study arm. Hopefully, other therapies based on our improving

Further reading

Apte MV, Phillips PA, Fahmy RG, *et al*. Does alcohol directly stimulate pancreatic fibrogenesis? Studies with rat pancreatic stellate cells. *Gastroenterology* 2000; 118: 780–794.

Chen X, Baoan JI, Han B, *et al*. NF-kB activation in pancreas induces pancreatic and systemic inflammatory response. *Gastroenterology* 2002; 122: 448–457.

Hamano H, Kawa S, Joriuchi A, *et al*. High serum IgG4 concentrations in patients with sclerosing pancreatitis. *N Eng J Med* 2001; 344: 732–738.

Keck T, Balcom JH, Fernandez-del Castillo C, *et al*. Matrix metalloproteinase-9 promotes Neutrophil migration and alveolar capillary leakage in pancreatitis-associated lung injury in the rat. *Gastroenterology* 2002; 122: 188–201.

Steer M. Pancreatitis severity: who calls the shots? *Gastroenterology* 2002; 122: 1168–1172.

Yekebas E, Eisenberger CF, Ohnesorge H, *et al*. Attenuation of sepsis-related immunoparalysis by continuous venovenous hemofiltration in experimental porcine pancreatitis. *Crit Care Med* 2001; 29(7): 1423–1430.

Chapter 15

Diagnosis of Pancreatitis

William B. Long

CHAPTER OUTLINE

This chapter will review the diagnosis of acute and chronic pancreatitis, focusing on clinical presentation, serologic tests, and radiographic evaluation. Testing to assist differential diagnosis and testing for prognostic purposes will also be discussed.

Acute pancreatitis

Clinical history and physical examination may suggest acute pancreatitis but these investigations are never adequate to establish the diagnosis. Any patient suspected of having acute pancreatitis should have a laboratory test to detect elevation of pancreatic enzyme in serum or urine, and an abdominal film or CT scan. These studies will either confirm the diagnosis or suggest other abdominal disease.

Difficulties in diagnosis arise in the unusual patient with severe disease who does not have abdominal pain, whose serum amylase is normal and in whom computed CT of the abdomen is not performed. Mild pancreatitis may not be diagnosed because the symptoms are atypical or very mild, serum amylase is not measured or has returned to normal, and the pancreas appears normal on CT. Since there is no definitive test, no "gold standard" for acute pancreatitis, it is impossible to know precisely how often particular tests are normal in patients with acute pancreatitis. However, normal CT is probably rare in serious disease.

Clinical presentation

The most common signs and symptoms of acute pancreatitis reported in large series of patients are shown in Table 15.1.

Abdominal pain usually begins and is most intense in the epigastrium. It may radiate to the left upper or right upper quadrants. In about half of patients the pain radiates through to the mid-back. Less commonly pain radiates to the right or left lower quadrants, perhaps reflecting extension of pancreatic exudates along the right or left colon. Most commonly pain begins abruptly but may increase in severity over several hours. It is usually severe, requires narcotics for relief, fluctuates little in intensity, and persists for more than 24 hours. Patients may lean forward or lie on the side with knees drawn up in an attempt to obtain some relief. Infrequently

Table 15.1 Common signs and symptoms of acute pancreatitis

Sign or symptom	Frequency of occurrence
Abdominal pain	> 95%
Nausea and vomiting	70%–90%
Epigastric tenderness	> 95%
Low-grade fever	70%
Hypertension	30%
Hypotension	20%–40%
Mental changes	20%

acute pancreatitis can occur without a history of pain in patients with shock or altered mental state, and in postoperative patients.

Rapid onset of pain simulating acute pancreatitis is seen with biliary colic, perforated ulcer, mesenteric ischemia, and stranglulated or obstructed bowel. Pain that resolves in a few hours is consistent with biliary colic or obstructed bowel but is not typical of acute pancreatitis. Pain that fluctuates in intensity suggests intestinal obstruction rather than pancreatitis. Pain limited to the right upper quadrant is unusual in acute pancreatitis and is more consistent with acute cholecystitis.

Most patients with acute pancreatitis are nauseated and many vomit. Vomitus is usually non-bloody and may contain bile but, in contrast to vomiting associated with small bowel obstruction, is not feculent. Vomiting does not relieve pain as it might if caused by intestinal obstruction.

The epigastrium is tender in almost all patients and this tenderness exceeds that of other areas of the abdomen. Abdominal rigidity is unusual but may develop if the attack is severe. Bowel sounds are diminished in most patients and may be absent.

Fever is unusual at the outset but develops in about 70% of patients during the first few days of illness. Most fevers in the first week of pancreatitis are the result of inflammation. Fever over 102 °F and fever associated with rigor suggest infection. Tachycardia, hypertension, and hypotension all occur and reflect more severe disease. Respiratory rate increases on account of inflammation below the diaphragm, pleural effusion, or acute respiratory distress syndrome. Jaundice reflects biliary obstruction from gallstone, biliary compression from pancreatic edema or cyst, or concomitant liver disease.

Unusual findings include lipemia retinalis reflecting markedly elevated serum triglycerides, ecchymosis in the flank (Grey Turner sign) or peri-umbilical region (Cullen's sign) associated with hemorrhagic pancreatitis, and the very rare finding of subcutaneous fat necrosis, characterized by tender red nodules over the extremities.

Laboratory tests

All patients suspected to have acute pancreatitis should have measurement of blood amylase or lipase, hemoglobin, white cell count, urea nitrogen/creatinine, liver-associated enzymes, bilirubin, calcium, glucose and triglycerides, and determination of oxygen saturation. These tests are needed to assist in the differential diagnosis, to predict potential severe disease and as a baseline for further management. Certain investigators use other tests such as C-reactive protein for prognostic purposes.

Initial hemoconcentration elevates hematocrit and indicates more severe disease. As fluid losses are replaced hemoglobin often falls. Moderate leukocytosis is the rule, and, infrequently, leukemoid reactions are observed. Hyperglycemia can reflect underlying diabetes, severe necrosis, or a transient dysfunction of the pancreas. Serum electrolytes, blood urea nitrogen and creatinine are needed to detect acidosis and renal failure. Previously non-diabetic patients who have acute pancreatitis and hyperglycemia seldom develop ketoacidosis. Therefore, patients with ketoacidosis and elevated amylase may not have pancreatitis. On the other hand, patients with hyperosmolar coma may have severe pancreatitis. Mesenteric ischemia masquerading as pancreatitis should be considered in any patient with an unexplained metabolic acidosis.

A decrease in serum calcium in the first few days of pancreatitis may be an indication of severe disease. This decrease is often associated with a fall in serum albumin, reflects a decrease in non-ionic calcium, and does not usually produce neurologic signs. Binding of calcium by fatty acids produced by peripancreatic lipolysis may lower ionic serum calcium and cause neuromuscular irritability. Hypomagnesemia may aggravate hypocalcemia.

Measurement of serum triglyceride is important because elevated triglyceride may be the cause of the pancreatitis, acute respiratory distress is more common in these patients, and because of the tendency for serum amylase assay to remain normal with lactescent serum.

Elevations of serum bilirubin less than 2 mg/dL may reflect hemolysis but direct hyperbilirubinemia suggests biliary obstruction or concomitant liver disease. Serum alanine aminotransferase over 80 IU/L has been observed in 80% of gallstone pancreatitis but in only 10% of non-gallstone pancreatitis.

Amylase

Serum amylase determination has been a cornerstone in the diagnosis of acute pancreatitis for decades. Even though improved assays have now made serum lipase a readily available test and some investigators have proposed other screening tests such as urinary trypsinogen, the extensive experience with serum amylase has solidified the central role of serum amylase in evaluating patients. Amylase as an aid in the diagnosis of pancreatic disease will, therefore, be discussed in detail.

Amylase metabolism Amylase is an enzyme that hydrolyzes the internal alpha 1–4 linkages of starch producing maltose, isomaltose, and larger fragments containing 1–6 linkages which amylase cannot break. Traditional amylase assays relied on production of maltose, or on the reduction in starch, but newer automated methods employ synthetic saccharide substrates that release dyes or activate coupling enzymes when digested. Since different methods may be used, levels of amylase may not correlate exactly between different clinical laboratories. With the possible exception of hypertriglyceridemic serum, no significant amylase inhibitors are present in serum, urine, or other body fluids. Pancreatic and salivary cells and secretions contain amylase many orders of magnitude greater than that of serum. Although pancreatic and salivary amylases have about the same molecular weight (55 000 Da) they can be separated with electrophoresis or isoelectric focusing. Specific plant inhibitors are also employed to measure isoforms. Small amounts of amylase with characteristics similar to salivary amylase are present in milk, tears, fallopian tube, and lung. Some tumors, most notably lung and ovarian tumors produce a salivary-type isoamylase. For practical purposes the liver and intestine produce no amylase.

Normal serum contains about equal amounts of pancreatic and salivary types of amylase. The pancreas is the only source of the pancreatic-type amylase and this isoenzyme disappears from blood after total pancreatectomy. It is suspected that salivary-type amylase in the blood originates mainly from the salivary glands. A small percentage of amylase synthesized by the pancreas and salivary glands enters blood perfusing these organs. With glandular inflammation or obstruction of their ducts, a substantially larger amount of amylase enters either the venous blood or lymphatic drainage of the pancreas or salivary glands. Disease of the pancreas gives rise to elevated serum pancreatic amylase and disease of the salivary glands to elevated salivary isoamylase.

Healthy esophageal and intestinal mucosa prevents back diffusion of amylase into the blood. Disruption of this mucosal barrier by perforation or ischemic injury permits small amounts of amylase to pass from the lumen to the blood. Therefore, disease causing mucosal disruption may be associated with increases in salivary or pancreatic serum amylase. Examples are elevated salivary amylase in pleural fluid and serum associated with esophageal perforation and elevated pancreatic amylase associated with intestinal perforation, obstruction or ischemia.

Lipase is produced in the pancreas but not in the salivary glands and serum lipase serves as a surrogate for pancreatic isoamylase. Tumors and organs such as fallopian tubes that can produce salivary-type amylase do not produce lipase. Elevated serum lipase indicates that the elevated serum amylase is pancreatic type. Although amylase isoenzyme analysis is available it is relatively expensive and rarely needed.

Amylase is cleared from the blood quite rapidly. The major site of amylase catabolism is unknown. In the baboon the half-life of serum amylase is about 2 hours, with 20% of intravenously infused amylase being excreted in the urine. In man the half-life of amylase has been estimated as several hours and, as in the baboon, only a portion is excreted in the urine. Some amylase filtered through the glomerulus is catabolized by the renal tubules and does not appear in the urine. That there is also a non-renal site for amylase catabolism is evident since serum amylase may be normal and is infrequently more than twice normal in bilaterally nephrectomized patients. Nevertheless, mild (twofold) increases in serum amylase in patients with chronic renal failure may reflect decreased amylase clearance.

Urinary clearance of amylase Proteins with molecular weights less than 35 000 Daltons are freely filtered through the renal glomerulus, but proteins as large as albumin (molecular weight 68 000 Da) are minimally filtered. Amylase with an intermediate molecular weight of 55 000 Da is filtered at an intermediate rate. Filtered amylase that is not catabolized by renal tubules appears in the urine. The normal urinary clearance of serum amylase is about 3% of creatinine clearance. Pancreatic isoamylase is cleared about twice as fast as salivary amylase. Calculation of amylase clearance requires a timed collection of urine. It is easier to calculate the ratio of amylase to creatinine clearance by determining amylase and creatinine concentrations in samples of serum and urine obtained simultaneously; a timed urine collection is not needed. The formula is

amylase/creatinine clearance%
= (urine amylase × serum creatinine) × 100
÷ (serum amylase × urine creatinine)

In acute pancreatitis urinary clearance of amylase and amylase to creatinine clearance increase about threefold and this increased clearance gradually returns to normal as the patient recovers. The increased clearance usually persists longer than the elevation in serum amylase and may be useful diagnostically later in the course of pancreatitis. The initial enthusiasm for the diagnostic utility of amylase clearance has waned as it has been learned that elevated amylase clearance is not specific for acute pancreatitis. Amylase clearance also increases in diabetic acidosis, cardiopulmonary bypass, abdominal surgery, multiple myeloma, and renal failure.

Amylase clearance in acute pancreatitis is increased, in part, on account of an increase in the percentage of pancreatic amylase in the serum, but, especially, on account of decreased renal tubular absorption of filtered amylase. As mentioned, pancreatic amylase is cleared into the urine twice as fast as salivary amylase and about half of normal serum amylase is salivary. A marked increase in pancreatic amylase could increase serum amylase clearance by only 50%. In acute pancreatitis renal tubular absorption of low-molecular-weight proteins is defective and this is the probable explanation for the threefold increase in amylase clearance. Urinary clearance of both salivary and pancreatic amylases is increased in acute pancreatitis.

Clearance of amylase is lower than normal when elevated serum amylase is caused by salivary amylase or macroamylase. In each of these situations serum lipase will be normal. The reason for the lower clearance of salivary as opposed to pancreatic amylase is unclear. Macroamylase is too large to pass through the glomerulus. Since assays for macroamylase are not available in most clinical laboratories, suspicion of macroamylase is probably the major indication for calculating amylase to creatinine clearance ratios. For macroamylase to be considered the ratio should be less than 1%.

Conditions associated with hyperamylasemia Serum amylase is increased in many conditions. It is helpful to separate these conditions into those with elevated pancreatic isoamylase, salivary isoamylase, or both (serum lipase may be used as a surrogate for pancreatic amylase) (Table 15.2).

Serum amylase in acute pancreatitis Serum amylase increases within a few hours of the onset

Table 15.2 Conditions associated with hyperamylasemia

Pancreatic isoamylase	Salivary isoamylase	Both

Pancreatic disease
  pancreatitis
  carcinoma
  trauma
  ERCP
  pseudocyst
  pancreatic ascites
  abscess
	Salivary disease
	  infection
	  radiation
	  trauma
	  duct obstruction
		Renal failure
		Diabetic acidosis
		Burns

	Lung disease
	  pneumonia
	  tuberculosis	

Intestinal disease
  perforated ulcer
  mesenteric infarction
  intestinal obstruction
	Ovarian/fallopian tube
	  ruptured ectopic pregnancy
	  ovarian cyst	

Biliary disease
  cholecystitis
  common duct stone
	Malignancies
	  lung
	  ovary
	  prostate
	  pancreas
	Alcoholism
	Bulimia	

of symptoms of acute pancreatitis and usually peaks in the first 48 hours. Serum amylase that is at least three times the upper limit of normal is found in about 90% of patients with acute pancreatitis if tested within the first 36 hours of the disease. Serum amylase tends to be lower in alcoholic than in non-alcoholic pancreatitis. Although high serum amylase may be seen in many conditions, lesser elevations are more typical of diseases other than pancreatitis. The increase in serum amylase in acute pancreatitis is caused by an increase in pancreatic-type amylase and there is no increase in salivary amylase. Since serum lipase will be elevated in nearly all of these patients, serum lipase is an appropriate test in any patient in whom etiology of elevated amylase is uncertain.

Total serum amylase returns to the normal range in nearly all patients by the second week of disease. In patients with persistently elevated amylase complications of pancreatitis including pseudocyst or pancreatic fistula should be considered. Other conditions causing persistent elevation of amylase including malignancies and macroamylase will be discussed below (see p. 287).

The height of serum amylase does not correlate with the severity of disease. Acute pancreatitis-associated mortality, need for surgery, or artificial ventilation is just as great in patients whose serum amylase on admission is less than three times normal as in those whose serum amylase is greater than three times normal.

Situations in which total serum amylase may be normal or less than three times the upper limit of normal in acute pancreatitis include hypertriglyceridemia, alcoholic pancreatitis, and measurement of amylase days after onset of disease. The reason for normal amylase in association with elevated triglycerides is often attributed to a hypothetical inhibitor in serum, but no inhibitor has been identified and urine amylase is similarly reduced. Because serum lipase may be elevated in pancreatitis associated with hyperlipidemia, it is a more reliable indicator of pancreatitis in these patients than is amylase. In a series of alcoholic pancreatitis diagnosed by CAT scan or ultrasound, 32% of patients had normal serum amylase. Many of these patients may have had pain associated with chronic pancreatitis masquerading as acute pancreatitis. Serum amylase is usually lower in acute alcoholic pancreatitis than in biliary pancreatitis. Patients with bouts of abdominal pain from chronic pancreatitis frequently have normal serum amylase.

And finally, it is important to measure amylase during the first day of disease if possible. Serum amylase returns to the normal range in about a third of patients by the second or third day of pancreatitis. Serum lipase, pancreatic isoamylase, and urinary clearance of amylase elevations persist longer than elevation of total serum amylase, and these tests may be diagnostically useful in patients seen after the first days of pancreatitis.

Other causes of elevated pancreatic amylase in serum
Perforated abdominal viscus, mesenteric infarction, acute cholecystitis, and common duct gallstone may produce abdominal pain and elevate serum pancreatic amylase. Serum amylase associated with intestinal perforation or infarction may increase to several times the upper limit of normal and probably originates from absorption of amylase that has leaked into the peritoneal cavity. Elevated amylase associated with biliary disease is also pancreatic in type and may reflect a subtle abnormality in the pancreas. Abdominal film, CT, and ultrasound help distinguish these conditions. A normal-appearing pancreas on CT in a severely ill patient suggests disease other than acute pancreatitis. Surgical exploration of the abdomen may be needed if non-invasive studies do not exclude intestinal infarction.

More than half of patients have elevated pancreatic-type serum amylase in the several hours following ERCP, even if clinical pancreatitis is not present. Mild elevations of serum amylase have been reported infrequently in association with bowel obstruction, gastroenteritis, appendicitis, and carcinoma of the pancreas.

Traumatic rupture of the pancreatic duct, or spontaneous rupture of a pancreatic pseudocyst into the peritoneum or pleural space, produces a moderate increase in serum amylase. Amylase in the associated ascites or pleural fluid is substantially higher than serum amylase. Lipase will be markedly elevated in the ascites or pleural fluid.

Elevated serum amylase of non-pancreatic or mixed origin
As listed in the above table, multiple non-pancreatic conditions may acutely or chronically elevate serum amylase. Appreciation of this fact is important lest one assume that elevated amylase implies pancreatic disease. Amylase isoenzyme or lipase determination is often helpful in the evaluation of such patients. Except for the rare pancreatic carcinoma that produces salivary-type amylase, normal lipase or pancreatic isoamylase indicate that the elevated serum amylase is not of pancreatic origin.

Elevated amylase in ascites or pleural fluid, and lesser increases in serum amylase, may be caused by lung disease (e.g. tumors), ovarian tumors, or ruptured ectopic pregnancy. These conditions often simulate chronic pancreatic ascites or pancreatic–pleural fistulas. Ruptured ectopic pregnancy must be distinguished from other acute abdominal emergencies. Since the amylase is not pancreatic, serum and fluids associated with these conditions will not contain lipase or pancreatic-type amylase.

Mild and often persistent elevation in serum salivary amylase occurs in about 10% of chronic alcoholics, perhaps because of disease of the salivary gland.

Although acute pancreatitis occurs in about 10% of patients with diabetic ketoacidosis, another 10% to 30% of these patients have elevated serum amylase or lipase in the absence of clinical or CT evidence of pancreatitis. Generally, if the serum amylase or lipase is greater than three times the upper limit of normal, pancreatitis is likely. Conversely, acute pancreatitis as verified by CT but with normal serum amylase and lipase is seen in a small percentage of patients, usually in the setting of hyperlipidemia. The lack of significant abdominal pain in occasional patients is another reason that pancreatitis may be difficult to diagnose in the setting of ketoacidosis.

Renal failure is often, but not invariably, associated with elevation of either salivary or pancreatic amylase. Chronic pancreatitis is found in many patients who have died of renal failure, and pancreatic disease should be suspected if either pancreatic amylase or lipase is at least three times the upper limit of normal.

Serum lipase

The list of conditions causing elevated serum lipase is shorter than that causing elevated serum amylase (Box 15.1).

Box 15.1 Conditions that cause elevated serum lipase

Acute pancreatitis
Pancreatic ascites/effusion
Intestinal perforation
Intestinal infarction
Diabetic ketoacidosis
Renal failure
Acute cholecystitis
Pancreatic carcinoma
Macrolipasemia
Idiopathic

The pancreas is the source of serum lipase in the great majority of situations in which it is elevated. In general, serum lipase is somewhat more sensitive and specific than serum amylase in making an early diagnosis of acute pancreatitis. As is the case with serum amylase, sensitivity and specificity depend on the assay used, the population studied, and the threshold above which the diagnosis is made. At values of serum lipase above five times the upper limit of normal, specificity for diagnosing pancreatitis approaches 100%. But at this level sensitivity for acute pancreatitis may be reduced to 60%. Most investigators using recent rapid and specific tests for serum lipase report that values above two or three times the upper limit of normal are consistent with acute pancreatitis. Unfortunately, serum lipase may be significantly increased in intestinal perforation and mesenteric infarction and, like serum amylase, does not distinguish these emergency conditions from acute pancreatitis.

More than 99% of the lipase produced by the pancreas is secreted into the pancreatic duct and little diffuses from the basolateral portion of acinar cells into pancreatic lymph and capillaries and then into the peripheral circulation. Lipase has a molecular weight of about 50 000 Da and is filtered by the renal glomerulus, but much is absorbed by the proximal tubules. Serum lipase may increase to three times normal in patients after nephrectomy or in renal failure. The half-life of serum lipase is estimated to be between 7 and 14 hours and lipase remains elevated longer than serum amylase in acute pancreatitis. The degree of elevation of serum lipase does not correlate with severity of disease.

Alcoholic pancreatitis Serum lipase tends to become more elevated in acute alcoholic pancreatitis than does serum amylase. In a series of 29 patients with acute alcoholic pancreatitis diagnosed by CT, mean serum lipase tested within the first 24 hours increased twenty-seven-fold but mean serum amylase increased only fivefold above the upper limit of normal. An increase in serum amylase or lipase up to threefold was noted in some chronic alcoholics without clinical evidence of pancreatitis. In 45% of pancreatitis patients serum amylase overlapped with values found in non-pancreatitis alcoholic patients. On the other hand, all pancreatitis patients had serum lipase elevated above values seen in alcoholic patients without pancreatitis.

Lipase:amylase ratio

Serum amylase may increase more dramatically in biliary than in alcoholic pancreatitis. This observation lead to studies comparing the ratio of admission serum lipase and amylase, expressed as multiples of the upper limit of normal, in patients with biliary and alcoholic pancreatitis. Although two studies suggested that admission lipase/amylase ratio above two or five indicated alcoholic pancreatitis, two other groups of investigators reported that the ratio did not clearly differentiate alcoholic and biliary etiology. Reasons for the conflicting results are unclear but lipase/amylase ratio is not accepted as a reliable method of determining the etiology of pancreatitis.

Chronically elevated serum amylase or lipase

Chronically elevated serum amylase may be caused by elevated pancreatic or salivary amylase and by macroamylasemia. Serum lipase elevation indicates the amylase is of pancreatic origin. Persistent pancreatic hyperamylasemia is seen with pseudocyst, pancreatic ascites, or pancreatic–pleural fistulas. In these situations amylase is always elevated, and often greatly elevated, in the cyst, ascites, or pleural fluid, and is lower and perhaps normal in the serum.

Chronically increased salivary amylase may arise from many types of tumors (especially lung and ovary), chronic parotid disease, alcoholism, and bulimia.

Evaluation of 47 subjects seen in a referral center with persistent, asymptomatic hyperamylasemia and no clinical history of pancreatic disease revealed that 8 had macroamylasemia, 11 had salivary hyperamylasemia, 9 had mixed salivary and pancreatic hyperamylasemia, and 19 had hyperamylasemia of exclusively pancreatic origin. All but three of the patients with elevated pancreatic amylase also had elevated serum lipase. Serum amylase was only mildly or moderately elevated. After thorough evaluation excluded pancreatic disease the patients with elevated pancreatic amylase were followed for a mean of 8 years and did not develop clinical or imaging evidence of pancreatic disease.

Macroamylase and macrolipase

Macroamylase and macrolipase are complexes of amylase or lipase with larger proteins in serum. These are usually chronic conditions that have no clinical significance other than causing confusion. Occasionally these macromolecules have been associated with certain diseases (see below). Macroamylase and macrolipase are rarely present in the same individual, therefore they should be considered in patients in whom either amylase or lipase, but not both, is elevated. The large size of the enzyme complexes prevents renal glomerular filtration and markedly reduced urinary clearance suggests their presence. Serum levels of amylase or lipase are often much higher than those seen in renal failure, indicating that reduced urinary clearance is not the sole reason for chronicity or elevation in serum.

Macroamylase has been found in the serum of 0.5% to 5% of patients with elevated serum amylase. Among patients with unexplained chronic elevation of amylase, macroamylase accounts for about 20% of patients. The proteins binding amylase include immunoglobulins and non-immune glycoproteins. Hallmarks of macroamylasemia include chronicity, normal serum lipase, and a very low urinary clearance of amylase. Urinary amylase/creatinine clearance ratio is usually less than 1%. Since salivary amylase clearance may also be about 1% of creatinine clearance, elevation of salivary amylase should also be considered in patients with moderately depressed amylase clearance. Definitive diagnosis depends upon determination of molecular size by gel filtration. Presumptive evidence of macroamylase is provided by a test that takes advantage of enhanced precipitation of macroamylase by polyethylene glycol. Since the presence of macroamylase has no adverse clinical implications, molecular identification is usually not important. Diagnosis is helpful, however, to avoid confusion with significant disease.

Macroamylase has been described in healthy individuals and in association with alcoholism, chronic pancreatitis, liver disease, autoimmune disorders, systemic lupus erythematosis, lymphoma, inflammatory bowel disease, and celiac disease. Macroamylasemia has been reported in 17% of celiac disease patients and infrequently has disappeared in such patients treated with a gluten-free diet. Celiac disease should be excluded in any patient with macroamylasemia.

Macrolipasemia is an even rarer phenomenon, with only a handful of cases reported. Macrolipasemia should be considered in patients in whom the serum lipase is chronically elevated and serum amylase is normal. However, a case of simultaneous macrolipasemia and macroamylasemia associated with systemic lupus erythematosis has been reported.

Other laboratory tests: diagnostic and predictive value

Intrapancreatic activation of trypsin and cytokines is believed to be the initial event in the pathogenesis of acute pancreatitis, and serum and urine tests reflecting their activation have been found to be of diagnostic and prognostic value. Urinary trypsinogen, serum trypsinogen, and serum trypsin-2-alpha-antitrypsin complexes are elevated in over 95% of patients with acute pancreatitis, with a negative predictive value at least comparable to that of serum lipase or amylase.

Two isoenzymes of trypsinogen, trypsinogen-1 (cationic) and trypsinogen-2 (anionic), are normally secreted by the pancreas, and inappropriately enter the serum in acute pancreatitis. Trypsinogen in the serum remains unbound, but if converted to trypsin, the trypsin is inactivated by complexing with alpha-2-macroglobulin or alpha-1-antitrypsin. Trypsinogen has a molecular weight of only 25 000 Da and, because of its small size, is readily filtered through the renal glomerulus. For unknown reasons, tubular absorption of trypsinogen-1 is greater than that of trypsinogen-2, and urinary trypsinogen-2 exceeds urinary trypsinogen-1.

A rapid dipstick test for trypsinogen-2 was positive on admission in 50 of 53 patients (94%) with acute pancreatitis; positive tests were found in 21 of 447 patients (5%) with other abdominal disorders; the test was normal in each of 5 patients with intestinal perforation. Paradoxically, one false-negative result was caused by an extremely high concentration of urinary trypsinogen that saturated antibodies on the test strip. Another group of investigators found elevated urine trypsinogen in only 53% of acute pancreatitis, although urine trypsinogen was significantly higher in patients with severe disease than in those with mild disease. Urine trypsinogen was not elevated in 30 patients with non-pancreatic acute abdomen, indicating that the test may be very specific. Since trypsinogen should be rapidly converted to trypsin in the intestine, it is possible that urine trypsinogen would not become elevated in patients with intestinal ischemia or perforation in whom differentiation from acute pancreatitis is very important. More experience is needed with urinary trypsinogen in patients with acute abdomen. The test is not yet available in the USA.

Predictors of severity

Laboratory tests to assist the clinical diagnosis of severely ill patients have been sought to determine which patients need intensive care and thorough radiographic study (such as serial CT scans). Several tests have been reported to be early predictors of severe acute pancreatitis. These include serum trypsinogen-2, trypsin-2-alpha-1-antitrypsin, pro-inflammatory cytokines such as TNF, IL-1, IL-6 and IL-8, C-reactive protein, and urinary trypsinogen activation peptide.

In a series of 63 patients with acute pancreatitis diagnosed in the emergency department by elevated serum amylase, typical pain, and abnormal CT or ultrasound, serum trypsinogen-2 and trypsin-2-alpha-1-antitrypsin were significantly more elevated in severe than in mild disease, but there was overlap of values. C-reactive protein, lipase, and amylase did not correlate with the severity of disease. Other investigators have also found that C-reactive protein levels peak after the first 2 days and, therefore, this test may not be useful as a prognostic test.

Tumor necrosis factor and IL-1, IL-6, and IL-8 are more elevated during the first day of disease in patients who develop severe pancreatitis than in those developing mild acute pancreatitis, with accuracy rates of 72% to 88% for prediction of severe disease. The accuracy of these tests is similar to that of the APACHE II (Acute Physiology and Chronic Health Evaluation) score. The early elevation of inflammatory cytokines supports the hypothesis that they are involved in the pathogenesis of acute pancreatitis.

Trypsinogen activation peptide is a peptide split from trypsinogen during activation to trypsin. Trypsinogen activation peptide is increased in the urine of patients with acute pancreatitis and may be predictive of severe disease. Twenty-four hours after pain onset mean urinary trypsinogen activation peptide was reported as 37 nM in 35 patients with severe acute pancreatitis and 15 nmol in 137 patients with mild pancreatitis. At a cut off of 35 nmol urinary trypsinogen activation peptide had a negative predictive value of 86% and a sensitivity of 58%. This test is not yet commercially available in the USA.

Laboratory tests to determine etiology of pancreatitis

Distinguishing gallstone pancreatitis from pancreatitis of other causes may affect patient management. A meta-analysis revealed that a serum alanine aminotransferase of at least three times the upper limit of normal has a positive predictive value of 95% for acute gallstone pancreatitis. However, the sensitivity of alanine aminotransferase for gallstone pancreatitis is low, and only half of patients with gallstone pancreatitis have a threefold elevation.

A recent study indicates that serum trypsinogen-1 is preferentially increased in biliary pancreatitis. Conversely, serum trypsin-2-alpha-1-antitrypsin is usually higher in patients with alcohol-induced pancreatitis. The trypsin-2-alpha-1-antitrypsin to trypsinogen-1 ratio is proposed as a promising marker for discriminating biliary and alcohol-induced pancreatitis, but there is overlap between groups and further evaluation is needed.

As discussed previously, a serum lipase: amylase ratio above 2.0 or 5.0 has been reported to indicate alcoholic pancreatitis but conflicting reports suggest that this is not a reliable method of determining etiology.

Serum carbohydrate-deficient transferin identifies nearly all alcoholic patients and is very sensitive for detecting potential alcoholic pancreatitis, but a positive test is not specific for pancreatitis. Investigators also reported significantly higher serum trypsin activity and younger age (mean age 39 versus 65 years) in alcoholic than in biliary pancreatitis. Combining carbohydrate-deficient transferin, serum trypsin, and patient age enabled correct prediction of alcoholic etiology of pancreatitis in 98% of cases. Further experience is needed.

Diagnostic and prognostic imaging

Diagnostic imaging is required during initial evaluation in all patients suspected of having acute pancreatitis. Minimal assessment should include chest and abdominal films and an ultrasound of the biliary tree and pancreas. Severely ill patients and patients in whom the diagnosis is uncertain will usually require abdominal CT scans with oral and, perhaps, intravenous contrast. Computed tomography with intravenous contrast identifies areas of necrosis in the pancreas and has prognostic significance. Follow-up CT is important in patients at risk of complications such as pseudocyst or abscess. Magnetic resonance imaging with intravenous gadolinium is probably as useful as CT with intravenous contrast, but is not as readily available. Endoscopic ultrasound is appropriate in specialized situations.

Chest films detect abnormalities in about a third of patients with acute pancreatitis. Changes include elevation of the diaphragm, pleural effusion, atelectasis, and acute respiratory distress syndrome. Abdominal films may reveal localized ileus of bowel adjacent to inflamed pancreas or give clues of intestinal perforation or obstruction. Ultrasound examination is the most sensitive non-invasive test for gallbladder stones and may also reveal a dilated biliary tree indicating biliary obstruction and an enlarged edematous pancreas. Unfortunately, overlying intestinal gas obscures the pancreas in about a third of patients. Ultrasound cannot distinguish edematous and necrotic pancreas.

Computed tomography

Computed tomography (CT) scan with oral and intravenous contrast is the most accurate radiographic test to diagnose acute pancreatitis, but intravenous contrast should not be used if there is evidence of renal dysfunction. There is conflicting experimental evidence that early intravenous contrast increases pancreatic necrosis. Although there is no convincing clinical evidence that intravenous contrast aggravates pancreatitis, avoidance of intravenous contrast in the first few days of disease may be appropriate unless there is a clinical indication for its use. Routine CT is probably not necessary in mild pancreatitis.

CT without intravenous contrast provides limited evidence that reflects the severity of acute pancreatitis but necrosis can only be determined if CT is enhanced with intravenous contrast. Areas of the pancreas that do not perfuse with contrast are assumed to be necrotic. A CT severity index includes features of the unenhanced study and post-contrast estimate of the amount of necrosis (Box 15.2). To calculate the CT severity index, points of the unenhanced and enhanced CT are combined. Balthazar reported 3% mortality with a CT severity index of 0 to 3 and 17% mortality if the CT severity index was over 7.

The value of follow-up CT after the first week of disease is appropriate only in patients with severe disease or clinical deterioration. A prospective series of 102 patients that had CT with intravenous contrast performed during the first 2 days of illness and then again at 7 days revealed that radiographic complications developed in only 8% of those with Ranson score of zero or one, and that complications were clinically suspected correctly in 92% of patients. The authors concluded that there is "little justification for systematic early CT, especially in patients with Ranson score < 2 and late CT does not need to be performed routinely".

Magnetic resonance imaging

Magnetic resonance imaging depicts necrosis and peripancreatic fluid collections as well as CT does. Intravenous gadolinium is required to detect necrosis but this contrast does not have the nephrotoxi-

Box 15.2   CT severity index. The total index is the sum of unenhanced and intravenous contrast enhanced CT points

Unenhanced CT points

0   normal pancreas
1   focal or diffuse enlargement of the pancreas
2   grade B plus peripancreatic inflammation
3   grade C plus single fluid collection
4   grade C plus more than one fluid collections or air in inflammation

Intravenous contrast-enhanced CT points

0   no necrosis
2   less than 30% necrosis
4   30% to 50% necrosis
6   greater than 50% necrosis

city of the intravenous contrast used in CT. Although high quality MRI studies are not as widely available as CT studies are, high-speed MRI and other advances in MRI technique may make this test increasingly attractive.

Endoscopic ultrasound

Endoscopic ultrasound (EUS) is superior to extracorporeal ultrasound (US) for the detection of gallbladder and bile-duct stones. In a series of 18 patients with idiopathic acute pancreatitis, gallbladder stones (1–9 mm) were revealed by EUS in 14 patients, even though all had one transcutaneous US, 9 had repeat US, 6 had CT and 13 had ERCP which failed to reveal the cause. Another study of gallstone pancreatitis (36 patients) reported that the accuracies of US, ERCP (Endoscopic retrograde cholangiopancreatography), and EUS were 83%, 89%, and 97% respectively. Endoscopic ultrasound has the advantage of having fewer complications than ERCP, but the disadvantage that there are fewer individuals who are skilled in performing EUS.

ERCP

Therapeutic ERCP is used infrequently in acute gallstone pancreatitis if there is evidence of continued biliary obstruction, but there is no role for diagnostic ERCP during the attack. Diagnostic ERCP may be appropriate in patients with idiopathic recurrent acute pancreatitis.

Idiopathic recurrent acute pancreatitis

In 10% to 30% of patients with acute pancreatitis the etiology is not evident by history or after initial testing, including abdominal ultrasound. As many as 50% of these patients have recurring acute attacks. In patients with recurrent pancreatitis further testing is appropriate. Tests employed include bile analysis for crystals, EUS, ERCP, biliary manometry, and serologic tests for hereditary pancreatitis.

Crystals are found in bile in a majority of patients with idiopathic recurrent pancreatitis and recurrent attacks are usually prevented by cholecystectomy or sphincterotomy. Crystals may be identified microscopically in bile collected by duodenal intubation or endoscopy after cholecystokinin stimulation of gallbladder contraction. Bile is centrifuged and examined by polarized microscopy. Repeated transabdominal ultrasound may also reveal sludge or minute stones missed on the first examination. Endoscopic ultrasound is more sensitive than US and may be performed at the time of bile collection.

Other causes of recurrent pancreatitis should be considered. Using ERCP, EUS, or MRI, unsuspected changes of chronic pancreatitis, choledocholithiasis, or congenital abnormalities such as pancreas divisum or choledochocele may be detected. Because they provide accurate structural information without the risk of inducing pancreatitis, EUS and MRI are reducing the usefulness of diagnostic ERCP. Drug-induced pancreatitis should always be considered. In appropriate circumstances intestinal ascariasis may be found. In young patients testing for inherited causes is appropriate, especially if there is a family history of pancreatitis; mutation of the cationic trypsinogen gene or cystic fibrosis transmembrane conductance regulator gene may be identified

In patients in whom crystals are not found, sphincter of Oddi dysfunction has been reported in as many as a third of patients seen at referral centers. It is less clear how many patients with elevated pressure have durable relief with sphincterotomy or sphincteroplasty and whether the frequency of sphincter dysfunction seen at referral centers reflects experience in most practices. Sphincter pressure measurement is technically difficult and is associated with a 20% risk of precipitating acute pancreatitis. For all these reasons, sphincter manometry is performed in only a few centers, but should be considered if a patient persists in having significant attacks. Empiric biliary sphincterotomy in selected patients may be appropriate but even complete ablation of the biliary sphincter does not exclude disease caused by a hypertensive pancreatic sphincter.

Chronic pancreatitis

Severe chronic pancreatitis may cause pain, steatorrhea, and diabetes mellitus. Diabetes or steatorrhea caused by chronic pancreatitis develops only if there is loss of 85% to 90% of pancreatic endocrine or exocrine function. These patients are said to have exocrine or endocrine pancreatic "insufficiency". The major symptom of milder disease is pain, but the chronic pancreatitis may be painless, and even severe disease is painless in about 20% of patients. The pain is characteristically epigastric, often boring into the mid-back, severe, of long duration, and exacerbated by eating or alcohol consumption. Unusual presentations include biliary obstruction, occlusion of the splenic vein with formation of gastric varices, and fistulas from the pancreatic duct producing ascites or pleural effusion.

Diagnosis is based on structural or functional studies. Functional tests other than Sudan stain of stool for fat are performed infrequently in most centers. Computerized tomography, magnetic resonance imaging, EUS, and ERCP are the major tests to determine structural alterations in parenchyma or pancreatic ducts.

Functional tests include assays to detect undigested fat in the stool (microscopic examination of Sudan-stained stool and 72-hour fecal fat determination), collection of duodenal secretion following pancreatic stimulation to analyze for bicarbonate or enzymes, and "tubeless" tests (such as the benzoyl-tyrosyl-p-aminobenzoic acid (pABA), flourescein dilaurate, dual-labeled Schilling, and ^{14}C-labeled triglyceride tests) which measure urinary or breath output of products absorbed following digestion. The functional tests are generally abnormal in patients with advanced disease and steatorrhea but are less reliable in mild disease (see p. 293).

Blood tests are occasionally helpful in evaluating chronic pancreatitis. Serum amylase is usually normal unless there is associated acute pancreatitis, pseudocyst, pancreatic ascites, or pancreatic pleural effusion. Although fluid in chronic pseudocysts is always high in amylase, serum amylase is elevated in only half of these patients. Similarly, amylase is always increased in ascites or pleural effusions caused by pancreatic fistulas but serum amylase is less elevated. Blood glucose may be elevated if chronic pancreatitis has destroyed most of the pancreatic islets, as occurs in at least 80% of patients with exocrine insufficiency.

Serum IgG4 has been reported to be markedly elevated in patients with autoimmune sclerosing pancreatitis.

Genetic tests

Major advances have been achieved in understanding the genetic defects underlying some forms of chronic pancreatitis. Defects in genes regulating production of cationic trypsinogen, CFTR, and SPINK1 have been identified. Genetic testing should be considered in idiopathic pancreatitis, especially if the patient developed pancreatitis at a young age or if there is a family history of idiopathic pancreatitis. Informed consent is usually required before obtaining tests for genetic abnormalities.

The described defects in cationic trypsinogen gene produce trypsin that is resistant to autolysis. The R122H mutation of cationic trypsinogen is reported in 80% to 90% of affected families and the N29I mutation in about 10% to 20%. Rarer defects have also been described. Phenotypic expression (penetrance) occurs in about 80% of the R122H defect.

Heterozygous mutations in the CFTR gene or the 5T allele on intron 8 occur about 2.5 times the expected rate in the general population. One study reported an abnormal CFTR allele in 37% of patients with idiopathic chronic pancreatitis. Another study found abnormal CFTR genes in 13.4% of consecutive patients with chronic pancreatitis (eleven times the expected frequency). Abnormality of the CFTR gene was not increased in patients with alcoholic pancreatitis. The 5T allele, which may result in a reduction of CFTR messenger RNA, was found twice as often as expected. Patients with these heterozygous mutations developed pancreatitis at an earlier age (average 33 years) than those with normal CFTR gene, had no lung disease suggestive of cystic fibrosis, and had normal sweat chloride tests. Since hundreds of abnormalities have been described in the CFTR gene and most laboratories test only for the most common, some gene abnormalities may be missed on routine testing. Although an abnormal gene may suggest a cause of pancreatitis, the meaning of such a finding is not definite. Furthermore, there is no specific therapy for CFTR-related pancreatitis.

Sequence alterations in the SPINK1 gene have been found in about 25% of chronic pancreatitis patients and in 2% of control individuals. It is thought that abnormality in SPINK1 may affect the course of the pancreatitis but is insufficient by itself to cause pancreatitis.

Structural tests

In the past ERCP has been considered the most sensitive and specific test for structural abnormalities of chronic pancreatitis, but CT, EUS, and MRI are challenging its role as a first-line test. Simple X-ray of the abdomen and transabdominal ultrasound are occasionally diagnostic. X-ray detects calcifications pathognomonic of chronic pancreatitis in about 30% of patients. The ability of ultrasound to satisfactorily visualize the pancreas is often limited by intervening air or structures.

The major problems of ERCP are the risk of provoking acute pancreatitis in about 5% of examinations (especially if pressure sufficient to fill side branches and the pancreatic tail are used), lack of visualization of the parenchyma, and inability to examine ducts proximal to an obstruction. Computed tomography, EUS, and MRI provide information about the parenchyma and peripancreatic structures as well as the pancreatic duct. There are some advantages to ERCP over CT, MRI, and EUS. Subtle abnormalities of side branches are visualized more adequately and communication between the pancreatic duct and a cyst is discernable since contrast is injected into the duct. ERCP also allows therapeutic maneuvers such as stenting, sphincterotomy, and stone removal. Determining which test is most sensitive or specific is difficult because of an inability to obtain pathologic confirmation in most patients. It is also difficult to distinguish between benign and malignant disease in many patients without pathology. Although cytologic brushing during ERCP reveals malignant cells in about 25% of malignant strictures, positive cytology is more often obtained by EUS, CT, or ultrasound-guided needle aspirate.

ERCP

ERCP diagnosis of chronic pancreatitis is based on demonstrating irregularity or dilation of the main pancreatic duct or its side branches. The Cambridge classification of abnormalities is often used to grade severity of chronic pancreatitis (Table 15.3).

Differentiation of a stricture caused by chronic pancreatitis and carcinoma may be difficult. The side branches and main duct are typically dilated upstream of a malignant stricture; ducts downstream of the malignant stricture are usually normal. Calcification and cysts that communicate with the main pancreatic duct indicate benign disease

Computerized tomography

Changes of chronic pancreatitis seen with CT are dilation of the main pancreatic duct, pancreatic calcifications, pseudocyst, atrophy, and occasionally parenchymal swelling caused by extensive fibrosis or inflammation. Thin cuts through the pancreas and intravenous and oral contrast are needed for high-quality scans. Tumors may be difficult to distinguish from focal areas of chronic pancreatitis and tissue diagnosis is often needed. An advantage of CT over MRI is its ability to detect calcification. As mentioned, calcification indicates benign disease and regression of calcification may be a sign of carcinoma developing in chronic pancreatitis. Sensitivity and specificity for diagnosis of chronic pancreatitis are about 75% to 85%, but the pancreas may appear normal in mild disease.

Magnetic resonance imaging

Newer techniques allow MRI pancreatogram and cholangiogram to visualize the pancreatic and biliary ducts nearly as well as ERCP does. Advantages over ERCP include the lack of a need for sedation, lack of iodinized intravenous contrast, no risk of

Severity	ERCP findings
Normal	normal main pancreatic duct and side branches
Equivocal	normal main pancreatic duct, fewer than three abnormal side branches
Mild	normal main pancreatic duct, three abnormal (ectatic) side branches
Moderate	abnormal main pancreatic duct
Severe	ductal filling defect or calculus, or main pancreatic duct more than 10 mm, obstructed or severely irregular main pancreatic duct, or cavity more than 10 mm

Table 15.3 Severity of chronic pancreatitis evaluated by ERCP, Cambridge classification

inducing acute pancreatitis, ability to easily perform the examination in patients in whom ERCP is technically difficult, demonstration of ductal anatomy upstream of obstruction, and visualization of other abdominal structures. Comparisons between MRI and ERCP have revealed agreement of 83% to 100% for ductal dilation, 70% to 92% for ductal narrowing and 92% to 100% for ductal filling defects. ERCP is considered superior for subtle disease.

Endoscopic ultrasound

Three studies comparing EUS with ERCP and secretin test indicate that EUS should be considered a first-line test for diagnosing chronic pancreatitis. Endoscopic ultrasound criteria for diagnosing chronic pancreatitis are given in Table 15.4.

As the number of EUS criteria for diagnosing chronic pancreatitis is increased the sensitivity decreases and the specificity of the test increases. If three or more criteria are present, EUS has 84% to 87% sensitivity and 57% to 98% specificity, using either abnormal ERCP or secretin testing to indicate chronic pancreatitis. The sensitivity and specificity of EUS for diagnosing chronic pancreatitis are estimates and the most important factor is probably the experience of the endoscopist.

Unfortunately ERCP and secretin testing are also fallible. Determination of minor irregularities of the pancreatic duct on ERCP relies greatly on the interpretation by the endoscopist and secretin testing is insensitive for mild disease. Surgical experience indicates that patients with clinical characteristics of chronic pancreatitis occasionally have histologic evidence of chronic pancreatitis in spite of non-diagnostic changes on CT or ERCP. We do not know if EUS will accurately detect such subtle abnormalities. Advantages of EUS include avoiding inducing pancreatitis, visualization of the entire gland, and ability to biopsy areas suggestive of tumor. Disadvantages are the relative lack of endoscopists skilled in EUS, the need for sedation, and rare instances of perforation.

Table 15.4 Endoscopic ultrasound criteria for diagnosing chronic pancreatitis

Ductal abnormalities	Parenchymal abnormalities
Echogenic duct walls	Inhomogeneity
Irregular duct contour	Echogenic foci (calcification)
Dilated side branches	Echogenic strands (fibrosis)
Ductal stones	Lobularity

Functional tests

Since the advent of ERCP, CT, MRI, and EUS the importance of pancreatic function testing has waned. The most well-studied pancreatic function test is the secretin test. It is performed following intubation of the duodenum and stomach. Secretin is administered intravenously and pancreatic secretions are collected for bicarbonate analysis via a double lumen (Dreiling®) tube. Gastric secretion is aspirated to avoid neutralization of bicarbonate. In its heyday in the 1960s, David Dreiling published his findings from 10 000 tests. Currently the secretin test, which has been inappropriately called one of the "gold standards" for diagnosing chronic pancreatitis, is rarely performed, even in major centers. Modifications of the secretin test such as the Lundh meal or secretin-CCK tests have fared no better. These tests have several problems. Most important, they are insensitive and a negative test does not exclude the diagnosis of chronic pancreatitis. Intubation of the duodenum is unpleasant, production of secretin has been curtailed, "normal" levels of bicarbonate vary in different laboratories from 80 to 100 mmol/L, distinction of chronic pancreatitis and pancreatic cancer is usually impossible and few individuals are experienced in performing the tests are now few.

Indirect "tubeless" tests of pancreatic function have been devised. These tests depend upon altered digestion and reduction of products of digestion in blood, urine, or breath. Since alteration in digestion does not take place until there is advanced disease, tubeless tests are insensitive for mild disease. The plethora of tubeless tests probably reflects their ineffectiveness. Tests include the pABA, pancreolauryl, dual-labeled Schilling, and ^{14}C-labeled triglyceride tests. Each involves the absorption of a marker following digestion and measurement of the marker. In the pABA, pancreolauryl, and dual-labeled Schilling tests, para-aminobenzoic acid, flourescein and B12, respectively, are measured in the urine. In the C14 triglyceride test, ^{14}C is measured in the breath. In addition to being insensitive except for severe disease, abnormal gastric emptying or renal disease may cause false-positive tests.

Fecal analysis for fat or proteolytic enzymes may be useful. By definition steatorrhea is excess fat in the stool and reflects advanced disease. A 72-hour fecal fat determination is the best quantitative evaluation to detect steatorrhea. A normal value is less than 7 grams of fat per day while the patient is consuming 100 grams of fat per day. The test is infrequently performed. Cost considerations usually prevent a 72-hour collection in hospital and collection is repugnant to patients and staff.

Fecal analysis for chymotrypsin or elastase concentrations may be useful. Chymotrypsin analysis is used most often in children with cystic fibrosis. Oral enzyme supplements must be stopped several days prior to the test. The test is abnormal in about 85% of patients with severe disease and is less sensitive in milder disease. A monoclonal antibody test for human elastase has been developed and appears more sensitive than the chymotrypsin assay. These tests are of limited availability.

Because of its simplicity, Sudan stain of stool for fat is the most useful of the stool tests. Stain of stool without acidification identifies triglycerides, and stain following acidification identifies both fatty acids and triglycerides. Over 100 fat droplets per high-power field is abnormal. All patients with daily fecal fat over 15 grams, and most with 10 grams of fat, will have an abnormal Sudan stain.

Further reading

Cohn J, Freidman K, Noone P, Knowles M, Silverman L and Jowell P. Relation between mutations of the cystic fibrosis gene and idiopathic pancreatitis. *N Engl J Med* 1998; 339: 653.

Elmas N. The role of diagnostic radiology in pancreatitis. *Eur J Radiol* 2001; 38: 120.

Hawes R. Comparison of diagnostic modalities: EUS, ERCP, and fluid analysis. *Gastrointest Endosc* 1999; 49: S94.

Hedstrom J, Kemppainen E, Andersen J, Jokela H, Stenman U. A comparison of serum trypsinogen-2 and trypsin-2-alpha1-antitrypsin complex with lipase and amylase in the diagnosis and assessment of severity in the early phase of acute pancreatitis. *Am J Gastroenterol* 2001; 96: 424.

Levy M, Geenen J. Idiopathic acute recurrent pancreatitis. *Am J Gastroenterol* 2001; 96: 2540.

Munoz-Bongrand N, Panis Y, Soyer P, Riche F, Laisne M, Boudiaf M, Valleur P. Serial computed tomography is rarely necessary in patients with acute pancreatitis: a prospective study in 102 patients. *J Am Coll Surgeons* 2001; 193: 146.

Smotkin J and Tenner S. Laboratory diagnostic tests in acute pancreatitis. *J Clin Gastroenterol* 2002; 34: 459.

Chapter 16

Management of Acute and Chronic Pancreatitis

Alphonso Brown and William B. Long

CHAPTER OUTLINE

This chapter provides an overview of the management of patients with acute and chronic pancreatitis.

Acute pancreatitis

The management of acute pancreatitis requires accurate diagnosis, an estimation of disease severity, and aggressive therapy. In the past two decades, in spite of a lack of specific therapy to abort the inflammatory and necrotizing process in the pancreas, improved management appears to have reduced the mortality in patients with severe disease from 50% to about 15%. Reduction in mortality has been attributed to early identification of severe disease and aggressive therapy for organ failure, infection, and other complications.

Acute pancreatitis is an acute inflammatory condition of the pancreas usually manifest by acute upper abdominal pain. A serum amylase or lipase greater than three times normal is consistent with acute pancreatitis. The elevation of serum lipase is more specific than amylase for pancreatic inflammation, but amylase is the more traditional assay. Computed tomography scan with intravenous contrast can also provide a definitive diagnosis of acute pancreatitis, distinguishing it from other causes of abdominal pain. In addition to its ability to aid in the diagnosis of acute pancreatitis, contrast-enhanced CT can detect pancreatic necrosis and, thereby, predict the severity of disease. Using a combination of these clinical, serologic, and radiological criteria, almost all cases of severe acute pancreatitis can be accurately diagnosed. (See Chapter 15 for further discussion of diagnosis).

Disease stratification

Once acute pancreatitis has been diagnosed the next important step is the accurate stratification of patients based on disease severity (Tables 16.1–16.4). The most widely used severity stratification systems are Ranson's, Glasgow (or Imrie), APACHE-II, and Balthazar CT scores. A Ranson or Glasgow score greater than 3 or an APACHE-II score greater than 8 have negative predictive values of over 90% and identify most, but not all, seriously ill patients on admission. Ranson's scoring system has separate scores for alcohol and

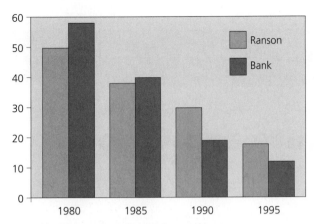

Figure 16.1 Mortality % in severe acute pancreatitis (from data of Ranson and Bank, reported in *J Clin Gastroenterol* 2002; 35:50).

Table 16.1	Ranson's prognostic criteria	
	Acute pancreatitis	
	Alcohol induced	Biliary
On admission or diagnosis		
Age	> 55 years	> 70 years
White blood cell count	> 16 000/mm³	>18 000/mm³
Blood glucose	> 200 mg/dL	> 220 mg/dL
Serum LDH	> 350 U/L	> 400 U/L
Serum SGOT	> 250 U/L	> 250 U/L
During initial 48 h		
Hematocrit decrease	> 10%	> 10%
BUN	> 5 mg/dL	> 2 mg/dL
Serum calcium level	< 8 mg/dL	< 8 mg/dL
Arterial PO₂	< 60 mmHg	
Base deficit	> 4 mmol/L	5 mmol/L
Estimated fluid sequestration	> 6 L	> 4 L

biliary pancreatitis and, like the Glasgow score, includes data obtained over the first 48 hours.

Serologic assays are also used in the early prediction of disease severity. A hematocrit over 44% on admission reflects volume contraction and usually indicates severe disease. Serum glucose less than 150 mg/dL in a previously non-diabetic patient with biliary pancreatitis is reported in one study to have a negative predictive value for severe pancreatitis of 95%. Although hematocrit and glucose as predictors of severe disease have not been evaluated as well as the scoring systems mentioned above, glucose over 150 mg/dL or hematocrit over 44% may justify initial admission to an intensive care unit. Elevated C-reactive protein may reflect severe

disease, but elevation may not be present initially. Urinary trypsinogen activation peptide and certain serum cytokines (IL-6, IL-8, and TNF) are more elevated in severe than mild disease, but these tests are not generally available.

Additional predictors of severity include a Balthazar score greater than 7, chest X-ray evidence of pulmonary edema or pleural effusion, morbid obesity, and elevated serum creatinine. Clinical judgment should not be overlooked. A patient in shock needs care in an intensive care unit no matter what the hematocrit or Ranson score.

Accurate and early disease stratification is important because management of patients with severe disease may be dramatically different than that of patients with mild disease. Patients with severe acute pancreatitis should be admitted to an intensive care unit and managed by a multidisciplinary team.

In the first several days the most serious systemic complications of acute pancreatitis are respiratory failure, shock, and renal failure. According to a 1992 Atlanta symposium on severity in acute pancreatitis, the presence of any of these systemic complications is referred to as "organ failure" and is associated with increased mortality. Organ failure is seen in approximately 30% of subjects with severe acute pancreatitis. After the first week, infection, pseudocysts, and bleeding are additional severe complications and causes of mortality.

Therapy

Unfortunately, no specific therapy based on the pathophysiology of pancreatitis has been shown to be effective. Improved outcomes depend on meticulous supportive care. The pathology of acute pancreatitis is thought to result from activation of trypsin in the pancreas and a local and systemic inflammatory response. Some drugs that are effective in experimental pancreatitis have been tried clinically, so far without success. Randomized prospective studies investigating the anti-proteases aprotinin and gabexate, failed to show significant reduction in the development of systemic complications in patients with severe acute pancreatitis. Platelet activating factor is an inflammatory mediator that is elevated in experimental pancreatitis and therapy with a platelet activating factor inhibitor (Lexipafant®) has lessened the severity of experimental pancreatitis. Lexipafant® was tested in a large placebo controlled study but treated patients did as poorly as placebo-treated patients.

Table 16.2   Acute physiology and chronic health evaluation (APACHE-II)

Physiologic variable	+4	+3	+2	+1	0	+1	+2	+3	+4
Rectal temperature (°C)	≥ 41	39–40.9	–	38.5–38.9	36–38.4	34–35.9	32–33.9	30–31.9	≤ 29
Mean arterial pressure (mmHg)	>160	130–159	110–129	–	70–109	–	50–69	–	≤ 49
Heart rate	>180	140–179	110–139	–	70–109	–	55–69	40–54	≤ 39
Respiratory rate	> 50	35–49	–	25–34	12–24	10–11	6–9	–	≤ 5
Oxygenation									
FiO$_2$ ≥ 0.5	> 500	350–499	200–349	–	< 200	–	–	–	–
FiO$_2$ ≤ 0.5	–	–	–	–	PO$_2$ > 70	61–70	–	55–60	< 55
Arterial pH	≥ 7.7	7.6–7.69	–	7.5–7.59	7.33–7.49	–	7.25–7.32	7.15–7.24	< 7.5
Serum sodium (mmol/L)	≥ 180	160–179	155–159	150–154	130–149	–	120–129	111–119	<110
Serum potassium (mmol/L)	≥ 7	6–6.9	–	5.5–5.9	3.5–5.4	3–3.4	2.5–2.9	–	< 2.5
Serum creatinine (mmol/L)	≥ 3.5	2–3.4	1.5–1.9	–	0.6–1.4	–	< 0.6	–	–
Hematocrit (%)	≥ 60	–	50–59.9	46–49.9	30–45.9	–	20–29.9	–	< 20
White blood count	≥ 40	–	20–39.9	15–19.9	3–14.9	–	1–2.9	–	< 1
Glasgow coma score	–	–	–	–	–	–	–	–	–
Serum HCO$_2$ (use if no arterial blood gas)	≥ 52	41–51.9	–	32–40.9	22–31.9	–	18–21.9	15–17.9	< 15

A Total acute physiologic
Score: sum of points for each physiologic variable.

B Age points

Age (yrs)	Points
<=44	0
45–44	1
45–54	2
55–64	3
65–74	4
>=75	5

C Chronic Health Points
a. Five points for non-operative or emergency post-operative patients.
b. Two points for elective post-operative patients, end stage liver disease, severe congestive heart failure (CHF), end stage lung disease, end stage renal disease, and chronic immunosuppression.

APACHE-II score = A+B+C
Total score >8 is consistent with severe disease

Table 16.3 Glasgow severity score

Age	> 55 years
Serum uncorrected calcium	< 2.00 mmol/L
Serum urea	> 16 mmol/L
LDH	> 600 U/L
Blood glucose(no diabetes)	> 10 mmol/L
WBC	>15 × 10⁹/L
Serum albumin	< 32 g/L
PaO₂	< 60 mmHg (7.5 kPa)

Table 16.4 Balthazar computed tomography severity staging system for acute pancreatitis

CT score

0. normal pancreas
1. focal or diffuse enlargement of the pancreas
2. peri-pancreatic inflammation
3. as 2 plus an ill-defined fluid collection in or near the pancreas
4. as 2 plus two or multiple fluid collections or the presence of gas in or adjacent to the pancreas.

If necrosis is present on contrast-enhanced images, the following scores are added to the CT scores above to calculate a total score.

Necrosis score

0. no necrosis
2. less than 33%
4. 33%–50%
6. more than 50%

A total score greater than 7 indicates severe disease.

Other unsuccessful therapies include peritoneal lavage, somatostatin, and anticholinergic medication.

Pancreatic necrosis

Necrosis of the pancreas occurs in a minority of cases of acute pancreatitis but is responsible for more than 70% of the associated mortality. Damage to the pancreatic microcirculation may be the key injury leading to the development of pancreatic necrosis. Impairment of pancreatic microcirculation is an early injury in experimental models of severe acute pancreatitis. The impairment in the pancreatic microcirculation is probably multifactorial. Possible causes include systemic hypovolemia with decreased pancreatic blood flow, thrombosis, and constriction of pancreatic vessels and vascular endothelial damage. Techniques utilized to improve pancreatic circulation in experimental acute pancreatitis include anti-inflammatory agents and early aggressive fluid resuscitation. Most investigators feel that vigorous fluid replacement is essential in acute pancreatitis but such therapy has not been proven to diminish necrosis. Dextran 60 improves pancreatic microcirculation and reduces damage to the pancreas in experimental pancreatitis but its clinical effectiveness has not been established.

Mild disease

Acute pancreatitis may be mild or severe. Mild disease is defined as acute pancreatitis without systemic complications or predictors of severe disease. By these criteria 90% of acute pancreatitis attacks are mild and these attacks produce less than 1% of all mortality associated with acute pancreatitis. Most patients with mild disease can be managed safely on the general medical floor. Hospital stay is usually no more than 7 days.

Imaging

Patients should have abdominal films to detect ileus and intestinal obstruction. Chest X-ray is appropriate to diagnose associated atelectasis, effusion, and pulmonary infiltrates indicative of respiratory distress syndrome. Abdominal ultrasound is performed in most patients to detect gallstones or evidence of acute cholecystitis and to visualize the pancreas. Unfortunately, about a third of abdominal ultrasounds obtained in this setting will not adequately visualize the pancreas because of overlying bowel gas. Abdominal CT scan is rarely needed in mild acute pancreatitis and is not routinely performed.

Fluid resuscitation

Early and aggressive fluid resuscitation is extremely important because of extensive "third spacing" of fluid. Most patients with mild disease require the repletion of 3 to 4 liters of fluid in the first 24 hours. When necessary, plasma expanders such as blood and albumin may be given, but these are usually needed only in severe disease.

Pain management

Abdominal pain is usually managed with parenteral narcotics. High doses are often needed and, when first seen, patients tend to be under-medicated. The

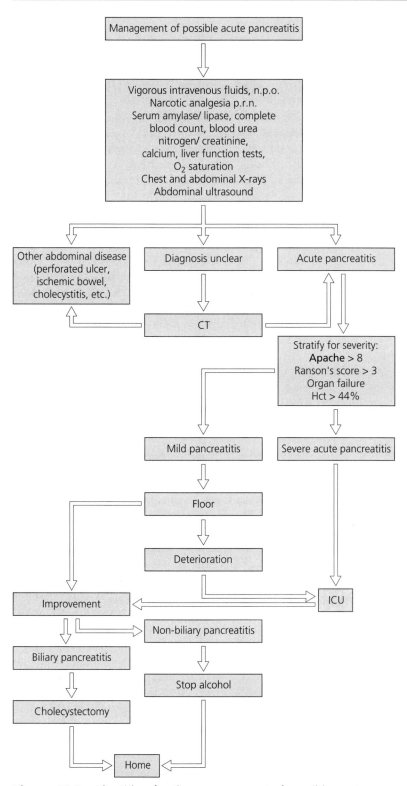

Figure 16.2 Algorithm for the management of possible acute pancreatitis.

first few doses may be given intravenously every 15 minutes until the patient is comfortable. Thereafter, narcotics should be administered every 2 to 3 hours as needed; every 4 hours is often inadequate. Analgesia administered via a patient controlled pump is the optimal method to ensure adequate dosing and avoid indiscriminate use of narcotics. Although there has been concern that morphine-induced sphincter

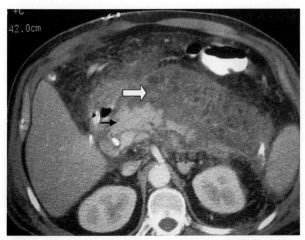

Figure 16.3 Computed tomography with intravenous contrast: pancreatic necrosis (white arrow) is not enhanced by contrast; viable pancreas (black arrow) enhances.

of Oddi spasm could aggravate pancreatitis, there is no clinical evidence that this occurs. Sphincter pressure may be unimportant since pancreatic secretion is curtailed in acute pancreatitis. Because of a small risk of seizures with meperidine use, morphine is probably the preferred analgesic.

Nutrition

Initially, patients receive nothing by mouth. Nasogastric suctioning may be of benefit if there is nausea or vomiting. Patients may begin to receive oral nutrition when they are no longer having abdominal pain and ileus has abated.

Prognosis

Most patients with mild acute pancreatitis will have a full recovery and will not suffer serious long-term sequelae of their disease. In individuals with multiple episodes of acute pancreatitis, the initial episode tends to be the most severe, but this is not predictable. Patients with alcoholic pancreatitis should abstain from further alcohol ingestion. Patients with biliary pancreatitis should have cholecystectomy, usually before leaving the hospital, in order to prevent recurrent disease.

Severe acute pancreatitis

Individuals with severe acute pancreatitis are at significant risk of death or long-term morbidity from this disease. It is a medical emergency and patients should be triaged promptly to specialized care in an intensive care unit.

Imaging

Computed tomography scan of the abdomen should be performed in patients with severe acute pancreatitis. Optimal timing is unclear, but scans should probably be obtained within the first few days to assess complications such as pancreatic necrosis or peripancreatic fluid collections. Limited experimental, but no reliable clinical evidence, suggests that intravenous iodinated contrast at the initiation of pancreatitis may exacerbate the disease. Because of this, some clinicians believe that intravenous iodinated contrast should be avoided in the first day or two of pancreatitis. Radiologists experienced in pancreatic disease advocate the use of intravenous contrast for more informative CT scans and usually recommend non-ionic contrast. Non-ionic contrast has less risk of precipitating renal failure than does ionic contrast. If the diagnosis is unsure, CT should be performed immediately to confirm pancreatitis and rule out other disease such as bowel infarction or perforation that might simulate pancreatitis.

Although CT without intravenous contrast will reveal pancreatic swelling and peripancreatic collections, intravenous contrast is needed to detect pancreatic necrosis. Non-enhancing parenchyma with diameter greater than 3 centimeters on dynamic intravenous contrast CT or MRI scan indicates necrosis. Necrosis is detected in 10% to 20% of patients with acute pancreatitis and in a much higher percentage of those with severe acute pancreatitis. Patients found to have necrosis should have follow-up scanning about a week after the first scan and then at increasing intervals until resolution or stabilization of disease.

Findings on CT scanning may be graded according to the Balthazar severity score (Table 16.4). A Balthazar score greater than 7 indicates severe pancreatitis and increased mortality.

In patients with renal dysfunction, a MRI scan with intravenous gadolinium will provide information similar to that obtained with CT and does not carry the risk of exacerbating renal function associated with CT contrast dye.

Fluid resuscitation

Restoration of intravenous volume and prevention of hypovolemic shock are essential. Daily fluid deficits may be as great as 10 liters. Plasma expanders, such as blood or albumin, are often required. Swan–Ganz catheterization is useful to monitor central venous pressure in patients in whom adequate volume resuscitation is difficult. Vasopressor agents may be necessary to maintain renal perfusion or blood pressure. Peripheral vasodilatation and hyperdynamic circulation may simulate the circulatory pattern of sepsis and empiric antibiotic coverage is appropriate until blood culture results are available.

Pain management

Pain management is the same as that used in cases of milder disease but patients may be too ill for patient-controlled analgesia.

Nutrition

Patients should receive nothing by mouth until ileus and pain have resolved. The majority will require total parenteral nutrition. Total parenteral nutrition is continued until adequate oral nutrition is tolerated and may be needed for weeks if feeding exacerbates pain or disease. Some studies have indicated that jejunal feeding decreases the risk of infection (from infected total parenteral nutrition catheters or from intestinal bacterial translocation) and may reduce mortality. Further study of such enteral feeding is needed.

Infection

Infection develops in about half of severe acute pancreatitis patients ill for more than 2 weeks. Infection occurs in or adjacent to the pancreas or at systemic sites, such as the lungs (pneumonia), urinary tract, or at intravenous punctures. Many of the infecting organisms are thought to translocate from the intestines. Decreased systemic resistance to infection may also dispose to infection. Gram-negative, gram-positive, aerobic, anaerobic, and fungal organisms may be found on culture. In recent years with more widespread use of potent antibiotics, fungal infections or antibiotic resistant bacterial infections have become more common.

Infection may occur in areas of pancreatic necrosis or in fluid collections adjacent to the pancreas. Patients with more than 30% necrosis are at increased risk compared with those having lesser necrosis. Infection of necrotic pancreas requires surgical debridement and procrastination increases mortality. Percutaneous drainage procedures usually fail to adequately drain the viscous material found in infected necrosis, at least during the first few weeks of pancreatitis. Contents of pancreatic abscesses occurring after several weeks may be liquid enough for percutaneous large-bore catheter drainage. Percutaneous drainage by interventional radiology should be done in conjunction with surgical consultation and depends on local expertise. The prognosis in patients with abscesses occurring after the first 2 weeks is often better because of the lack of organ failure.

Clues to the presence of infected necrotic tissue include high fever, sustained tachycardia, and leukocytosis, but each of these is non-specific and may reflect inflammation without infection. Infection should be considered in patients who do not continue to improve clinically. Blood cultures and CT scan to detect gas within the pancreas are helpful. The most reliable method for distinguishing sterile from infected necrosis is CT-guided needle aspiration of necrotic areas, with gram stain and culture of the aspirate.

Antibiotic therapy depends upon the organism identified. Initial therapy with a broad-spectrum antibiotic such as imipenem may be appropriate. Antifungal therapy may be needed since fungal infections have become more common, but should usually await culture results. Optimal duration of antibiotic therapy is unclear and consultation with infection disease specialists is helpful.

Prophylactic antibiotics

Because of the serious implications of infection in patients with severe acute pancreatitis, prophylactic antibiotic use has been proposed. Although clinical trials suggest lessened infection with the use of potent broad-spectrum antibiotics, evidence of effectiveness is not convincing. None of the trials was blinded, all were underpowered, and the statistically significant reduction in mortality seen in one small trial was not reproduced in others (Table 16.5). Nevertheless, antibiotic prophylaxis was associated with trends toward reduced mortality and infection in these studies and many clinicians advocate prophylactic antibiotics such as imipenem or ciprofloxan beginning with the first evidence of severe disease. Further study is needed in this area.

Sterile necrosis

Individuals with sterile necrosis have increased mortality depending on the extent of necrosis. In general, however, the mortality from sterile necrosis is much less than that associated with infected necrosis. Extensive necrosis may produce diabetes or exocrine insufficiency, but mortality correlates more with development of infection or systemic complications such as respiratory failure rather than with necrosis *per se*.

The role of surgery in patients with sterile necrosis is controversial. Surgical debridement may be considered in patients who are deteriorating clini-

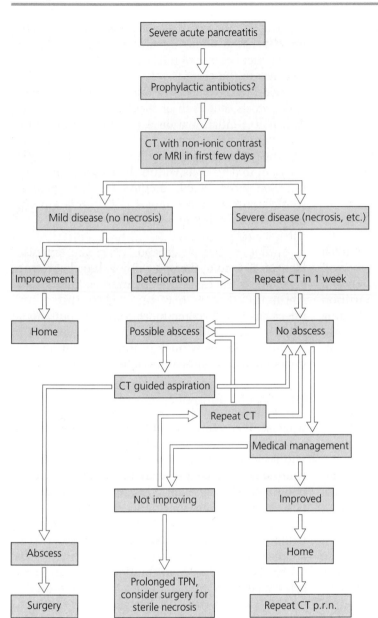

Figure 16.4 Algorithm for the management of severe acute pancreatitis.

Table 16.5 Antibiotic prophylaxis in severe acute pancreatitis (from Buchler *et al. Gut* 1999; 45: 311–316)

Reference	Drug	Patients		Infection (%)		Mortality (%)	
		Control	*Case*	*Control*	*Case*	*Control*	*Case*
Luiten *et al.*	cefotaxime, colistin amphotericin, norfloxacin	52	50	38	18	35	22
Pederzoli *et al.*	imipenem	33	41	30	12	12	7
Sainio *et al.*	cefuroxime	30	30	40	30	23	3
Delcenserie	ceftazadime, amikacin, metronidazole	12	11	58	0	25	9
Schwarz *et al.*	ofloxacin, metronidazole	13	13	53	61	5	0
Bassi *et al.*	pefloxacin (P) vs imipenem (I)	30(P)	30(I)	34(P)	10(I)	24(P)	10(I)

cally, but most surgeons prefer prolonged observation, only using surgery for infected necrosis.

Pulmonary and renal dysfunction

The systemic inflammatory response of acute pancreatitis may produce organ dysfunction within the first several days. Pulmonary and renal dysfunctions are the most common and are associated with increased mortality.

Hypoxia should be evaluated and an etiology determined in all patients with severe acute pancreatitis. Tachypnea and hypoxia may reflect diaphragmatic splinting because of abdominal pain, atelectasis, pleural effusion, coexistent pulmonary disease, or acute respiratory distress syndrome. Oxygen supplementation is recommended when oxygen saturation falls. Severe or worsening disease may require mechanical ventilation and positive end-expiratory pressure as in other forms of acute respiratory distress syndrome. No specific therapy is available.

Deteriorating renal function is initially managed with volume resuscitation and maintenance of adequate blood pressure. There is no data to support prophylactic or therapeutic "renal-dose" dopamine to prevent acute tubular necrosis in pancreatitis. In patients with deteriorating renal function intravenous CT dye should be avoided. Hemodialysis may be needed

Cholecystectomy and early endoscopic sphincterotomy

Biliary pancreatitis recurs in a significant proportion of patients discharged with intact gallbladders. Therefore, elective cholecystectomy is often advised before discharge from the hospital. Benefit from early endoscopic sphincterotomy is more controversial. Three randomized trials of sphincterotomy within the first 72 hours of disease have suggested benefit, but probably only if there is cholangitis or persistent jaundice.

Pancreatic pseudocyst

Pseudocysts are fluid-filled collections with well-defined inflammatory and fibrotic walls. Most develop in the first few weeks of pancreatitis. Pseudocysts may be asymptomatic or they may cause symptoms such as pain. Cysts may rupture into the peritoneal cavity (producing chronic pancreatic ascites) or into adjacent bowel. Pressure on the stomach or duodenum may produce nausea and early satiety, and compression of the bile duct pro-

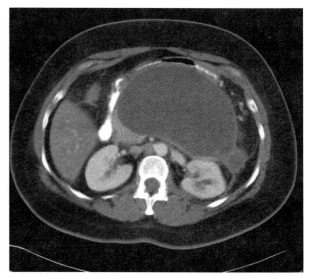

Figure 16.5   Contrast-enhanced computed tomography showing large pancreatic pseudocyst.

duces biliary obstruction. Arterial aneurysms in the cyst wall may bleed and produce hemosuccus pancreaticus.

Pseudocysts resolve spontaneously in about half of cases. Drainage is usually reserved for cysts that are greater than 5 centimeters in diameter after several weeks observation and are enlarging or causing symptoms. Pseudocysts may be drained surgically, endoscopically, or radiographically. No randomized trials have been done to demonstrate the advantage of one therapy over another and choice of procedure usually depends on local expertise. Follow-up CT or ultrasound a few weeks after drainage is appropriate to assure successful drainage. Recurrence of cysts is not infrequent.

Endoscopic drainage of pseudocysts may be performed by direct puncture through the stomach or duodenal wall or by stenting the pancreatic duct. Direct puncture may be considered if the cyst abuts the stomach or duodenum. Endoscopic ultrasound is advisable to exclude intervening arteries. Cysts that communicate with the pancreatic duct may be drained by transpapillary stents. Even large transpapillary stents will occlude and should be removed or replaced within a few weeks.

Percutaneous pigtail catheter drainage of sterile, or even infected, pseudocysts may be performed. The fluid in an infected pseudocyst is often less viscous than that in an area of infected necrosis and may, therefore, be drained via a large-bore catheter. Many surgeons advocate percutaneous rather than surgical drainage if possible.

Surgical drainage of pseudocysts is by cystgastrostomy or Roux-en-Y cystojejunostomy. Preoperative

ERCP is often recommended to determine if the cyst communicates with the main pancreatic duct and that there is no downstream obstruction, but effect of ERCP on outcome has not been demonstrated. When cysts are associated with pancreatic necrosis surgical evacuation will usually be needed because of the viscous nature of the cyst contents.

Other complications and therapies

Rare complications of severe acute pancreatitis include chronic pancreatic ascites, pancreatic pleural effusion, pancreatic fistulas to the skin, splenic artery aneurysm, and splenic vein occlusion. Pancreatic ascites or fistulas to the pleural space indicate a disrupted pancreatic duct; they are treated initially with pancreatic "rest" (nothing by mouth, total parenteral nutrition, and perhaps octreotide intravenously) for a few weeks but usually need surgical therapy. Preoperative ERCP is needed to identify the site of leak (this is one situation in which MR pancreatogram has not replaced diagnostic ERCP). Drainage by ERCP-placed transpapillary stent has also been successful.

Splenic artery aneurysm may be treated by arterial embolization if bleeding occurs. Splenic vein occlusion is not treated unless bleeding gastric varices develop, in which case surgical splenectomy is appropriate.

Metabolic abnormalities of acute pancreatitis include elevated hypertriglyceridemia, hypocalcemia, and hypomagnesemia. Severe pancreatitis with persistent and markedly elevated triglyceride may respond to plasmapheresis to lower triglyceride levels. Hypocalcemia is most often non-ionic and the result of low serum albumin and does not need therapy. Low serum ionic calcium may cause neuromuscular irritability and responds to intravenous calcium. Low serum magnesium may intensify hypocalcemia and should be corrected.

Chronic pancreatitis

Chronic pancreatitis is an inclusive term describing a group of pancreatic diseases in which there is persistent injury to the endocrine and exocrine parenchyma or ducts of the pancreas. The changes may be atrophic or involve chronic inflammation and fibrosis of parenchyma, strictures, or dilation of ducts, and precipitation and calcification in ducts. Chronic or intermittent pain is the most common symptom of chronic pancreatitis. Severe disruption of pancreatic function may result in maldigestion or diabetes mellitus.

Etiologies and possible pathophysiology of chronic pancreatitis are discussed in other chapters. For purposes of management it is important to identify etiologies such as alcoholism, hypercalcemia, medications (e.g. Imuran®), congenital abnormalities (pancreas divisum, choledochocele), parasites (e.g. ascariasis), and autoimmune disease that may be treated. Unfortunately, in many patients the disease is idiopathic. Even if the disease is idiopathic, oral enzyme replacement and insulin provide reasonably effective therapy for maldigestion and diabetes. Pain control may be more difficult. Separation of patients with markedly dilated ducts from those with relatively normal-size ducts is important in some aspects of pain management, as is outlined on the algorithm below (Figure 16.6). It is possible that dilation of ducts implies duct obstruction with resultant increased duct pressure and that pain will respond to relief of obstruction.

Pain

Pain is the most common complication of chronic pancreatitis, occurring in about 80% of all patients. Pain is usually epigastric, may radiate to the back, and be constant or intermittent. Pain may be exacerbated by eating or alcohol consumption. The etiology of the pain associated with chronic pancreatitis is unclear. Hypotheses for the etiology of pain include increased pressure in the pancreatic duct and parenchyma, parenchymal inflammation, and neural inflammation.

Since alcohol is a potential pancreatic toxin, all patients in whom pain is a problem should abstain from alcohol consumption. Avoidance of large meals, especially fatty meals, may be helpful in some patients. Painful attacks may gradually abate as the disease "burns out". The possibility of spontaneous improvement over months, or even years, should be considered before undertaking radical surgical procedures.

Evaluation of the pancreas with CT, MR pancreatogram, or EUS should be performed in all patients with pain to determine if there are dilated ducts, pseudocysts, calcification, biliary obstruction, or splenic vein occlusion. If less invasive tests do not reveal evidence of chronic pancreatitis ERCP may be appropriate. See Chapter 15 on diagnosis of pancreatic disease for further discussion of diagnostic testing.

Non-narcotic analgesics such as non-steroidal anti-inflammatory drugs (NSAIDs) or acetaminophen may be tried but many patients will require narcotics. Concern for development of narcotic

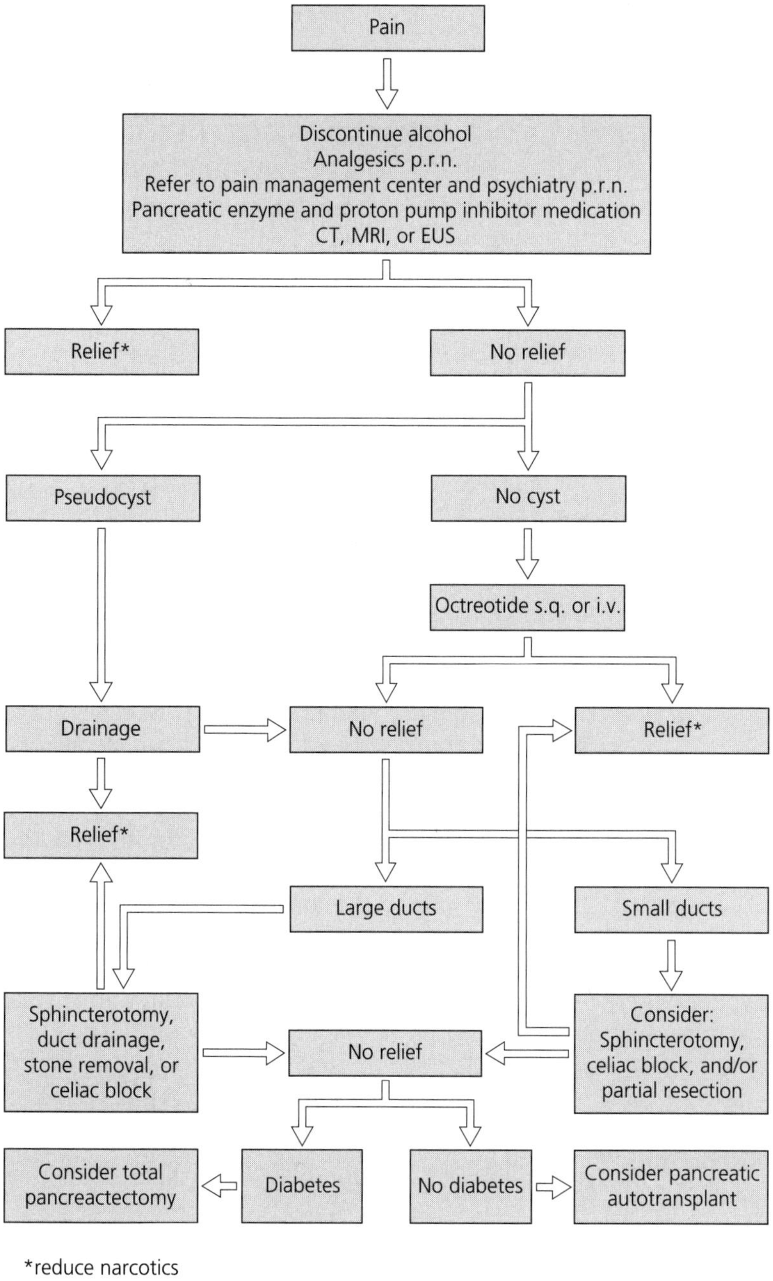

Figure 16.6 Algorithm for the management of pain.

*reduce narcotics

abuse or dependence is appropriate and often patients should be referred to a pain management center. Psychiatric evaluation may be helpful, not only in limiting narcotic use, but also in treating alcoholism. Antidepressant medication may have a synergistic effect with analgesic therapy. Patients should be urged to reduce narcotics whenever pain improves.

Limited data indicate that large doses (e.g. 32 000 non-enteric coated lipase units every 4 hours while awake) of pancreatic enzymes by mouth may lessen pain. A trial of such therapy for a few weeks is appropriate. The hypothesis for effectiveness of this therapy is that intraduodenal trypsin inhibits CCK release and, thereby, reduces pancreatic secretion. Patients with non-dilated ducts and mild parenchyma disease may respond better than other patients. Non-enteric-coated enzyme preparations (Table 16.6) are used because they are active in the proximal duodenum where much CCK release occurs. A proton pump inhibitor is given with enzyme therapy to reduce gastric acid inactivation of enzymes.

Subcutaneous or intravenous ocreotide may be tried. Two small, uncontrolled, clinical trials suggested that octreotide at a dose of 100 micrograms subcutaneously every 8 hours decreased the pain of chronic pancreatitis, but this benefit was not observed in a small controlled study. Octreotide has

Table 16.6 Pancreatic enzyme preparations

		Lipase (USP)	Protease (USP)	Amylase (USP)
Enteric coated enzymes				
Cotazym-S	capsules	5 000	20 000	20 000
Creon 5	capsules	5 000	18 750	16 600
Creon 10	capsules	10 000	37 500	32 200
Creon 20	capsules	20 000	75 000	64 400
Pancrease	capsules	4 500	25 000	20 000
Pancrease MT4	capsules	4 000	12 000	12 000
Pancrease MT 10	capsules	10 000	30 000	30 000
Pancrease MT 16	capsules	16 000	48 000	48 000
Pancrease MT 20	capsules	20 000	44 000	56 000
Zymase	capsules	12 000	24 000	24 000
Non-enteric coated enzymes				
Cotazym	capsules	8 000	30 000	30 000
Viokase	tablets	8 000	30 000	30 000
	powder	16 800	70 000	70 000

been found to reduce output from pancreatic fistulas and might ameliorate pain by reducing pancreatic secretion.

More aggressive therapy for pain

If pain has not responded to the measures outlined above, more aggressive measures may be needed. Unfortunately, these aggressive measures are effective in only some patients and each measure involves significant risk. Surgical or endoscopic therapy should be performed only by highly skilled consultants and after thorough discussion of the risks with patients. Patients in whom pseudocysts may be the cause of pain may benefit from drainage of the cyst.

Patients with dilated pancreatic ducts are candidates for duct decompression. Endoscopic sphincterotomy, stenting, and duct-stone removal may be tried but are less likely to be effective than surgical duct drainage and stone removal. Extracorporeal shock wave lithotrypsy is used in some centers to fragment stones and facilitate their removal. Longitudinal pancreaticojejunostomy is the most commonly performed drainage procedure. Initially it gives relief to 80% of patients, but many have recurrence of pain in subsequent years. When disease is most severe in the pancreatic head, a Whipple-type resection may be appropriate (see Chapter 18 on surgery for pancreatic disease for further discussion). Endoscopic or surgical sphincterotomy may be helpful in patients with pancreas divisum or, rarely, in other patients with non-dilated ducts. Measurement of pancreatic sphincter pressure is performed in a few centers to evaluate these difficult patients. Resection

of an area of focal pancreatic disease may give relief.

Celiac block performed with radiographic, endoscopic, or surgical guidance may provide relief but is often only transiently effective and carries significant risks. The most radical therapies are total pancreatectomy and pancreatic autotransplant. Total pancreatectomy should be considered only if the patient is already diabetic. Pancreatic autotransplant may preserve endocrine function and has provided pain relief in a few patients. Autotransplantation involves moving the pancreas to another area in the abdomen with new vascular and enteric anastomoses; in the process nerves to the pancreas are severed.

Pancreatic insufficiency

Steatorrhea or diabetes mellitus may develop after severe deterioration of pancreatic function. Pancreatic steatorrhea usually is seen when less than 10% of the exocrine functional capacity of the pancreas remains. It may take several years for steatorrhea to develop. In patients with idiopathic chronic pancreatitis (CP) the mean latency from first evidence of disease to onset of steatorrhea is 20 to 30 years. A simple qualitative stain of the stool for fecal fat can confirm a clinical suspicion of steatorrhea. The classic, and quite repugnant, 72-hour stool fecal fat determination is rarely needed.

Pancreatic enzyme supplements are the mainstay of therapy in pancreatic steatorrhea. Enteric-coated preparations may be more effective because the enteric coating reduces inactivation of enzymes by gastric acid. Studies have shown that approximately 25 000 to 40 000 units of lipase must be delivered per meal in order to ensure the proper digestion of fats. Enzymes should be given with the meal so that good mixing with food occurs. Table 16.6 lists non-enteric and enteric enzyme preparations.

If adequate calories are not absorbed following enzyme replacement, medium chain triglycerides may be substituted for some of the fat in the diet. Medium chain triglycerides are more easily hydrolyzed than long chain-fats. Reduction of total fat intake may be needed to reduce foul-smelling fatty stools.

Approximately 30% of patients with chronic pancreatitis will develop diabetes after 10 years of disease, and diabetes is present in about 80% of those with steatorrhea. Diabetes caused by chronic pancreatitis may be very labile and insulin therapy is directed at maintaining "loose" but acceptable control of blood sugar. Chronic pancreatitis reduces glucagon as well as insulin production by the pancreas, and patients lacking the protective effect of glucagon are at increased risk for severe episodes of hypoglycemia. Rarely the appearance of diabetes in patients with CP heralds the onset of pancreatic cancer. It is currently unknown which individuals with CP and diabetes will develop pancreatic cancer and this area remains under active investigation.

Other complications of chronic pancreatitis

Chronic pancreatitis, like severe acute pancreatitis, may be associated with the development of pseudocysts, pancreatic ascites, pancreatic pleural effusion, splenic vein occlusion, and splenic artery aneurysms. Management of these conditions is discussed in the section on severe acute pancreatitis (see p. 304).

Chronic biliary obstruction can occur in chronic pancreatitis because of fibrosis or cysts in the pancreatic head. Such obstruction is often slow in onset and dilation of bile ducts with marked elevation of alkaline phosphatase may precede the development of jaundice. Once bilirubin is elevated surgical relief is usually needed. Stenting is unlikely to be effective since the pathology is chronic and non-removable metal stents should never be employed. Cirrhosis, cholangitis, and liver abscesses secondary to the obstruction are unusual, but can occur.

Further reading

Balthazar EJ. Acute pancreatitis: assessment of severity with clinical and CT evaluation. *Radiology* 2002; 223(3): 603–613.

Bank S Singh P, Pooran N and Stark B. Evaluation of factors that have reduced mortality from acute pancreatitis over the past 20 years. *J Clin Gastroenterol* 2002; 35: 50–60.

Butturini G, Salvia R, Bettini R *et al*. Infection prevention in necrotizing pancreatitis: an old challenge with new perspectives. *J Hospital Infection* 2001; 49: 4–8.

Hawes RH. A clinician's perspective on chronic pancreatitis. *Reviews in Gastroenterological Disorders* 2002; 2(2): 57–65.

Meek K, Toosie K, Stabile BE and de Virgilio. Simplified admission criteria for predicting severe complications of gallstone pancreatitis. *Archives of Surgery* 2000; 135: 1048–1052.

Lankisch PG. Natural course of chronic pancreatitis. *Pancreatology* 2001; 1(1): 3–14.

Thompson DR. Narcotic analgesic effects on the sphincter of Oddi: a review of the data and therapeutic implications in treating pancreatitis. *Am J Gastroenterol* 2001; 96: 1266–1272.s

Chapter 17

Pancreatic Neoplasms

Nuzhat A. Ahmad

Pancreatic cancer

Cancer of the pancreas is the fifth leading cause of cancer-related deaths in the US. Ductal adenocarcinoma and its variants make up more than 90% of all malignant pancreatic exocrine tumors. The remainder are acinar cell carcinomas, sarcomas, lymphomas, and other tumors of uncertain histogenesis. Surgical resection is the only potentially curative treatment for pancreatic cancer. Unfortunately, only a minority of patients are eligible for resection at the time of diagnosis. Almost all patients with pancreatic cancer will die from the disease.

Epidemiology

Approximately 28 000 new cases of pancreatic cancer are diagnosed in the US every year. Men are slightly more susceptible to the disease. African Americans have a higher incidence of pancreatic cancer than white Americans or any other ethnic population, with an incidence of 14.8 per 100 000 compared to 8.8 per 100 000 in the general population. The peak incidence of pancreatic cancer is in the seventh and eight decades of life. It is extremely rare before the age of 40 years. Because of the aggressiveness of this cancer, the inability to diagnose it early, and the current lack of outcome-altering therapies, mortality rates from pancreatic cancer are almost identical to incidence rates.

Risk factors

Smoking

The risk factor most strongly linked to pancreatic cancer is cigarette smoking. Numerous studies have reported an increased risk of pancreatic cancer for smokers. The risk increases with the amount of cigarettes consumed. It has been estimated that

30% of cases of pancreatic cancer are due to smoking and that cessation of smoking could eliminate approximately 25% of pancreatic cancer deaths in the US.

Diet and exercise

A high intake of meat and fat in the diet has been linked to the development of pancreatic cancer while a protective effect has been suggested by the consumption of fruits and vegetables. Obesity has also been linked to pancreatic cancer.

Coffee and alcohol consumption

There is no evidence at present to support a definite link between coffee or alcohol consumption and the development of pancreatic cancer.

Diabetes mellitus

An association between diabetes mellitus and pancreatic cancer has been reported in numerous studies, but the exact nature of the relationship is not clearly defined. It has also been suggested that diabetes may be a consequence rather than a cause of pancreatic cancer.

Chronic pancreatitis

There are data suggesting that patients with chronic pancreatitis are at increased risk of developing pancreatic cancer. Studies have found that 1.8% of patients with chronic pancreatits developed pancreatic cancer during a mean follow-up of 7.4 years.

Hereditary factors

Familial aggregation and genetic susceptibility play a role in as many as 10% of patients with pancreatic cancer. It has been estimated that patients with hereditary pancreatitis have a 40% risk of developing pancreatic cancer by the age of 70. In several population studies 7% to 10% of patients with pancreatic cancer have a first-degree relative with the disease. The risk of pancreatic cancer is also increased in patients with certain familial cancer syndromes such as Peutz–Jeghers syndrome and Von Hippel–Lindau syndrome.

Surgery

A two- to five-fold increased risk of developing pancreatic cancer 15 to 20 years after partial gastrectomy has been described.

Clinical features

About two thirds of ductal adenocarcinomas occur in the pancreatic head, the rest occur in the body or tail, or diffusely throughout the pancreas. A diagnosis of pancreatic cancer is usually suspected based on the clinical presentation, which can include symptoms of pain, weight loss, or jaundice.

Jaundice

Jaundice is seen in pancreatic-head cancers and results from obstruction of the common bile duct by the tumor. Accompanying symptoms of pruritis, acholic stools, and dark urine can be present. Jaundice is unusual in tumors of the pancreatic body.

Pain

Pain is present in up to 80% to 85% of patients with locally advanced or distant disease. Pain is most commonly felt in the epigastrium but it may also be felt on either side of the abdomen or in the lower quadrants. Persistent severe back pain, caused by tumor invasion of the nerves, is usually indicative of unresectability.

Weight loss

Weight loss can be profound and is usually associated with anorexia, early satiety, diarrhea, and steatorrhea.

Other symptoms

These can include recent onset of diabetes mellitus, unexplained thrombophlebitis, depression, or an attack of pancreatitis.

On physical examination an abdominal mass or ascites can be demonstrated in 20% of patients with pancreatic cancer. A non-tender gallbladder can also be palpated in those with jaundice. Infrequently, an epigastric bruit caused by tumor invasion of an adjacent artery is audible. Rarely, malignant supraclavicular or umbilical ("Sister Mary Joseph") adenopathy is present and, if so, indicates unresectability. However, confirmatory physical findings are usually absent.

Diagnosis and staging

The two main issues in a patient with suspected pancreatic cancer are to establish the diagnosis and to determine whether the patient is a candidate for surgical resection. If the patient is deemed a surgical candidate, histologic proof of malignancy is usually not required. However, in patients with unresectable disease (i.e. distant metastases or major vessel involvement on radiographic studies), a histologic diagnosis is usually required prior to proceeding with any kind of palliative therapy.

The all-important determination of resectability is made using a variety of radiographic tests. With the advanced imaging technology now available, it is uncommon for unsuspected vascular involvement to be found at laporotomy. It is more common to find unsuspected peritoneal metastases or small liver metastases.

The imaging tests available include the following.

Abdominal ultrasound

Ultrasound is usually the first study in patients who present with jaundice. Dilated extrahepatic and intrahepatic bile ducts or the presence of a mass in the pancreas suggest the presence of a pancreatic malignancy. The reported sensitivity and specificity of ultrasound in diagnosing pancreatic cancer are up to 89% and 99%, respectively. Although ultrasound can delineate the relationship of the mass with the surrounding structures, it is not an optimal staging tool.

Computed tomography

Conventional CT provides information about the nature, site, and extent of the lesion. Currently, helical CT scan, which provides more complete and rapid image acquisition compared to conventional CT, is considered the most useful preoperative radiographic study in the diagnosis and staging of pancreatic cancers. Helical CT scan is able to detect tumors 2 centimeters or greater with a sensitivity and specificity of up to 90% and 95%, respectively. It also provides extraordinary detail about vascular anatomy and vascular invasion by tumor. In experienced hands, CT scan has an accuracy of 98% for determining unresectability and 80% for determining resectability of pancreatic tumors. However, it is suboptimal in the evaluation of lymph nodes and peritoneal metastases.

Magnetic resonance imaging

Magnetic resonance imaging offers little additional information to an optimal, good-quality helical CT scan. Recent studies have demonstrated the superiority of MRI over CT in the detection of peritoneal metastases. Magnetic resonance imaging may be useful when the index of suspicion is high and CT scan is normal or equivocal.

Endoscopic retrograde cholangiopancreatography

Endoscopic retrograde cholangiopancreatography has a sensitivity and specificity of 95% and 85%, respectively, for diagnosis of pancreatic cancers. It can detect some tumors not identified on CT scan. The classic finding that suggests the presence of a mass in the pancreas is a stricture in both the common bile duct and the pancreatic duct in the head of the pancreas, the so-called "double-duct sign". In pancreatic body and tail tumors, only the pancreatic duct appears abnormal. Endoscopic retrograde cholangiopancreatography permits brushings of the pancreatic duct which have a sensitivity of 30% to 79% and a specificity of 92% to 100% for diagnosis of pancreatic cancer. Another advantage of ERCP is direct access to the common bile duct that permits placement of a stent for biliary obstruction, particularly if complicated by cholangitis. Endoscopic retrograde cholangiopancreatography has no role in staging of pancreatic cancers.

Endoscopic ultrasound

Endoscopic ultrasound can detect tumors smaller in size than those currently detectable by CT scan. It also provides valuable information about vascular and nodal involvement by pancreatic tumors, thereby assessing resectability. In addition, EUS also permits fine-needle aspiration of pancreatic masses with a sensitivity of 75% to 90% depending on the tumor size. The reported accuracy of EUS in staging of pancreatic cancer is variable, which in part reflects the operator dependency of EUS.

Laproscopy

Laproscopy alone or in combination with laproscopic ultrasound is emerging as a new staging modality for pancreatic tumors. Occult metastases in the liver and peritoneum, which are rarely visible by CT scan or MRI, can be detected via this modality. Overall, the reported sensitivity, specificity, and accuracy of staging laproscopy and ultrasonography are 92%, 88%, and 89%, respectively.

Serum tumor markers

Several tumor markers for pancreatic cancer have been evaluated. The most widely used marker is cancer-associated antigen 19–9 (CA19–9). The sensitivity and specificity of CA19–9 is 80% and 90%, respectively. However, CA19–9 values are closely related to tumor size and are almost never elevated in tumors less than 1 centimeter in size. Postoperative monitoring of CA19–9 may have a role in assessing prognosis, recurrence, and response to therapy. Use of tumor markers has not been shown to reduce mortality of pancreatic cancer.

Cytology

Fine-needle aspiration of pancreatic mass can be performed using US or CT guidance. The sensitivity and specificity of this procedure is dependent on the tumor size and the operator expertise. However, a preoperative histological diagnosis of pancreatic cancer is not required prior to proceeding with surgical resection.

Approach to a suspected pancreatic tumor

Patients with suspected pancreatic cancer usually come to attention because of symptoms. The initial study performed is usually an abdominal ultrasound or a conventional CT scan (Figure 17.1).

If a mass is not visualized on CT scan, an EUS and/or an ERCP is indicated to assess for small lesions that can be missed on CT scan. If a mass in the pancreas is found on the initial studies in a symptomatic patient, it is reasonable to conclude that a malignant process is present. If the patient is a surgical candidate, resectability status of the mass needs to be determined. A helical CT scan usually determines this. If helical CT scan is equivocal about the resectability of the mass, then further studies including MRI/magnetic resonance arteriogram (MRA) and/or an EUS are warranted to preclude unnecessary surgical exploration. However, in a small percentage of patients, a preoperative determination of resectability of the mass can not be made and these patients usually undergo a surgical laparotomy or laparoscopy.

If the patient is not a surgical candidate, then a histological diagnosis needs to be made to allow palliation by endoscopic, chemotherapeutic, or radiotherapeutic means. Histological diagnosis can usually be made with either EUS- or CT-guided fine-needle aspiration.

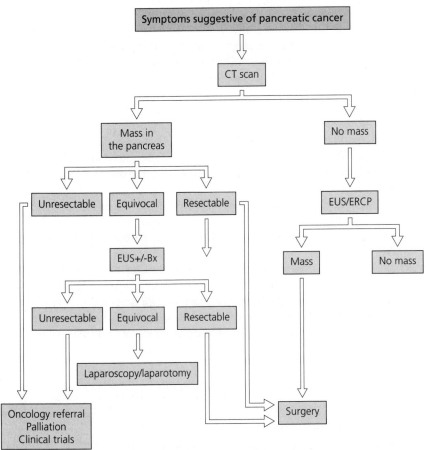

Figure 17.1 Suggested algorithm for the work-up of pancreatic cancer.

Treatment

Surgical resection is the only potentially curative treatment for pancreatic cancer. Unfortunately only 15% to 20% of patients are resectable at the time of initial diagnosis. The assessment of resectability is usually made preoperatively by various imaging studies as described above. In general, pancreatic cancers are considered unresectable if any of the following are present.

1. Distant metastases.
2. Encasement or invasion of the superior mesenteric vein, spleno-portal confluence, superior mesenteric artery, aorta or celiac axis. Some centers, however, are practicing technical resection in cases with superior mesenteric vein, and portal vein involvement, although curability in these cases is questionable.

The standard operation for pancreatic head cancers is a Whipple resection. The Whipple resection involves a partial gastrectomy, cholecystectomy, and removal of the distal common bile duct, head of the pancreas, duodenum, proximal jejunum, and regional lymph nodes. Reconstruction requires a pancreaticojejunostomy, hepaticojejunostomy, and a gastrojejunostomy. In the hands of experienced surgeons, the operative mortality is 2% or less. Pyloric-sparing pancreaticoduodenectomy was developed to decrease the incidence of postoperative dumping, marginal ulceration, and bile-reflux gastritis that can occur in many patients undergoing partial gastrectomy.

Resectable tumors in the body and tail of the pancreas require a distal pancreatectomy and splenectomy. Morbidity and mortality rates are lower than after a Whipple resection, but cures are much less frequent than those for cancer of the pancreatic head.

Adjuvant therapy with 5-flourouracil and radiotherapy confers a survival advantage in patients following curative resection for pancreatic cancer as well as for patients with locally advanced pancreatic cancer. There has been no demonstrated survival advantage or improvement in resectability with preoperative (neoadjuvant) chemoradiotherapy.

Palliative treatment

Alleviation of obstructive jaundice, pain, and gastric-outlet obstruction may be required in patients who are not resectable.

Surgical palliation of both biliary obstruction and duodenal obstruction (which can occur in 15% to 20% of patients) can be managed surgically with bypass procedures. The biliary obstruction can be bypassed by creating an anastamosis between the gallbladder and jejunum (cholecystojejunostomy) or between the common bile duct and the jejunum (choledochojejunostomy). Jaundice is relieved in 90% of cases with this technique. A duodenal obstruction can be bypassed by creating a gastrojejunostomy.

Non-surgical palliation of biliary obstruction can be performed with endoscopic placement of biliary plastic stents or expandable metal stents. Randomized trials have demonstrated that endoscopically placed metal stents are as successful as surgical bypass procedures in relieving obstructive jaundice. Metal stents have the advantage of staying patent for a longer duration than plastic stents. Currently, most patients with biliary obstruction are managed with endoscopic palliation.

Similarly, duodenal obstruction can be managed non-surgically with endoscopic placement of duodenal stents.

Pain can be treated with opioid and non-opioid analgesia. However, in selected cases celiac axis nerve block may be required to alleviate the pain. This can be performed by a surgical, radiographically guided percutaneous or endosonographically guided approach. Pain is relieved in up to 90% of patients with celiac plexus block.

Prognosis

Almost all patients with pancreatic cancer are expected to die from their disease. For patients with distant disease at presentation, the median survival is 3 to 6 months. For patients with locally advanced, unresectable disease, the median survival is 8 to 12 months. Surgical resection offers the only chance for a cure but the median survival after resection is only 18 to 20 months and the overall 5-year survival is 10%. However, in patients with clear surgical margins and no lymph node metastasis, the 5-year survival can be as high as 25% to 30%.

Pancreatic cystic neoplasms

The spectrum of cystic neoplasms of the pancreas encompasses biologically diverse diseases which range from benign to malignant lesions. These include serous cystadenomas, mucinous cystadenomas, and adenocarcinomas, solid and papillary epithelial neoplasms, and intraductal papillary mucinous tumor. Also included are other rarer entities such as acinar cell cystadenocarcinomas, cystic choriocarcinomas, cystic teratomas, and cystic lymphangiomatous neoplasms. These are all so unusual that they will not be mentioned further in this chapter.

Serous cystadenomas

These are cystic lesions that account for about 1% of neoplastic pancreatic lesions and are composed primarily of a collection of multiple small (< 2 cm), thin-walled cysts lined by a single layer of benign-appearing, glycogen-rich, serous cells. Serous cystadenomas usually occur in elderly females in the sixth and seventh decades of life and are most often found incidentally when a cross-sectional imaging study is performed for some other reason. The lesions typically have a characteristic honeycomb appearance on imaging studies, and are usually large with well-demarcated borders. Although malignant transformation of these lesions can occur, these are considered to be benign lesions, and if diagnosed are usually managed with observation alone. Surgical resection is indicated if they cause symptoms or enlarge.

Mucinous cystic neoplasms

These lesions represent a continuum ranging from clinically and pathologically benign mucinous cystadenomas to the malignant mucinous cystadenocarcinomas that can mimic the aggressive biological behavior of ductal adenocarcinomas of the pancreas. Mucinous cystic neoplasms can be divided into three groups.

1. *Mucinous cystadenoma* These neoplasms comprise about 65% of the total number of mucinous tumors. They contain a single layer of benign columnar mucinous cells.
2. *Proliferative mucinous cystic neoplasms* These comprise about 30% of the total number of mucinous tumors. This group contains varying degrees of atypia, dysplasia, papillary epithelial infolding, and even carcinoma *in situ* without any tissue invasion.
3. *Mucinous cystadenocarcinomas* These lesions comprise less than 10% of all mucinous cystic neoplasms. They may have areas of objective stromal invasion beyond the epithelial basement membrane, i.e. an invasive cancer.

Preoperative differentiation between these groups can be difficult because malignant changes in the cystic lining may be focal and thus may be missed on fine-needle aspiration or biopsy.

Mucinous cystic neoplasms are also rare, comprising about 1% to 2% of exocrine tumors. They occur predominantly in women but at a somewhat earlier age (mean age 53 years) compared to serous cystadenomas. These lesions are found incidentally or can present with non-specific or vague abdominal complaints. Symptoms usually are a result of local mass effect rather than neoplastic invasion. About 10% of these patients can present with a history of pancreatitis.

The majority (77%) of mucinous cystadenomas are found in the body or tail of the pancreas. Mucinous cystic neoplasms may be multicystic but may also present as a single macrocystic lesion, are usually large (> 5 cm) and are lined with columnar, mucin-containing epithelium which may contain foci of dysplastic cells or invasive carcinoma.

The recognition and differentiation of mucinous cystic neoplasms from other cystic neoplasms of the pancreas is crucial because of their premalignant potential. The presence of papillary fronds, septae within the cystic structure, peripheral calcification, or an eccentric solid component within the wall of the cystic mass on imaging studies is suggestive of mucinous cystic neoplasms. Once the suspicion of a mucinous cystic neoplasm is entertained, operative resection is indicated. When mucinous cystic neoplasms are located in the head of the pancreas, a Whipple resection is required. When these occur in the body and tail of the pancreas, a distal pancreatectomy is required. Mucinous cystadenocarcinomas have a better prognosis than ductal pancreatic cancer; the 5-year survival after a curative resection of a mucinous cystadenocarcinoma approaches 50%. Resected lesions that prove to be mucinous cystadenomas or proliferative mucinous cystic neoplasms are cured by resection and almost always do not recur. Therefore, follow-up for patients with completely resected, non-malignant groups of mucinous cystic neoplasms may be unnecessary.

Intraductal papillary mucinous tumor of the pancreas

Intraductal papillary mucinous tumor consists of dilated pancreatic ductal segments that are lined by mucous-secreting cells, which have a high malignant potential. Unlike other cystic neoplasms of the pancreas which are generally asymptomatic, intraductal papillary mucinous tumor often presents as idiopathic recurrent pancreatitis of the elderly. The episodes of pancreatitis are triggered by obstruction of the pancreatic duct by the thick inspissated mucus and intraductal tumor growth.

Computed tomography scans demonstrate a dilated main pancreatic duct, while ERCP reveals the characteristic appearance of thick mucus emanating from the orifice of the papilla of Vater. The ampullary orifice has a "fish-mouth" appearance. Endoscopic retrograde cholangiopancreatography also demonstrates dilated pancreatic duct and intraductal filling defects, which represent mucus, intraductal papillomatous growths, or areas of malignant degeneration or invasion. At the time of diagnosis, approximately 30% to 40% of intraductal papillary mucinous tumor patients already have an invasive malignancy; the remainder of patients have intraductal micropapillary changes with atypia, dysplasia, or carcinoma *in situ*, confirming the premalignant potential of intraductal papillary mucinous tumor. Intraductal papillary mucinous tumor represents a multifocal disorder of the pancreatic ductal epithelium usually necessitating a total pancreatectomy.

Diagnosis

It is critical to distinguish benign cystic lesions of the pancreas from those that are malignant or have malignant potential. The major challenge is the differentiation between a pseudocyst, serous cystadenoma, and mucinous cystic lesions.

Clinical history cannot always discern between the different types of lesions. A good quality CT scan usually permits discrimination between pseudocysts, serous cystadenomas, and mucinous cystadenoma.

1. Serous cystadenomas characteristically appear as microcystic with a honeycomb appearance with an area of central fibrosis or calcification. The individual cysts that comprise the cystadenoma are less than 1 cm in size and are separated by a thin wall or septum. Debris or solid component is unusual.
2. Mucinous cystadenomas/adenocarcinomas appear as macrocystic lesions. Septations, solid component, and peripheral calcifications may be seen.
3. Pseudocysts appear as unilocular fluid collections with well-defined walls. Floating debris may be present. Parenchymal changes of pancreatitis may also be seen.

These criteria are fallible, however, and distinction between the lesions may not always be possible. Endoscopic ultrasound may be helpful in this setting but its accuracy is still being determined. Aspiration of the intracystic fluid percutaneously or endosonographically with analysis of cystic fluid for cytology and tumor markers may help discriminate between the various lesions (Table 17.1). However, a false-negative diagnosis is not unusual.

Management

Cystic lesions of the pancreas should be managed as follows.

1. Serous cystadenomas should be resected when symptomatic or enlarging. Small, asymptomatic and non-enlarging serous cystadenomas can be observed since the risk of malignant change is small.
2. Mucinous cystadenomas, when recognized, should be resected because of the high potential for malignant change.
3. Intraductal papillary mucinous tumors should be resected, even when patients are asymptomatic, because of the significant risk that these lesions may evolve into invasive

Table 17.1 Analysis of cystic fluid in cystic neoplasms of the pancreas

	Cytology	Amylase activity	CEA	Viscosity	Mucin
Serous cystadenomas	Glycogen-rich	↓	↓	↓	Negative
Mucinous cystic neoplasms	Mucinous	↓	↑↑	↑	Positive
Pseudocysts	Inflammatory	↑↑↑	↓	↓	Negative

cancer. Resection usually depends on the location and extent of the lesions but frequently requires a total pancreatectomy.

The management of patients whose cystic lesions cannot be characterized with certainty presents a greater problem. Resection is generally recommended for even moderately suspicious lesions.

Further reading

Cooperman AM. Pancreatic cancer: the bigger picture. *Surg Clin North Am* 2001; 81(3): 557–574.

Freeny PC. Pancreatic carcinoma: imaging update 2001 *Dig Dis* 2001; 19(1): 37–46.

Pisters PW, Lee JE, Vauthey JN, Charnsangavej C, Evans DB. Laparoscopy in the staging of pancreatic cancer. *Br J Surg* 2001; 88(3): 325–337.

Sarr MG, Kendrick ML, Nagorney DM, Thompson GB, Farley DR, Farnell MB. Cystic neoplasms of the pancreas: benign to malignant epithelial neoplasms. *Surg Clin North Am* 2001; 81(3): 497–509.

Shankar A, Russell RC. Recent advances in the surgical treatment of pancreatic cancer. *World J Gastroenterol* 2001; 7(5): 622–626.

Chapter 18

Surgery of the Pancreas

T. Sloane Guy and Ernest F. Rosato

CHAPTER OUTLINE

Acute pancreatitis

Indications for surgery

Surgery is not indicated for uncomplicated acute pancreatitis. The overall mortality rate for acute pancreatitis is 10%. Over 90% of patients with acute pancreatitis have an uncomplicated course and are therefore not candidates for surgery. On occasion, patients may present with an acute abdomen for which the diagnosis is unclear and may be taken for exploratory laparotomy. There are many causes of hyperamylasemia in acute surgical patients, including bowel obstruction and bowel perforation. Likewise, there are patients ultimately demonstrated to have acute pancreatitis with normal serum amylase and lipase levels on initial evaluation.

The decision to operate on a patient with severe acute pancreatitis requires careful judgment. Common, well-accepted indications for surgery include

1. the need to establish a diagnosis in a patient with an acute abdomen and no clear diagnosis
2. infected pancreatic necrosis (usually demonstrated by CT-guided percutaneous aspirate gram stain and culture, or demonstration of gas on CT scan)
3. biliary pancreatitis (see discussion in chapter 16) when endoscopic therapy fails
4. the need to drain a pancreatic abscess or infected pancreatic pseudocyst when percutaneous therapy fails.

Additional indications for surgery that are less well accepted include extensive sterile pancreatic necrosis as demonstrated by non-enhancement of over 50% of the pancreas on CT scan and persistent pancreatitis in the setting of a deteriorating patient despite aggressive medical therapy. Acceptable but uncommon indications include hemorrhagic pancreatitis, severe generalized peritonitis, and biliary or duodenal obstruction.

Surgical options

Surgery for severe acute pancreatitis usually involves open exploration of the abdomen with aggressive debridement of necrotic pancreatic tissue and surgical drainage of the abdomen. One approach includes placement of large sump drains in the area of greatest inflammation. Many of the patients (20%) treated with this approach will develop recurrent or persistent infection requiring reoperation or percutaneous drainage. Another approach involves carefully attaching the borders of the lesser sac (stomach and transverse colon) to the abdominal wall, leaving the lesser sac completely open and packed. This approach necessitates daily dressing changes and wound irrigation and is labor intensive. However, when the surgeon feels that he/she is unable to completely remove all necrotic tissue, this represents a good option. Subsequent closure of the abdomen can be undertaken when sepsis has resolved and granulation tissue appears.

Pancreatic abscesses usually occur 3 to 4 weeks following an episode of severe acute pancreatitis. The physiologic state of the patient varies but is often better than with the initiating episode of pancreatitis. Computed tomography scans demonstrate fluid collections that appear as either ascites or pancreatic pseudocyst. Infection is documented by the clinical status of the patient, and by either gas bubbles on CT scan or percutaneous aspirate demonstrating the presence of organisms. Percutaneous treatment is often attempted initially and may be successful if the fluid is thin and with minimal particulate matter. Surgical drainage is indicated if the material is thick and particulate, the patient fails to improve, or a large amount of devitalized tissue is observed on CT scan. Mortality is in the range of 20%.

The morbidity and mortality for patients undergoing surgery for severe acute pancreatitis is largely a factor of the severity of the disease and the adequacy of surgical debridement. Overall mortality rates range from 10% to 35%.

Biliary pancreatitis

In general, patients with gallstones and pancreatitis who lack an obvious cause for their pancreatitis should undergo cholecystectomy with cholangiogram, either intra-operative or by preoperative or postoperative ERCP. Any common bile duct stones should be removed, either endoscopically or surgically. Surgical common bile duct exploration can be done in an open fashion or laparoscopically, although the laparoscopic approach requires significant experience with the technique. Both techniques require decompression of the common bile duct with a "T" tube at the conclusion of the procedure. Surgical spincterotomy is generally not performed unless an impacted distal common bile duct stone cannot be removed endoscopically or via surgical choledochotomy. Surgical spincterotomy adds significant morbidity to the operation because of the need to open the duodenum. If the surgeon is uncomfortable with surgical spincterotomy, it is acceptable to leave the stone for future endoscopic attempts and rely on the "T" tube to decompress the bile duct. Another approach to this difficult situation is to perform a side-to-side choledochoduodenostomy above the obstructing stone.

With regard to the timing of surgery, patients with gallstone pancreatitis who present with uncomplicated biliary pancreatitis generally undergo surgery prior to discharge, frequently 3 to 6 days following admission. This period allows for the pancreatitis to resolve. In the past, such patients were discharged and returned 4 to 6 weeks later for elective cholecystectomy. However, such an approach is associated with a 60% to 80% chance of recurrence during the delay period, thus subjecting the patient to unnecessary complications.

However, patients with severe biliary pancreatitis generally should not undergo early cholectectomy but rather be treated endoscopically and be allowed to recover and be discharged. These patients are then returned to the operating room 4 to 6 weeks later when the severe inflammation has subsided, reducing the risk of operative complications. If the endoscopist is unable to perform the ERCP and associated stone removal and spincterotomy, the surgeon may be forced to operate. In the setting of severe inflammation, strong consideration should be given to simple removal of stones from the biliary tree and placement of a cholecystostomy tube, avoiding cholecystectomy in the setting of severe inflammation. One exception to this would be patients with concomitant acute gangrenous cholecystitis. The decision regarding timing of cholecystectomy is difficult and requires careful assessment of the patient's physiologic state.

Chronic pancreatitis

Indications for surgery

The most common indication for surgical treatment of chronic pancreatitis is intractable pain.

Other indications include suspicion for cancer, common bile duct stricture, duodenal or colonic obstruction, splenic or portal vein obstruction, and symptomatic pseudocysts.

All patients being considered for surgical treatment of chronic pancreatitis should undergo an abdominal CT scan and ERCP. Psychological evaluation of patients with chronic intractable pain is warranted and aids both the physician and patient in decision making.

Chronic pain and surgical options

Procedures for the relief of chronic pain in patients with chronic pancreatitits fall into two categories.

1. The first category of operations is designed to improve the drainage of pancreatic exocrine secretions on the premise that obstruction of these secretions contributes to the pathophysiology of pain associated with chronic pancreatitits. These operations are considered in the setting of dilated pancreatic ducts.
2. The second category of operations are designed to resect diseased portions of the pancreas with normal sized ducts.

The most commonly used drainage procedure for a patient with intractable pain secondary to chronic pancreatitis in the setting of a dilated pancreatic duct is the longitudinal pancreaticojejunostomy, or Puestow procedure (Figures 18.1 and 18.2). The duct should be 7 mm or greater in diameter. A

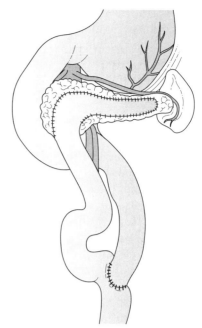

Figure 18.2 Completed Puestow procedure illustrating Roux-en-Y anastomosis

Puestow performed on a normal-sized duct will be unsuccessful. The main pancreatic duct is opened over its extent and a side-to-side Roux-en-Y pancreaticojejunostomy is performed. Immediate relief of pain is experienced by 80% to 90% of patients. However, 25% to 50% of patients will have recurrent pain within 5 years of the operation. The procedure caries a mortality of approximately 4% with minimal morbidity. Improvements in malabsorption are not seen but patients often gain weight because diminished pain improves eating.

In a minority of patients obstruction either at the pancreaticojejunostomy or more distally at the jejunojejunostomy (made to form the Roux-en-Y) can be demonstrated endoscopically and surgical revision may be helpful. However, in the vast majority of patients no cause for recurrence is identified.

Pancreatic resections for chronic pancreatitis are considered for pain relief in the setting of a normal-sized duct, failed prior drainage procedure, or when the pathologic changes of pancreatitis are more localized within the pancreas. Pancreatic resections are also performed for pancreatitis in the setting of localized stricture in which malignancy cannot be ruled out.

A pancreaticoduodectomy, identical to that done for malignancy, may be performed when disease is localized to the head of the pancreas. A majority of patients will achieve pain relief, weight gain, and improved quality of life. A 95% distal pancreatec-

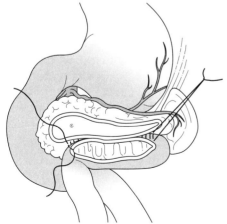

Figure 18.1 Pancreaticojejunostomy (Peustow procedure)

tomy can be performed. This procedure entails splenectomy and leaving only a small amount of pancreas adjacent to the duodenum. Total pancreatectomy can also be performed but results in brittle diabetes. Most surgeons will resect the duodenum as part of this procedure but some have managed to spare it. The reason for resecting the duodenum is the shared blood supply of the duodenum and the head of the pancreas.

A "Frey procedure" may also be performed. This involves a longitudinal Roux-en-Y jejunopancreatic anastomosis as in the Puestow procedure, but with the addition of resection of a core of tissue from the pancreatic head. The jejunum is then sewn to the entire open pancreatic head and ductal system. When involvement of the entire pancreas is seen in the setting of a large duct, this may be the procedure of choice.

The mortality of most pancreatic resections is less than 5%. However, a significant number of patients develop diabetes even when a good portion of the pancreas is left in place. Pain relief occurs in 80% to 90% of patients. Astonishingly, we have seen patients in whom the entire pancreas has been resected who continue to have severe pain identical to that which they experienced preoperatively.

Percutaneous chemical ablation of the celiac ganglion does have a role in relieving pain. Pain relief in the short-term is common, however, long-term pain relief is uncommon. This option might be considered in order to relieve a patient's symptoms temporarily while the patient and the surgeon consider surgical options.

Pancreatic transplantation has been utilized for these patients with the premise that this procedure will eliminate the complication of diabetes. However, because of the limitations of immunosuppression and the complications associated with pancreatic transplantation, this has not been very successful.

Pancreatic pseudocysts

A pancreatic pseudocyst is simply an extravasated collection of pancreatic secretions outside the pancreas. They most often occur as a complication of pancreatitis. They can also occur after trauma or surgery of the pancreas. Complications include hemorrhage (6%), rupture into the peritoneum or hollow viscous (7%), and infection (14%).

Roughly 40% of pseudocysts associated with acute pancreatitis will resorb as the pancreatic inflammation resolves. However, all pseudocysts in the setting of chronic pancreatitis should be considered mature and will persist. Small (< 5–6 cm), asymptomatic, mature pseudocysts do not require an operation and are associated with a lower rate of complications. Recent studies have demonstrated that even large asymptomatic pseudocysts may be followed with serial studies.

Indications for surgery include symptoms, growth in the size of the cyst, suspicion of cystic malignancy, or development of complications. Symptoms usually result from compression of adjacent structures such as the stomach. In the differential diagnosis of a pancreatic cystic structure is a cystic malignancy. When surgery is performed, it is important to send a biopsy of the cyst wall in order to demonstrate the lack of an epithelium that would indicate that the structure is a true cyst. Characteristics of cystic neoplasms include a lack of history of pancreatitis, internal septa on CT scan, wall calcification, and persistence. Presence of such characteristics favors a surgical approach to treatment.

The treatment options include resection and internal or external drainage; for example, cysts isolated in the distal pancreatic tail can be treated by distal pancreatectomy. External drainage may be indicated when an enterocyst anastomosis cannot be safely performed because the wall is not thick enough. Such drainage can be done surgically or percutaneously. Although 20% of patients treated with external drainage develop a pancreatic fistula most of these close spontaneously. Fistulas form more frequently when preoperative ERCP demonstrates communication between the cyst and the pancreatic duct. Endosopic retrograde cholangiopancreatography is not routinely indicated prior to surgery, but if performed, surgery should be performed within 24 hours to reduce the risk of sepsis from the introduction of bacteria into the cyst. Endosopic retrograde cholangiopancreatography would be indicated if evidence of concomitant biliary obstruction exists. If the ERCP demonstrates a clear communication of the cyst with the pancreatic duct, the cyst is less likely to resolve.

Internal drainage is commonly performed for pancreatic pseudocyst. Such drainage procedures include cyst gastrostomy or duodenostomy (if the cyst is adherent to the adjacent stomach or duodenum) and cyst Roux-en-Y jejunostomy. An infected pseudocyst adherent to the stomach can be drained by cyst gastrostomy. However, a cyst Roux-en-Y jejunostomy is generally not performed to an infected cyst given the increased risk of anastomotic dehiscence.

The results of drainage procedures are generally excellent. After drainage pseudocysts recur at a rate of approximately 10%. Most of these are associated with episodes of acute pancreatitis. Many patients do experience continued pain secondary to chronic pancreatitis.

Cystic neoplasms

Cystic neoplasms may be confused with pancreatic pseudocyst. Rare papillary cystic neoplasms of the pancreas are benign tumors found in young women less than 25 years of age. These are often large and locally invasive but are curable with resection and generally do not metastasize. Serous microcystic cystadenomas of the pancreas are the most common benign tumor of the pancreas. Mucinous cystadenomas are premalignant tumors that often develop into cystadenocarcinomas. These are large tumors most often found in the body and tail of the pancreas.

Surgery is indicated for either symptoms or inability to rule out malignancy. Benign microcystic serous adenomas have a honeycomb appearance on cut section and are generally resected if possible. Macrocystic mucinous adenomas are charactized by thick, viscous contents and are always resected. Outcomes for resection of malignant cystic neoplasms of the pancreas are much better than for adenocarcinoma.

Pancreatic ascites

Pancreatic ascites is caused by continuous free extravasation of pancreatic secretions into the abdomen. Given the retroperitoneal location of the pancreas, such fluid can turn up in a variety of places, including the pleura, pericardium, peritoneum, mediastinum, and inguinal region. Patients present with abdominal distension, weight loss, and protein malnutrition. Rarely do they present with acute pancreatitis. Most patients are alcoholics with chronic pancreatitis. Pancreatic ascites can occur after trauma and is seen after injury to the distal pancreas during splenectomy or adrenalectomy.

Diagnosis is straightforward with paracentesis revealing fluid with a high (< 3 gm/dL) protein level and amylase level greater than that of serum. Initial treatment is conservative and includes bowel rest, total parenteral nutrition, and use of octreotide, a somatostatin analog. Such treatment may be attempted for 1 to 2 weeks prior to consideration of surgery, which will be needed in a minority of patients. Prior to surgery, an ERCP is mandatory to demonstrate the location of the leak. Distal leaks may be eliminated by distal pancreatectomy while central leaks may require a drainage procedure.

Exocrine neoplasms of the pancreas

Ductal adenocarcinoma of the pancreas accounts for 90% of the 28 000 cases of pancreatic exocrine cancer in the US. Of these, only 10% will have tumors confined to the pancreas, while 40% have locally advanced tumors. The remainder have distant metastatic spread. This has important implications for surgical therapy as only a small fraction of patients with adenocarcinoma of the pancreas are curable by surgical means.

An algorithm for evaluation of patients with suspected adenocarcinoma of the pancreas reflects the desire to avoid operation in patients with a limited life expectancy. If the history, physical examination, and abdominal CT scan are consistent with a mass in the head of the pancreas and no metastatic disease, laparotomy is indicated and further studies are unnecessary. Resectability is best determined intraoperatively, although further tests such as EUS, MRA, or angiography may be used as a preoperative adjunct to confirm the diagnosis and predict feasibility of resection.

Endoscopic retrograde cholangiopancreatography has a 95% specificity and 85% sensitivity for diagnosis of pancreatic carcinoma. It is not mandatory in the setting of a clearly identified mass of the head of the pancreas on CT scan. There is no evidence of improved survival or decreased surgical morbidity with preoperative biliary stenting (via ERCP or percutaneous transhepatic cholangiography) in patients scheduled for exploration although it is often done as a temporizing measure for patient comfort while the work-up progresses.

Some centers will employ laparoscopy to identify the 20% of patients who have peritoneal surface metastasis not seen on preoperative studies. The laparoscopic approach is not entertained if the surgeon intends to perform biliary or gastric diversion regardless of the findings.

Pancreatic resection for pancreatic carcinoma is indicated when all tumor can be removed within the resected block of tissue. Palliative resection is generally contraindicated. A tumor is considered resectable if there are no distant metastases, no involved lymph nodes outside of the resectable field, and the tumor does not directly invade adjacent major vascular structures (i.e. portal vein, superior mesenteric artery, or hepatic artery). If a liberal approach to exploration is employed, only 20% of patients with carcinoma of the head of the pancreas will be resectable. However, more extensive use of preoperative testing can greatly increase this rate by reducing the number of unresectable patients who arrive in the operating room. However, no test confirms unresectability better than operative evaluation. Less than 5% of body or tail tumors are resectable.

A histopathologic diagnosis of carcinoma is not required. If fine needle aspiration (FNA) is performed intraoperatively (because of equivocal findings), it should be performed through the duodenum so that if a fistula occurs, it drains into the intestines. However, there is often a zone of inflammation around the tumor and a negative FNA does not eliminate the possibility of carcinoma. Most experienced pancreatic surgeons do not require a preoperative tissue diagnosis in the proper clinical setting.

The pancreaticoduodectomy (Whipple procedure) is the most common operation for carcinoma of the pancreas (Figure 18.3). The procedure removes the head of the pancreas (where almost all resectable tumors are found), the duodenum, the distal stomach, the distal common bile duct, and the gallbladder. Resectability depends heavily upon whether a clear plane between the tumor and the portal vein and superior mesenteric artery can be established. Also, no distal mestastases or nodal disease outside the block of resection should be seen. This includes liver metastases, celiac or SMA nodes, or peritoneal implants.

Reconstruction consists of a gastrojejunostomy, a choledochojejunostomy, and a pancreaticojejunostomy. A variety of ways to construct these anastomoses exists. The duodenal-sparing Whipple procedure involves leaving the first portion of the duodenum with the pylorus intact such that a duodenojejunostomy is performed instead of a gastrojejunostomy. This may prevent postgastrectomy syndromes but can lead to a higher incidence of gastric-outlet obstruction.

The 5-year survival rate for patients undergoing a Whipple procedure for carcinoma of the head of the pancreas is approximately 10%. If no positive nodes are found, a 5-year survival of 35% can be obtained. Neither total pancreatectomy nor extended Whipple resections (resection of a wider margin of tissue, nodes, and the portal vein and superior mesenteric artery) have led to improved survival.

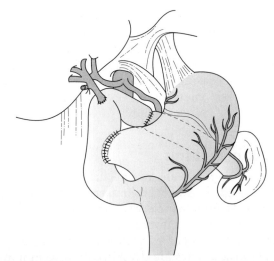

Figure 18.3 Pancreaticoduodenectomy (Whipple procedure)

Curative resection for adenocarcinoma of the body or tail of the pancreas is rare.

Palliative surgery

Most centers will perform palliative procedures when unresectable tumors are encountered intraoperatively, based on data suggesting a better quality of life after such surgery. However, this type of therapy remains controversial.

Roughly 70% of patients with unresectable cancer will experience biliary obstruction. Endoscopically placed stents are effective but need to be replaced every 3 months on average because of blockage. Also, less than one third of patients will experience significant duodenal obstruction in the natural course of their disease prior to death.

Endocrine neoplasms of the pancreas

Insulinoma

The diagnosis of insulinoma can be made on the basis of symptoms and laboratory studies alone. Whipple's triad of hypoglycemic symptoms with fasting, serum glucose less than 50mg/dL, and resolution of symptoms with administration of glucose supports the diagnosis. A fasting glucose can be checked every 6 hours up to 72 hours until symptoms develop. A plasma insulin to glucose ratio of greater than 0.3 confirms the diagnosis.

Only 10% of insulinomas are malignant, unlike most endocrine neoplasms of the pancreas.

With 10% to 20% of these tumors difficult to find intraoperatively, preoperative localization is important. Options for this include selective angiography, transportal venous sampling for insulin, CT, ultrasound (transabdominal or endoscopic), and MRI.

These tumors are evenly distributed throughout the pancreas. If the surgeon is unable to localize the tumor intraoperatively, an 80% chance of successful resection can be accomplished with distal pancreatectomy. However, one takes a 20% chance of leaving the tumor in the remaining pancreatic head that then has to be dealt with. It is acceptable to close the laparotomy without resection if localization is unsuccessful with hopes of re-exploration after better localization studies. However, this is not a situation most surgeons want to be in. A better approach is to exhaust all preoperative localization measures prior to operating.

Gastrinoma (Zollinger–Ellison syndrome)

Zollinger-Ellison syndrome is caused by gastric acid hypersecretion resulting from excessive gastric production by a gastrinoma. Symptoms of gastrinoma include diarrhea, peptic ulcer disease, and fat malabsorption. The diagnosis of gastrinoma is made by demonstrating a fasting gastrin level above 200 pg/mL, and a basal acid output above 15 mEq/h with an intact stomach or above 5 mEq/h after ulcer surgery. Most patients have a fasting gastrin level above 500 to 1000 pg/mL, which is diagnostic. However, patients with equivocal values of 200 to 500 pg/mL should undergo a secretin stimulation test which will result in a rise greater than 200 pg/mL in the basal gastrin level in patients with a gastrinoma. Computed tomography scans and sometimes angiography are used to localize the tumor. The differential diagnosis includes other causes of hypergastrinemia, such as gastric outlet obstruction, retained antrum following partial gastrectomy, and antral G-cell hyperplasia.

Most are found in the pancreas with the remainder mostly in the duodenum. The "gastrinoma triangle" represents the most likely location of the tumors and is defined by the cystic duct junction with the common bile duct, the neck of the pancreas, and the junction of the second and third portion of the duodenum. Within the pancreas, 60% of gastrinomas are islet cell carcinomas, 25% are soli-

tary adenomas, and 10% are microadenomas or hyperplasia. Roughly 25% of gastrinomas are associated with MEN I and are mostly benign and multifocal. Sporatic gastrinomas are mostly single and malignant. All of these tumors, even the malignant type, are slow growing and associated with prolonged survival. The severe gastric ulcer diasthesis associated with high gastrin secretion is the principle morbidity of these tumors.

The medical treatment of gastrinoma has been aided by the development of effective H_2 blockers and proton pump inhibitors. These drugs are particularly effective for patients with extensive metastatic disease or with MEN-I, where surgery is not helpful given the multifocal nature of the disease. Surgical treatment is indicated for sporatic tumors without evidence of extensive metastatic disease. Surgical treatment usually consists of enucleation. Intraoperative ultrasound may be used to localize the tumor. Rarely, a pancreaticoduodenectomy may be necessary. Distal pancreatectomy may also be employed, however, less than 10% of tumors are located outside the gastrinoma triangle (i.e. the distal pancreas).

Other endocrine tumors of the pancreas

Other endocrine tumors of the pancreas include VIPomas (Verner-Morrison sydrome, WDHA syndrome), glucogonomas, somatastatinomas, and others. The majority of these tumors are malignant and are treated similarly to gastrinomas. Any pancreatic endocrine neoplasm may be associated with MEN I (pancreatic endocrine neoplasms, pituitary adenomas, and parathyroid adenomas or hyperplasia).

Further reading

Azimuddin K, Chamberlain RS. The surgical management of pancreatic neuroendocrine tumors. *Surg Clin North Am* 2001; 81(3): 511–525.

Bowles MJ, Benjamin IS. ABC of the upper gastrointestinal tract: cancer of the stomach and pancreas. *BMJ* 2001; 323(7326): 1413–1416.

Brentjens R, Saltz L. Islet cell tumors of the pancreas: the medical oncologist's perspective. *Surg Clin North Am* 2001; 81(3): 527–542.

Cooperman AM. Pancreatic cancer: the bigger picture. *Surg Clin North Am* 2001; 81(3): 557–574.

Davis B, Lowy AM. Surgical management of hereditary pancreatic cancer. *Med Clin North Am* 2000; 84(3): 749–759.

Dolan JP, Norton JA. Occult insulinoma. *Br J Surg* 2000; 87(4): 385–387.

Kozuch P, Petryk M, Evans A, Bruckner. Treatment of metastatic pancreatic adenocarcinoma: a comprehensive review. *Surg Clin North Am* 2001; 81(3): 683–690.

Lieberman SM, Horig H, Kaufman HL. Innovative treatments for pancreatic cancer. *Surg Clin North Am* 2001; 81(3): 715–739.

Molinari M, Helton WS, Espat NJ. Palliative strategies for locally advanced unresectable and metastatic pancreatic cancer. *Surg Clin North Am* 2001; 81(3): 651–666.

Pisters PW, Lee JE, Vauthey, JN, *et al*. Laparoscopy in the staging of pancreatic cancer. *Br J Surg* 2001; 88(3): 325–337.

Poon RT, Fan, ST. Opinions and commentary on treating pancreatic cancer. *Surg Clin North Am* 2001; 81(3): 625–636.

Postier RG. Past, present, and future of pancreatic surgery. *Am J Surg* 2001; 182(6): 547–551.

Sarr MG, Kendrick ML, Nagorney DM, *et al*. Cystic neoplasms of the pancreas: benign to malignant epithelial neoplasms. *Surg Clin North Am* 2001; 81(3): 497–509.

Stanford P. Surgical approaches to pancreatic cancer. *Nurs Clin North Am* 2001; 36(3): 567–577.

Index